# Medical Embryology

# Medical Embryology

Editor: Leonard Roosevelt

AMERICAN
MEDICAL PUBLISHERS
www.americanmedicalpublishers.com

AMERICAN
MEDICAL PUBLISHERS
www.americanmedicalpublishers.com

**Cataloging-in-publication Data**

Medical embryology / edited by Leonard Roosevelt.
p. cm.
Includes bibliographical references and index.
ISBN 979-8-88740-249-9
1. Embryology, Human. 2. Abnormalities, Human. 3. Embryology.
4. Developmental biology. 5. Fetus--Development. I. Roosevelt, Leonard.
QM601 .M43 2023
612.64--dc23



American Medical Publishers,
41 Flatbush Avenue,
1st Floor, New York,
NY 11217, USA

ISBN 979-8-88740-249-9 (Hardback)

# Contents

# Preface

Embryology refers to the branch of biology concerned with the study of prenatal development of gametes, including fertilization and growth of embryos to the fetal stage. It is the foundation for understanding the intimate connection among structures in various organ systems, including muscles and the nervous system. It is integral for comprehending the developmental disorders that can manifest in humans as one of the congenital myopathies. One of the significant aspects of embryology comprises research on stem cells, as it helps to understand how genetic disorders progress and what effect does mutation have. Medical embryology is widely utilized for finding anomalies before birth. It investigates the various mechanisms and phases in which anomalies manifest in newborns. Appearance of abnormalities due to outside contributors results in disruptions. Teratogens are the outside disruptions. Retinoic acid, hyperthermic stress, alcohol and ionizing radiation are examples of common teratogens. The topics covered in this extensive book deal with the recent studies on medical embryology. It presents researches and studies performed by experts across the globe. This book aims to serve as a resource guide for students and experts alike and contribute to the growth of this discipline.

This book is the end result of constructive efforts and intensive research done by experts in this field. The aim of this book is to enlighten the readers with recent information in this area of research. The information provided in this profound book would serve as a valuable reference to students and researchers in this field.

At the end, I would like to thank all the authors for devoting their precious time and providing their valuable contribution to this book. I would also like to express my gratitude to my fellow colleagues who encouraged me throughout the process.

**Editor**

# 1

# A Novel Concept of Fundus-Ovary-Salpinx-Para-Aorta Implantation Promoting Unit during Human Embryo Implantation

Hiroshi Fujiwara, Yoshihiko Araki, Shigeru Saito, Kazuhiko Imakawa, Satoru Kyo, Minoru Shigeta, Masahide Shiotani, Akihito Horie and Takahide Mori

**Abstract**

Human embryo implantation is mainly regulated by the endocrine system. Since the ovary, fallopian tube, and fundus can directly communicate through the mesosalpinx and ovarian ligament, the local concentration of progesterone in the pathway of the developing embryo is considered to be higher than in systemic blood circulation. The immune system promotes embryo implantation by stimulating progesterone production of the ovary and by inducing endometrial differentiation. The recognition of the developing embryo in the fallopian tube by the immune system is achieved through the para-aortic lymph nodes. On the basis of the above evidence, the autologous immune cells activated in vitro were demonstrated to improve clinical pregnancy rates in patients with repeated implantation failures. In addition, the autonomic nerve system that innervates the fundus, the ovary, and the fallopian tube from the para-aortic region is proposed to regulate the environment of the pathway of the developing embryo. From these findings, we suppose that a unique unilateral functional unit to promote human embryo implantation exists in the pathway of the developing embryo including the para-aortic regions and propose naming this novel functional unit the Fundus-Ovary-Salpinx-Para-aorta Implantation Promoting unit (FOSPa-IP unit).

**Keywords:** embryo, FOSPa-IP unit, implantation

## 1. Introduction

In humans, the corpus luteum, which is formed from the ovulated follicle, produces progesterone that induces adequate endometrial differentiation for embryo implantation. During pregnancy, the embryo trophoblast cells secrete human chorionic gonadotropin (HCG) that stimulates the maternal corpus luteum to sustain progesterone production. In turn, it acts on the endometrium to maintain embryo implantation in the uterus. Thus, human embryo implantation is mainly regulated by the endocrine system.

In addition to this endocrine system, we have demonstrated that the immune system is involved in the process of promoting embryo implantation by stimulating progesterone production of the ovary and by inducing endometrial differentiation [1]. It is also suggested that recognition of the developing embryo in the fallopian tube by the immune system is achieved through the para-aortic lymph nodes from a very early stage of pregnancy. The intrauterine administration of autologous immune cells that was activated by HCG in vitro was demonstrated to improve embryo implantation rates in patients with repeated failure of in vitro fertilization and embryo transfer treatment [2].

These lines of evidence led us to conceive a novel concept that there is a unique unilateral functional unit to promote human embryo implantation among the fundus, the ovary, the fallopian tube, and the para-aortic regions. In this chapter, we propose naming this novel functional unit as the Fundus-Ovary-Salpinx-Para-aorta Implantation Promoting unit (FOSPa-IP unit) and describe its estimated characteristics.

## 2. The implantation pathway of the developing embryo

In humans, the ovulated oocyte is picked up by the fimbria of the fallopian tube and then the fertilized oocyte is transferred to the uterine cavity through the fallopian tube, causing embryogenesis to proceed toward the blastocyst stage (Figure 1). Recently, it has been widely accepted that a synchronized dialog between the developing embryo and the temporally and coordinately differentiated maternal endometriumis is necessary for successful embryo implantation [3]. Accordingly, the adequate preparation of endometrial receptivity as well as the quality of the embryo affects the success of the outcome of in vitro fertilization-embryo transfer (IVF-ET) therapy.

To support the significance of this period, the phenomenon of delayed implantation is well known in rodents and it has also been reported in humans [4]. Furthermore, in cows, this process continues for at least a few days and bovine early embryos become elongated during the pre-implantation period. Consequently, it can be speculated that embryonal signals locally induce further endometrial differentiation and/or an environment suitable for subsequent embryo implantation. We previously proposed that the Eph-ephrin system, which can induce a repulsive force between the epithelial cell layers, contributes to maintaining these crosstalk phases [5]. Several other systems may be involved in the molecular mechanisms of regulation of embryo-maternal crosstalk [4].

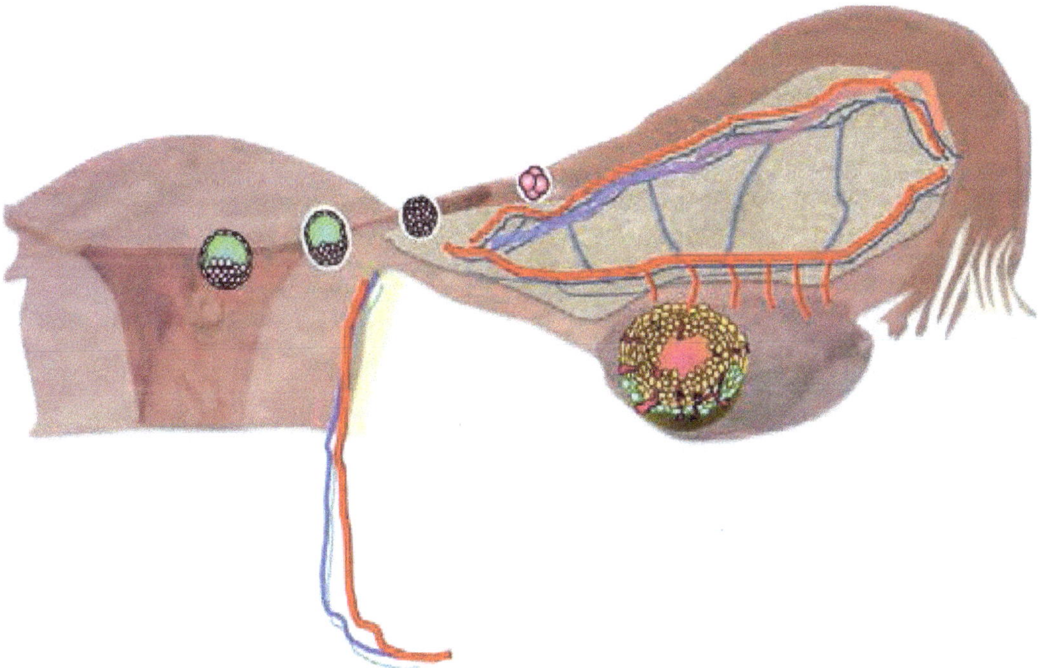

**Figure 1.** The implantation pathway of the developing embryo In humans, the ovulated oocyte is picked up by the fimbria of the fallopian tube and then the fertilized oocyte is transferred to the uterine cavity through the fallopian tube, causing embryogenesis to proceed toward the blastocyst stage.

In contrast to the majority of mammals with uterus bicornate bicollis, in humans, women have a single fused uterus derived from bilateral paramesonephric (Müllerian) ducts. From this perspective, the uterine fundus is a structure specific to primates among mammals. Shiotani et al. showed that the human uterus possesses a latent fluid-retaining space along the transversely communicating line (TCL) between the bilateral utero-tubal angles on the fundus [6]. To build on and confirm their findings, when we injected a small amount of contrast dye (70 μl) into the upper portion of the cavity, the dye spontaneously migrated toward the ceiling of the cavity, spread bilaterally to the utero-tubal angles, and formed along cylindrical space (TCL space) that was gently expanded by the dye (Figure 2A).This space communicated directly with the bilateral fallopian tubes (Figure 2B). When we observed the uterine cavity from a sagittal perspective using a surgically resected uterus, the TCL space was macroscopically manifested by innate tissue pressure of the muscle layer (Figures 3A and B). In contrast, macroscopic TCL space was not formed in the uterus with diffusion and firm enlargement by adenomyosis lesions (Figure 3C).

From these findings, we speculate that the main site of crosstalk between the human embryo and maternal tissues before implantation is the upper site of the uterine cavity in the fundus, that is, the TCL space. In support of this theory, Minami et al. reported that gestational sacs of patients in the early stage of spontaneous normal pregnancy were mainly observed on the right or left side of the upper third of the uterine cavity. They also reported that patients with gestational sacs in the upper region had a significantly lower miscarriage rate than those in the middle and lower regions, proposing that the endometrium at the uterine fundus, especially near the utero-tubal junction, is suitable for human blastocyst implantation under physiological conditions [7].

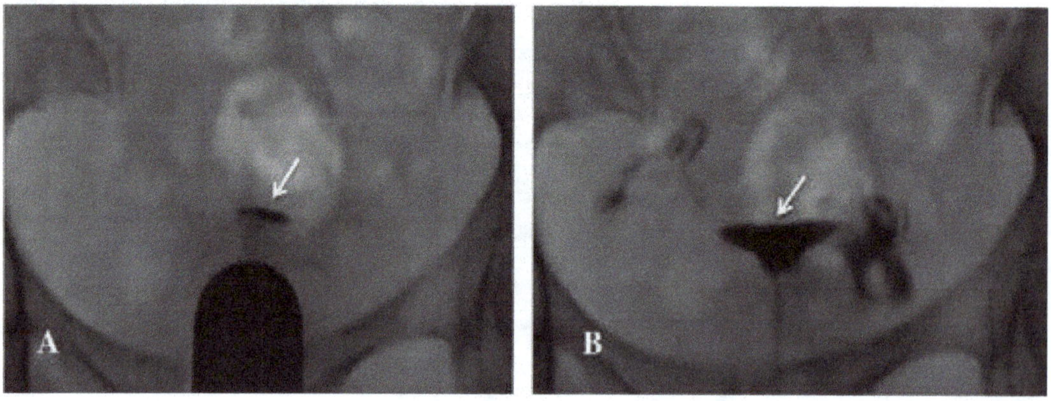


**Figure 2.** TCL space detected by hysterosalpingography A and B: The human uterus possesses a latent fluid-remaining space along the transversely communicating line (TCL, arrows) between the bilateral utero-tubal angles at the top of the cavity in the fundus. A: When a small amount of contrast dye was injected into the upper portion of the cavity, the dye spontaneously migrated toward the ceiling of the cavity, spread bilaterally to the utero-tubal angles, and formed along cylindrical space (TCL space) that was gently expanded by the dye. B: By subsequent conventional hysterosalpingography, this space communicated directly with the bilateral fallopian tubes.

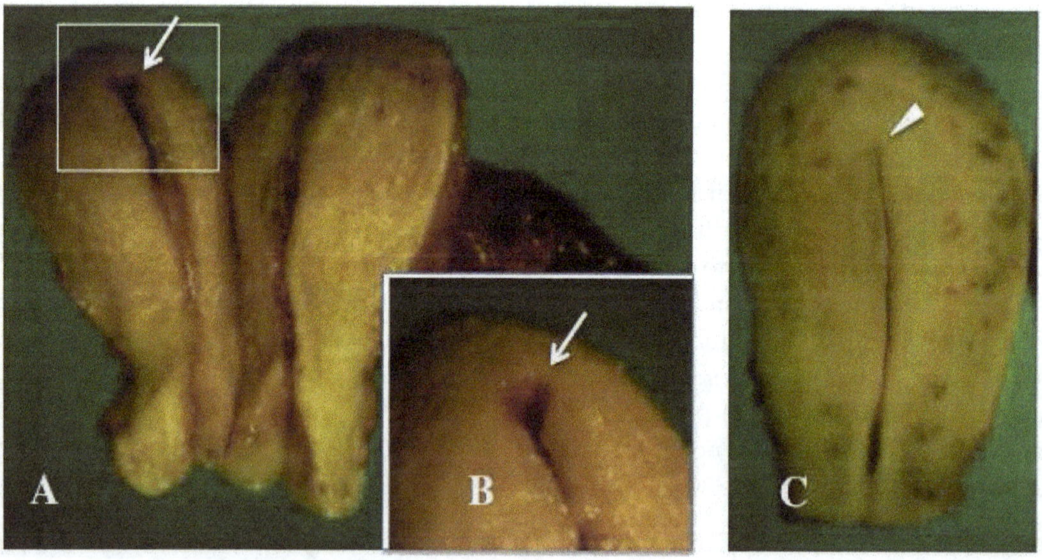


**Figure 3.** Macroscopic observation of TCL space A: When the uterine cavity was observed from a sagittal perspective using a surgically resected uterus due to carcinoma in situ lesion in the cervix, the TCL space was macroscopically manifested by innate tissue pressure of the muscle layer. B: A magnified figure of the square area of A. C: A uterine specimen that was resected due to adenomyosis. Macroscopic TCL space was not formed in the uterus with diffusion and firm enlargement by adenomyosis lesions.

## 3. The endocrine network around the implantation pathway

### 3.1. Local concentration of progesterone in the implantation pathway

Corpus luteum in the ovary is the main endocrine organ that produces progesterone. It has been widely accepted that progesterone prepares the uterus for embryo implantation, induces endometrial differentiation and decreases the contractility of uterine smooth muscle cells. Human endometrial decidualization is also induced by progesterone. The ovary is anatomically connected with the ipsilateral fallopian tube and the corneal region of the uterus. The vascular network is present among the fallopian tube as well as the ovary through the mesosalpinx and ovarian ligament. Therefore, it is speculated that the local concentration of progesterone is very high in the ipsilateral fallopian tube adjacent to the ovary that has an ovulated follicle.

Clinically, vaginal administration of progesterone is usually performed for luteal support for infertile patients receiving in vitro fertilization therapy. After vaginal administration, the uterine tissue concentration of progesterone has been found to exceed more than 10-fold the levels achieved by systemic administration. To explain this phenomenon, the "first uterine pass effect," that is, direct preferential vagina-to-uterus transport, was proposed [8]. By drug delivery analysis using tritiated progesterone, Bulletti et al. obtained experimental data to support this hypothesis [9]. Consequently, similar to the direct preferential vagina-to-uterus transport system, estrogen and progesterone produced by the corpus luteum in the ovary can be delivered to the corneal region of the uterus by a direct ovary-to-uterus transport system.

Using slice computed tomography (CT) scanning and vascular casting, it was demonstrated that both the intramuscular uterine artery and the ovarian artery had a typical ovarian branch connected as an arterial arch, that is, the ovarian artery-to-uterine artery anastomoses [10]. Importantly, these ovarian artery-to-uterine artery anastomoses are located in the mesosalpinx region. In mammals, the anatomical structure among the utero-ovarian vein and the ovarian artery is considered to be important to regulate the counter-current system of exchange from the uterus to the ovary and back again. In humans, the utero-ovarian vein forms a plexus around the ovarian artery. Therefore, it has been suggested that counter-current transfer facilitates local communication between the ovary, the fallopian tube, and the uterus [11]. Later, it was also reported that serum levels of estradiol and progesterone in the uterine vessels were more than 2–4 times higher than those in the systemic circulation, demonstrating the preferential transport of sex steroids produced in the ovary to the uterus [12]. Interestingly, the same group also suggested that the main blood supply to the uterine corneal region from uterine and ovarian arteries is shifted following ovulation [13]. This suggests the possibility that progesterone regulates counter-current blood flows in the mesosalpinx. Consequently, the local concentration of progesterone along the implantation pathway of the human embryo is speculated to be considerably high during its developmental process (Figure 4).

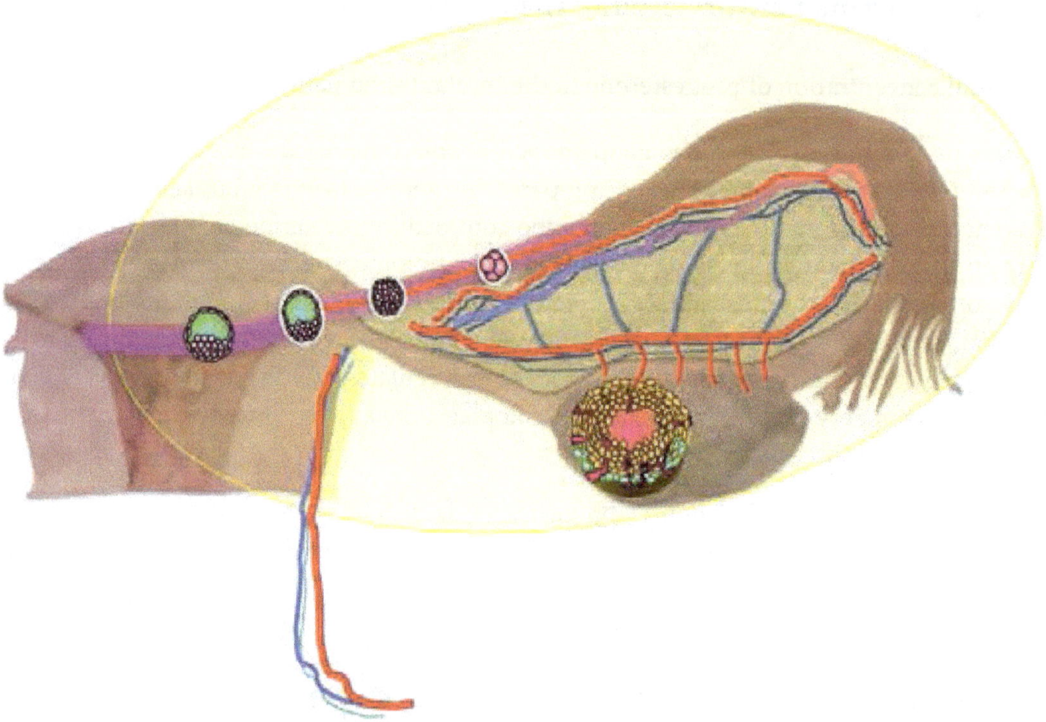

**Figure 4.** The local concentration of progesterone along the implantation pathway The local concentration of progesterone along the implantation pathway of the human embryo is speculated to be considerably high during its developmental process.

### 3.2. Hormonal regulation of the contractility around the implantation pathway by ovarian steroid hormones

Strict regulation of contractility in the uterus and the fallopian tube is essential for various reproductive functions including expulsion of menstrual debris, sperm transport, and adequate embryo placement during implantation [14]. More than half a century ago, the precise profiles of contractile activity of the non-pregnant uterus throughout the menstrual cycle were reported using an intrauterine pressure recording system [15, 16]. Recently, it has become possible for uterine contractility to be directly and non-invasively assessed using ultrasound scans and ultrafast magnetic resonance imaging techniques [17]. Accordingly, the inherent contractility of the uterus is classified into two patterns: a focal and sporadic bulging of the myometrium and a rhythmic and subtle stripping movement in the subendometrial myometrium, known as uterine peristalsis. Using these direct and non-invasive techniques, the precise profiles of several wavelike activity patterns throughout the menstrual cycle have been thoroughly analyzed, and it has been widely accepted that ovarian steroid hormones regulate contractions of the non-pregnant uterus. Clinically, uterine contractility has been demonstrated to influence the human embryo implantation process in both spontaneous cycles and assisted reproduction [18, 19].

Waves from fundus to cervix are dominant in the follicular phase, but diminish after ovulation. In contrast, waves from cervix to fundus were observed in the late follicular and luteal phases [20, 21], supporting implantation of the embryo at the upper region of the uterine cavity [22]. During the luteal phase, the movement of the upper fundal region is relatively quiescent facilitating embryo implantation [23]. By the sequential administration of estradiol (days 1–28) and progesterone (days 14–28), waves from fundus to cervix were induced by estradiol, but were immediately diminished after the administration of progesterone, whereas waves from cervix to fundus were observed in both the estradiol-only and the estradiol and progesterone combined phases [18]. It was also reported that there is horizontal movement at the fundus, often to and fro, not unidirectional [24]. Importantly, this horizontal movement can theoretically induce the migration of pre-implanted embryo back to the fallopian tubes along the TCL through the fluid by endometrial secretion (Figure 5).

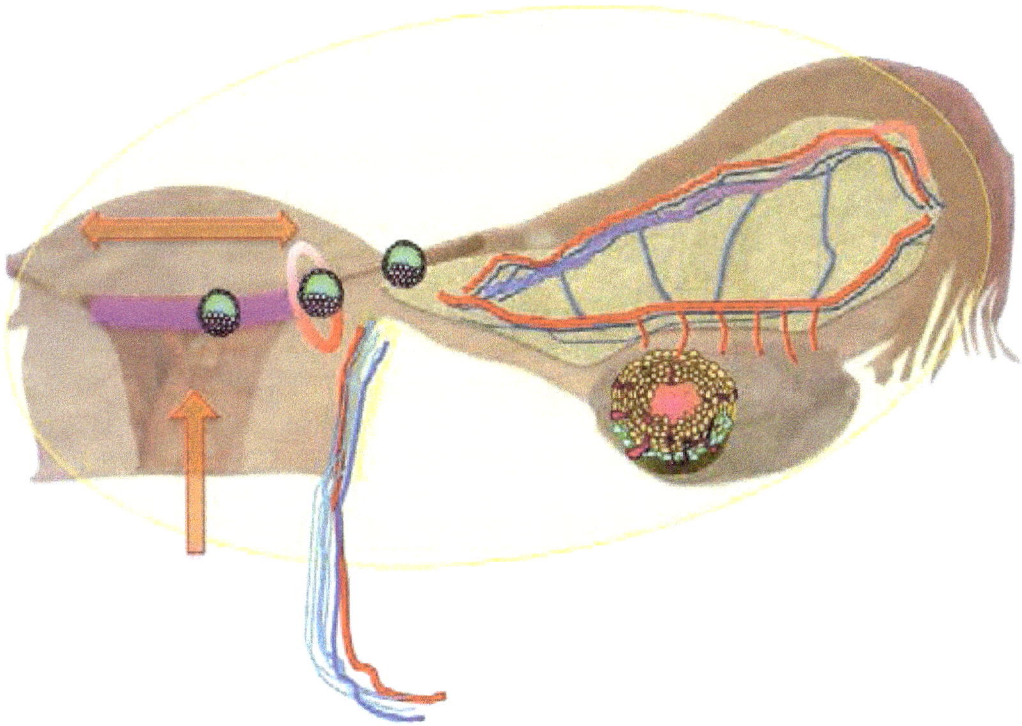

**Figure 5.** Hormonal regulation of the contractility around the implantation pathway by ovarian steroid hormones. Ovarian steroid hormones regulate contractions of the uterus. Waves from cervix to fundus were observed in the late follicular and luteal phases. There is also horizontal movement at the fundus, often to and fro, not unidirectional, which can theoretically induce the migration of pre-implantation embryo back to the fallopian tubes along the TCL.

Recently, it has been reported that a new population of c-kit-positive cells, interstitial Cajal-like cells, now called telocytes, had been found on the borders of smooth muscle bundles in human myometrium. These cells resemble interstitial cells of Cajal in the gut, which generate electrical slow waves to control peristalsis [14]. Telocytes in the myometrium are double-positive for c-kit and CD34, and have very long cellular extensions called telopodes that release extracellular vesicles, sending macromolecular signals to neighboring cells. It was proposed that they modulate spontaneous contractions of the non-pregnant human uterus, through a tyrosine-kinase-independent signaling pathway [25, 26]. Although the precise effects of ovarian steroid hormones on telocyte functions remain unclear, immunoreactive estrogen and progesterone receptors localized at the nucleus level of uterine telocytes suggested their involvement in the hormonal regulation of uterine contractility [27].

### 3.3. Hormonal regulation of immune environment around the implantation pathway by ovarian steroid hormones

During the implantation process, the semi-allogeneic embryo is not rejected by the maternal immune system. The mechanisms regarding how the fetus is tolerated by the maternal immune system are still not well understood. It is generally accepted that ovarian sex steroids regulate the function and population of endometrial and/or decidual immune cells in the uterus [28] and these immune–endocrine interactions contribute to fetal survival within the maternal uterus, suppressing adverse maternal immune responses and promoting immunotolerance pathways [29].

Progesterone regulates immune function by producing mediators such as the progesterone-induced blocking factor that induces Th2-dominant cytokine production [30] and glycodelin A that protects the embryo from maternal immune attack by inhibiting the proliferation of T cells and B cells and the activity of natural killer cells, or by deleting the monocytes [31]. The physiological effects of progesterone are mediated by its specific nuclear progesterone receptor (PR) that activates transcription factors. Nuclear PR has two main isoforms: PR-A and PR-B. PR-B acts as an activator of progesterone-responsive genes, while PR-A can inhibit the activity of PR-B. Using nuclear PR knockout mice, it has been shown that progesterone antagonizes estrogen-induced recruitment of macrophages and neutrophils into the uterus [32]. Recently, it has been demonstrated that progesterone at a relatively high concentration also acts on cells by a non-genomic mechanism through progesterone binding membrane proteins such as progesterone membrane components 1 and 2, and the membrane progestin receptors [33, 34]. Considering a local high concentration of progesterone, these non-genomic mechanisms may operate in the implantation pathway.

CD56(high+)CD16(–) uterine natural killer cells are the predominant population in the decidual tissues during the late secretory phase of the menstrual cycle and early pregnancy. They may be derived from natural killer cell progenitors and/or peripheral natural killer cells and are considered to contribute to the remodeling of maternal uterine vasculature in interaction with extravillous trophoblasts [29, 35]. Although the level of the expression of PR on uterine natural killer cells is very low [36], the progesterone-induced endometrial environment is an important factor for the in situ proliferation or differentiation of uterine natural killer cells in human endometrium, inducing reprogramming of their chemokine receptor profiles [37, 38]. Progesterone is also reported to reduce the antigen-presenting capacity of dendritic cells, monocytes, and macrophages and induce the recruitment of regulatory T (Treg) cells, contributing to local accumulation of pregnancy-protective cells [29]. These lines of evidence suggest the relationship between the endocrine and immune systems for establishing the embryo implantation environment.

## 4. The autonomic nerve network around the implantation pathway

In pigs, it was demonstrated that the oviduct is innervated by various efferent autonomic neurons such as the inferior mesenteric ganglion, ovarian ganglion, and celiac-superior mesenteric ganglion complex, forming discrete "oviductal centers" and implying that these nerve fibers regulate oviductal blood flow, non-vascular smooth muscle contraction, transmission of sensory information, and epithelial secretion [39, 40]. In monkeys, noradrenaline of the sympathetic nerves innervating the smooth musculature of the oviduct was demonstrated to change cyclically during the menstrual cycle, suggesting that the system of adrenergic nerves in the primate oviduct is under the control of endogenous estrogen and progesterone [41]. It was also reported that estrogen and progesterone affect not only the noradrenaline content of adrenergic nerves in the uterus and oviduct but also the turnover of noradrenaline, the activity of the enzymes that synthesize it, and the release of noradrenaline from nerve terminals [42]. By electron microscopic examination, non-vascular adrenergic nerves were found in smooth muscle bundles of human fallopian tube and electrical field stimulation of adrenergic nerves in the isthmic smooth muscle induced an alpha-receptor-mediated contractile response [43]. In rats, the sympathetic nerve fibers of the upper part of the uterus arise from the ovarian plexus nerve that mainly originates from neurons of the suprarenal ganglia and of the T10 to L3 ganglia of the paravertebral sympathetic chain, whereas most of the sympathetic innervation of the lower uterus arises from neurons of the paravertebral ganglia T13 to S2, principally at the L2–L4 levels, suggesting that regulation of myometrial activity by the sympathetic nerve system is functionally different between the oviduct and the cervical ends of the uterus [44].

Accordingly, the influence of the sympathetic nerve response on the female genital tract should be considered clinically. In fact, it was demonstrated that mock embryo transfer stimulation (injection of 20 μl of ultrasound contrast agent alone) evoked uterine peristalsis that could cause embryo migration and extrude the transferred embryo with fluid [45]. The density of nerve fibers in the oviduct isthmus in women with hydrosalpinx was revealed to be low compared with that in women without hydrosalpinx, suggesting the involvement of autonomous nerve system in the mechanism of hydrosalpinx-associated infertility [46]. A recent study showed that transcutaneous electrical acupoint stimulation significantly improved the clinical outcome of embryo transfer [47].

## 5. The immune network around the implantation pathway

### 5.1. Circulating immune cell contribution to embryo implantation

Mammals are a unique group of species in terms of accepting embryos within the maternal uterus (embryonal parasitic strategy). In this respect, maternal recognition of the developing embryo in the genital tract is a very important process to prepare a favorable maternal environment for subsequent embryo implantation. In humans, HCG secreted by the implanting embryo stimulates the corpus luteum of pregnancy to produce progesterone, maintaining embryo implantation in the uterus. Previously, we found that the immune system also contributes to this process and proposed that "corpus luteum function is maintained not only by HCG (endocrine system), but also by lymphocytes (immune system)" [48]. In mouse, implantation experiments, intravenous or intrauterine administration of splenocytes derived from early pregnant mice induced endometrial differentiation and successful implantation in pseudopregnant recipient mice [49, 50]. On the basis of these results, we proposed a new concept that "The immune system recognizes some information on the presence of the developing embryo around the implantation period and, thereafter, circulating immune cells transmit this information to the ovary and the uterus through blood circulation to induce adequate differentiation of pregnancy CL and endometrium to facilitate embryo implantation." Furthermore, we found that peripheral blood mononuclear cells (PBMC) promoted endometrial receptivity in vitro, while HCG affected PBMC function not through authentic HCG receptor, but sugar chain receptors, which is a primitive mechanism in the immune system [51, 52]. These experimental facts led us to pay attention to sugar chain moieties as candidate key structures of embryonal signals to the maternal immune system. These findings also suggest the important roles of circulating immune cells in embryo implantation from a very early stage [53].

### 5.2. Direct and functional communication between para-aortic lymph nodes and the implantation pathway of the developing embryo

What is the main immune organ for the first recognition of the developing embryo in the implantation pathway? From insight obtained from gynecologic oncology, para-aortic lymph nodes are classified as regional lymph nodes in patients with uterine corpus cancer. When we used a fluorescent indocyanine green to confirm the sentinel lymph nodes from the fundus lesion, rapid drainage into para-aortic lymph nodes, especially around the proximal site of the branch of the inferior mesenteric artery, from the uterine fundus through the suspensory ligament of the ovary and the meso-oviductal space, was initially detected using a PDA camera system (Figure 6). Theoretically, this supports the presence of direct communication between para-aortic lymph nodes and the implantation pathway of the developing embryo through the immune system.

Recently, Treg cells have been shown to facilitate maternal immune tolerance of the semiallogeneic conceptus and proposed to play a crucial role in embryo implantation and fetal development. During the pre-implantation period, factors in the seminal fluid delivered at coitus cause expansion of a CD4(+)CD25(+) putative Treg cell population in the para-aortic lymph nodes [54]. They were also reported to be rapidly recruited to para-aortic lymph nodes and activated in the first days after embryo implantation [55]. In mouse, implantation experiments, splenocytes derived from early pregnant mice (post-ovulation day 4) when the embryo had not yet attached to the endometrium could induce endometrial differentiation and successful implantation in the early stage of pseudopregnant recipient mice that had been

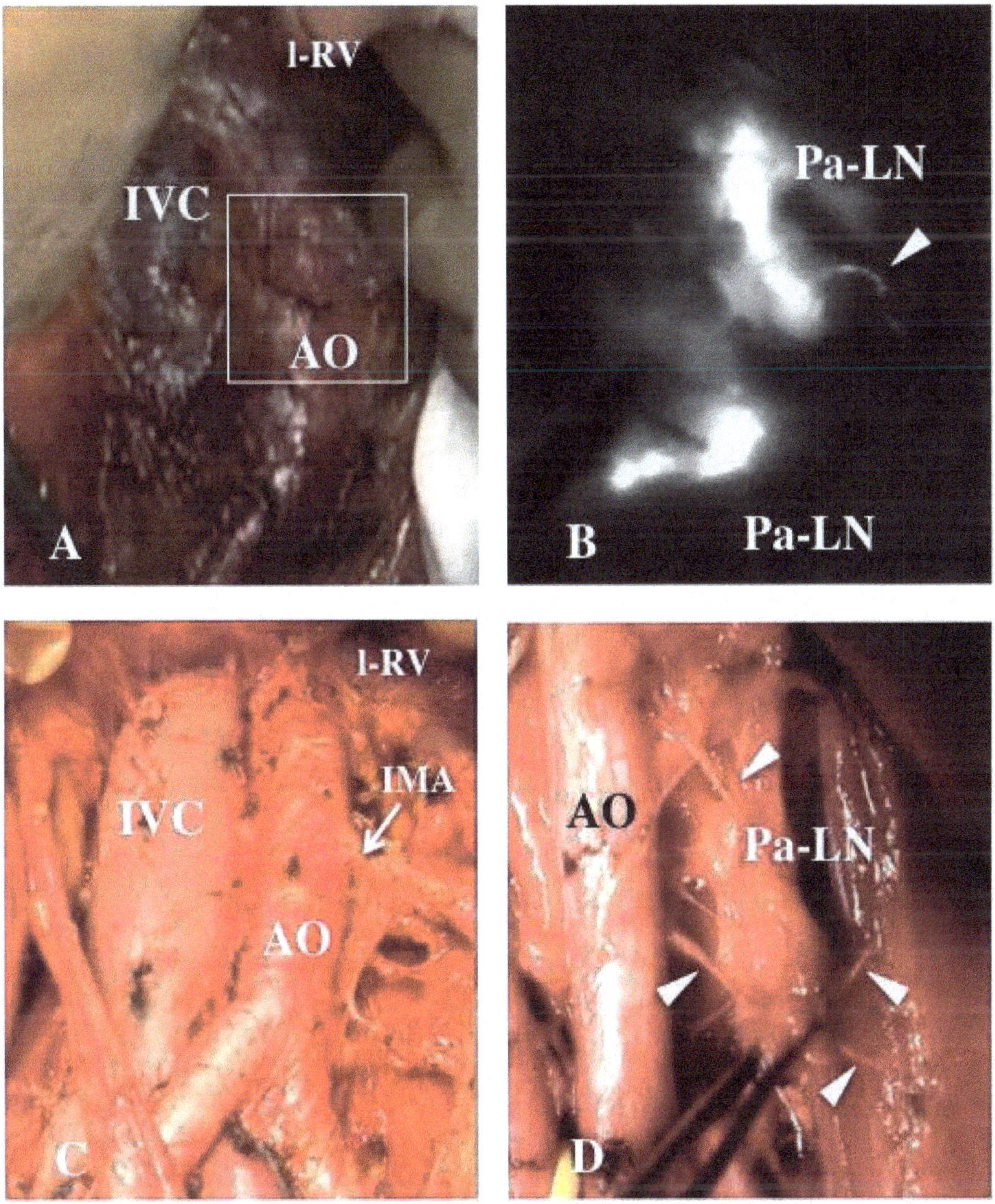


**Figure 6.** Direct communication between para-aortic lymph nodes and the embryo through the immune system. When fluorescent indocyanine green was injected into the uterine fundus that was affected by endometrial cancer cells in order to confirm the sentinel lymph nodes from the fundus lesion, rapid drainage into para-aortic lymph nodes, especially around the proximal site of the branch of the inferior mesenteric artery was detected by the PDA camera system. A: The retroperitoneal para-aortic region was opened. B: A magnified figure of the square area of A. Indocyanine green-positive para-aortic lymph nodes and an afferent lymph vessel (arrowhead) were clearly detected. C: A figure from after lymph node dissection. D: Para-aortic lymph nodes communicated by vessels and nerves (arrows). Pa-LN, para-aortic lymph nodes; Ao, aorta; IVC, inferior vena cava; IMA, inferior mesenteric artery; l-RV, left renal vein.

mated with vasectomized male mice, indicating that functional change of peripheral immune cells has already occurred before embryo implantation [49, 50]. Importantly, since the immune system of pseudopregnant recipient mice mated with vasectomized male mice was already sensitized with seminal plasma component of seminal fluid, the changes in splenocyte function were induced by the presence of developing embryos [56]. In addition, it was reported that functional changes in the endometrium could be induced in pregnant mice even when the uterotubal transition sites were ligated and entry of the developing embryos into the uterine cavity was inhibited [57], indicating that the developing embryo in the fallopian tube can influence maternal endometrial differentiation. Collectively, it is speculated that mothers can recognize the developing embryo during this early phase through the para-aortic lymph nodes.

The human para-aortic lymph nodes are rich in not only vascular but also automatic nerve networks (Figure 6D). Importantly, all primary and secondary immune organs receive substantial sympathetic innervation from sympathetic post-ganglionic neurons. This sympathetic nervous system either enhances or inhibits the activity of both acquired and adaptive immune systems [58]. Adrenergic nerve fibers were found following both afferent and efferent blood vessels as well as T areas, supporting a regulatory role of the sympathetic nervous system in human lymph nodes [59]. Intriguingly, amputation of autonomic nerves innervating the uterus was reported to cause on-time implantation failure in rats, increasing the population of uterine mast cells and facilitating the release of histamine by mast cells [60]. These findings support the concept that the neuro-immune network plays an important role in embryo implantation.

## 6. Fundus-Ovary-Salpinx-Para-aorta Implantation Promoting Unit (FOSPa-IP unit)

On the basis of the above evidence, we suppose that there is a unique unilateral functional unit to promote human embryo implantation among the fundus, the ovary, the fallopian tube, and the para-aortic regions (Figure 7). From an anatomical viewpoint, we here propose naming this novel functional unit as the Fundus-Ovary-Salpinx-Para-aorta Implantation Promoting Unit, that is, the FOSPa-IP unit. This functional unit seems to be co-operatively regulated by the endocrine, immune, and nerve systems.

Recently, increasing attention has been paid to patients with repeated implantation failures under IVF-ET treatment. It should be noted that the process of maternal recognition by the immune system in the FOSPa-IP unit is largely skipped in the treatment of IVF-ET. Considering the intrinsic function of the FOSPa-IP unit, we developed a novel therapy for patients with repeated implantation failures to complement the functions of the unit. Concretely speaking, PBMC are isolated from patients and incubated for two days with HCG in order to activate them. Thereafter, activated PBMC are administered into the uterine cavity to induce adequate endometrial differentiation. Three days later, blastocysts are transferred into the uterine cavity.

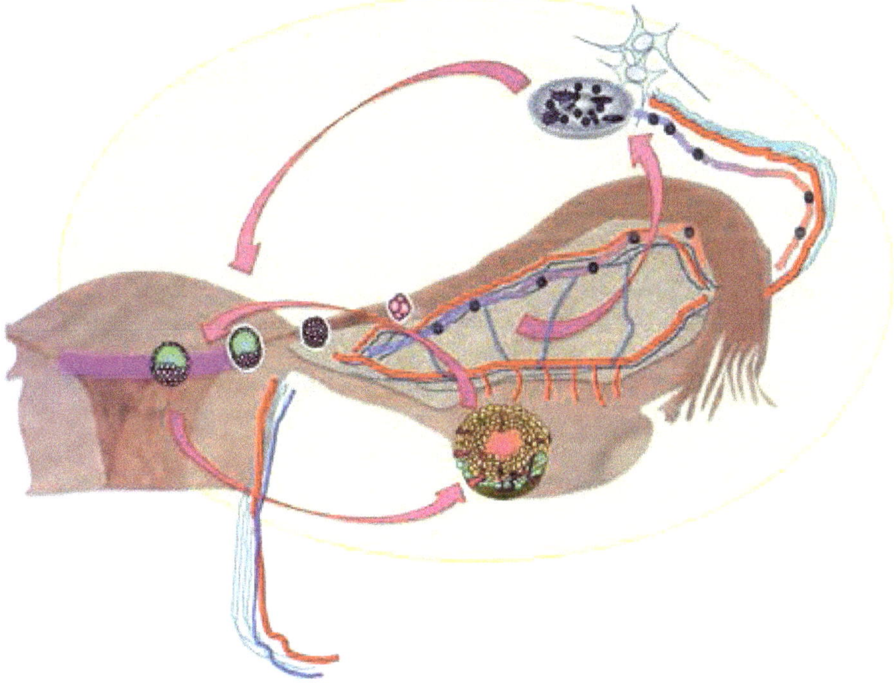

**Figure 7.** Proposal ofthe FOSPa-IP unit. We propose a unique unilateral functional unit that promotes human embryo implantation among the fundus, the ovary, the fallopian tube, and the para-aortic regions. This functional unit seems to be co-operatively regulated by the endocrine, immune, and nerve systems and can be named the Fundus-Ovary-Salpinx-Paraaorta Implantation Promoting Unit, that is, FOSPa-IP unit.

We applied this treatment to patients with 4 or more repeated failures in IVF therapy and it effectively improved the clinical pregnancy and implantation rates [2, 61].

## 7. Conclusion

In humans, the TCL space at the top of the uterine cavity in the fundus may be the main site of crosstalk between embryo and mother before implantation. Including this space, we propose the presence of a unique unilateral functional unit, named the FOSPa-IP unit, among the fundus, the ovary, the fallopian tube, and the para-aortic regions, which promotes human embryo implantation. The local concentration of progesterone along the implantation pathway of the human embryo is considered high, regulating uterine contractility and influencing human embryo implantation. On the other hand, the immune-endocrine interactions along the implantation pathway of the embryo generate an environment that promotes embryo implantation, contributing to fetal survival within the maternal uterus, suppressing adverse maternal immune responses and promoting immunotolerance pathways. In addition, circulating immune cells were shown to contribute to embryo implantation in a very early stage, probably after being activated in para-aortic lymph nodes. Furthermore, the influence of the sympathetic nerve response on the female genital tract has been clinically noticed, based on the concept that the neuro-immune network plays an important role in embryo implantation. Considering the intrinsic function of the FOSPa-IP unit, we developed a novel therapy for patients with repeated implantation failures to complement functions of this unit. Further understanding of reproductive organs from the viewpoint of the FOSPa-IP unit is expected to contribute to the development of new therapies, especially in the field of reproductive medicine.

## Author details

Hiroshi Fujiwara[1*], Yoshihiko Araki[2], Shigeru Saito[3], Kazuhiko Imakawa[4], Satoru Kyo[5], Minoru Shigeta[6], Masahide Shiotani[7], Akihito Horie[8] and Takahide Mori[9]

*Address all correspondence to: fuji@kuhp.kyoto-u.ac.jp

1 Department of Obstetrics and Gynecology, Kanazawa University Graduate School of Medical Science, Japan

2 Institute for Environmental and Gender-specific Medicine, Juntendo University Graduate School of Medicine, Japan

3 Department of Obstetrics and Gynecology, Faculty of Medicine, University of Toyama, Toyama, Japan

4 Laboratory of Animal Breeding and Reproduction, Veterinary Medical Sciences, Graduate School of Agricultural and Life Sciences, University of Tokyo, Japan

5 Department of Obstetrics and Gynecology, Faculty of Medicine, Shimane University, Japan

6 Advanced Fertility Center of Fuchu Nozomi, Osaka, Japan

7 Hanabusa Women's Clinic, Kobe, Japan

8 Department of Gynecology and Obstetrics, Kyoto University Graduate School of Medicine, Japan

9 Academia for Repro-Regenerative Medicine, Tokyo, Japan

## References

[1] Fujiwara H: Do circulating blood cells contribute to maternal tissue remodeling and embryo-maternal cross-talk around the implantation period? Mol Hum Reprod. 2009;15:335-43. doi: 10.1093/molehr/gap027.

[2] Yoshioka S, Fujiwara H, Nakayama T, Kosaka K, Mori T, Fujii S: Intrauterine administration of autologous peripheral blood mononuclear cells promotes implantation rates in patients with repeated failure of IVF-embryo transfer. Hum Reprod. 2006;21:3290-4.

[3] Cakmak H, Taylor HS: Implantation failure: molecular mechanisms and clinical treatment. Hum Reprod Update. 2011;17:242-53. doi: 10.1093/humupd/dmq037.

[4] Grinsted J, Avery B: A sporadic case of delayed implantation after in-vitro fertilization in the human? Hum Reprod. 1996;11:651-4.

[5] Fujii H, Tatsumi K, Kosaka K, Yoshioka S, Fujiwara H, Fujii S: Eph-ephrin A system regulates murine blastocyst attachment and spreading. Dev Dyn. 2006;235:3250-8.

[6] Shiotani M, Taniwa H, Hattori N, Nakamura K, Komatsu T, Hosino T, Shimada H, Ikeuchi M, Ihara Y: A specific uterine lumen for human embryo implantation educed from its configuration and implantation sites. Nihon Sanka Fujinka Gakkai Zasshi. 1999;51:S331. Japanese, Abstract.

[7] Minami S, Ishihara K, Araki T: Determination of blastocyst implantation site in spontaneous pregnancies using three-dimensional transvaginal ultrasound. J Nippon Med Sch. 2003;70:250-4.

[8] De Ziegler D, Bulletti C, De Monstier B, Jääskeläinen AS: The first uterine pass effect. Ann N Y Acad Sci. 1997;828:291-9.

[9] Bulletti C, de Ziegler D, Flamigni C, Giacomucci E, Polli V, Bolelli G, Franceschetti F: Targeted drug delivery in gynaecology: the first uterine pass effect. Hum Reprod. 1997;12:1073-9.

[10] Ouyang Z, Liu P, Yu Y, Chen C, Song X, Liang B, Zhong G, Liu C, Li Z: Role of ovarian artery-to-uterine artery anastomoses in uterine artery embolization: initial anatomic and radiologic studies. Surg Radiol Anat. 2012; 34:737-41.

[11] Einer-Jensen N, Hunter RH: Physiological and pharmacological aspects of local transfer of substances in the ovarian adnexa in women. Hum Reprod Update. 2000;6:132-8.

[12] Cicinelli E, Einer-Jensen N, Cignarelli M, Mangiacotti L, Luisi D, Schonauer S: Preferential transfer of endogenous ovarian steroid hormones to the uterus during both the follicular and luteal phases. Hum Reprod. 2004;19:2001-4.

[13] Cicinelli E, Einer-Jensen N, Barba B, Luisi D, Alfonso R, Tartagni M: Blood to the cornual area of the uterus is mainly supplied from the ovarian artery in the follicular phase and from the uterine artery in the luteal phase. Hum Reprod. 2004;19:1003-8.

[14] Hutchings G, Williams O, Cretoiu D, Ciontea SM: Myometrial interstitial cells and the coordination of myometrial contractility. J Cell Mol Med. 2009;13:4268-82. doi: 10.1111/j.1582-4934.2009.00894.x.

[15] Hendricks CH: A new technique for the study of motility in the nonpregnant human uterus. J Obstet Gynaecol Br Commonw. 1964;71:712-5.

[16] Hendricks CH: Inherent motility patterns and response characteristics of the non-pregnant uterus. Am J Obstet Gynecol. 1966;96:824-43.

[17] Togashi K: Uterine contractility evaluated on cine magnetic resonance imaging. Ann N Y Acad Sci. 2007;1101:62-71.

[18] Van Gestel I, IJland MM, Hoogland HJ, Evers JL: Endometrial wave-like activity in the non-pregnant uterus. Hum Reprod Update. 2003;9:131-8.

[19] Fanchin R, Ayoubi JM: Uterine dynamics: impact on the human reproduction process. Reprod Biomed Online. 2009;18 Suppl 2:57-62.

[20] Lyons EA, Taylor PJ, Zheng XH, Ballard G, Clifford CS, Kredentser JV: Characterization of subendometrial myometrial contractions throughout the menstrual cycle in normal fertile women. Fertil Steril. 1991;55:771-4.

[21] Kunz G, Beil D, Deininger H, Wildt L, Leyendecker G: The dynamics of rapid sperm transport through the female genital tract: evidence from vaginal sonography of uterine peristalsis and hysterosalpingography. Hum Reprod. 1996;11:627-32.

[22] IJland MM, Evers JLH, Dunselman GAJ, Van Katwijk C, Lo CR, Hoogland HJ: Endometrial wavelike movements during the menstrual cycle. Fertil Steril. 1996;65:746-9.

[23] Kunz G, Kissler S, Wildt L, Leyendecker G: In: Filicori M. editors, Endocrine Basis of Reproductive Function. Monduzzi. 2000.

[24] Fukuda M, Fukuda K: Uterine endometrial cavity movement and cervical mucus. Hum Reprod. 1994;9:1013-6.

[25] Cretoiu SM, Simionescu AA, Caravia L, Curici A, Cretoiu D, Popescu LM: Complex effects of imatinib on spontaneous and oxytocin-induced contractions in human non-pregnant myometrium. Acta Physiol Hung. 2011;98:329-38. doi: 10.1556/APhysiol.98.2011.3.10.

[26] Cretoiu SM, Cretoiu D, Marin A, Radu BM, Popescu LM: Telocytes: ultrastructural, immunohistochemical and electrophysiological characteristics in human myometrium. Reproduction. 2013;145:357-70. doi: 10.1530/REP-12-0369.

[27] Cretoiu D, Ciontea SM, Popescu LM, Ceafalan L, Ardeleanu C: Interstitial Cajal-like cells (ICLC) as steroid hormone sensors in human myometrium: immunocytochemical approach. J Cell Mol Med. 2006;10:789-95.

[28] Lea RG, Sandra O: Immunoendocrine aspects of endometrial function and implantation. Reproduction. 2007;134:389-404.

[29] Schumacher A, Costa SD, Zenclussen AC: Endocrine factors modulating immune responses in pregnancy. Front Immunol. 2014;5:196. doi: 10.3389/fimmu.2014.00196.

[30] Szekeres-Bartho J, Wilczynski JR, Basta P, Kalinka J: Role of progesterone and progestin therapy in threatened abortion and preterm labour. Front Biosci. 2008;13:1981-90.

[31] Alok A, Mukhopadhyay D, Karande AA: Glycodelin A, an immunomodulatory protein in the endometrium, inhibits proliferation and induces apoptosis in monocytic cells. Int J Biochem Cell Biol. 2009;41:1138-47. doi: 10.1016/j.biocel.2008.10.009.

[32] Tibbetts TA, Conneely OM, O'Malley BW: Progesterone via its receptor antagonizes the pro-inflammatory activity of estrogen in the mouse uterus. Biol Reprod. 1999;60:1158-65.

[33] Gellersen B, Fernandes MS, Brosens JJ: Non-genomic progesterone actions in female reproduction. Hum Reprod Update. 2009;15:119-38. doi: 10.1093/humupd/dmn044.

[34] Kowalik MK, Rekawiecki R, Kotwica J: The putative roles of nuclear and membrane-bound progesterone receptors in the female reproductive tract. Reprod Biol. 2013;13:279-89. doi: 10.1016/j.repbio.2013.09.001.

[35] Sharma S: Natural killer cells and regulatory T cells in early pregnancy loss. Int J Dev Biol. 2014;58:219-29.

[36] Henderson TA, Saunders PT, Moffett-King A, Groome NP, Critchley HO: Steroid receptor expression in uterine natural killer cells. J Clin Endocrinol Metab. 2003;88:440-9.

[37] Inoue T, Kanzaki H, Imai K, Narukawa S, Katsuragawa H, Watanabe H, Hirano T, Mori T: Progesterone stimulates the induction of human endometrial CD56+ lymphocytes in an in vitro culture system. J Clin Endocrinol Metab. 1996;81:1502-7.

[38] Carlino C, Stabile H, Morrone S, Bulla R, Soriani A, Agostinis C, Bossi F, Mocci C, Sarazani F, Tedesco F, Santoni A, Gismondi A: Recruitment of circulating NK cells through decidual tissues: a possible mechanism controlling NK cell accumulation in the uterus during early pregnancy. Blood. 2008;111:3108-15. doi: 10.1182/blood-2007-08-105965.

[39] Czaja K, Kaleczyc J, Sienkiewicz W, Majewski M, Lakomy M: Peptidergic innervation of the porcine oviduct studied by double-labelling immunohistochemistry. Folia Histochem Cytobiol. 1996;34:141-50.

[40] Czaja K, Kaleczyc J, Pidsudko Z, Franke-Radowiecka A, Łakomy M: Distribution of efferent neurones innervating the oviduct in the pig. Folia Morphol (Warsz). 2001;60:243-8.

[41] Sjöberg NO, Johansson ED, Owman C, Rosengren E, Walles B: Cyclic fluctuation in noradrenaline transmitter of the monkey oviduct. Acta Obstet Gynecol Scand. 1977;56:139-53.

[42] Marshall JM: Effects of ovarian steroids and pregnancy on adrenergic nerves of uterus and oviduct. Am J Physiol. 1981;240:C165-74.

[43] Sporrong B, Helm G, Owman C, Sjöberg NO, Walles B: Electron microscopic and pharmacologic evidence for a functional adrenergic innervation of the smooth musculature in the human fallopian tube. Brain Res Bull. 1982;9:695-9.

[44] Houdeau E, Rousseau A, Meusnier C, Prud'Homme MJ, Rousseau JP: Sympathetic innervation of the upper and lower regions of the uterus and cervix in the rat have different origins and routes. J Comp Neurol. 1998;399:403-12.

[45] Zhu L, Xiao L, Che HS, Li YP, Liao JT: Uterine peristalsis exerts control over fluid migration after mock embryo transfer. Hum Reprod. 2014;29:279-85. doi: 10.1093/humrep/det429.

[46] Zhu L, Chen J, Sun Y, Huang X, Xu H, Zhang X: Loss of nerve fibers in the oviduct isthmus in women with hydrosalpinx. Acta Histochem. 2013;115:609-15. doi: 10.1016/j.acthis.2013.01.008.

[47] Zhang R, Feng XJ, Guan Q, Cui W, Zheng Y, Sun W, Han JS: Increase of success rate for women undergoing embryo transfer by transcutaneous electrical acupoint stimulation: a prospective randomized placebo-controlled study. Fertil Steril. 2011;96:912-6. doi: 10.1016/j.fertnstert.2011.07.1093.

[48] Hashii K, Fujiwara H, Yoshioka S, Kataoka N, Yamada S, Hirano T, Mori T, Fujii S, Maeda M: Peripheral blood mononuclear cells stimulate progesterone production by luteal cells derived from pregnant and non-pregnant women: possible involvement of interleukin-4 and interleukin-10 in corpus luteum function and differentiation. Hum Reprod. 1998;13:2738-44.

[49] Takabatake K, Fujiwara H, Goto Y, Nakayama T, Higuchi T, Maeda M, Mori T: Intravenous administration of splenocytes in early pregnancy changes the implantation window in mice. Hum Reprod. 1997;12:583-5.

[50] Takabatake K, Fujiwara H, Goto Y, Nakayama T, Higuchi T, Fujita J, Maeda M, Mori T: Splenocytes in early pregnancy promote embryo implantation by regulating endometrial differentiation in mice. Hum Reprod. 1997;12:2102-7.

[51] Egawa H, Fujiwara H, Hirano T, Nakayama T, Higuchi T, Tatsumi K, Mori T, Fujii S: Peripheral blood mononuclear cells in early pregnancy promote invasion of human choriocarcinoma cell line, BeWo cells. Hum Reprod. 2002;17:473-80.

[52] Kosaka K, Fujiwara H, Tatsumi K, Yoshioka S, Sato Y, Egawa H, Higuchi T, Nakayama T, Ueda M, Maeda M, Fujii S: Human chorionic gonadotropin (HCG) activates monocytes to produce interleukin-8 via a different pathway from luteinizing hormone/HCG receptor system. J Clin Endocrinol Metab. 2002;87:5199-208.

[53] Fujiwara H: Immune cells contribute to systemic cross-talk between the embryo and mother during early pregnancy in cooperation with the endocrine system. Reprod Med Biol. 2006;5:19-29.

[54] Guerin LR, Moldenhauer LM, Prins JR, Bromfield JJ, Hayball JD, Robertson SA: Seminal fluid regulates accumulation of FOXP3+ regulatory T cells in the preimplantation mouse uterus through expanding the FOXP3+ cell pool and CCL19-mediated recruitment. Biol Reprod. 2011;85:397-408. doi: 10.1095/biolreprod.110.088591.

[55] Chen T, Darrasse-Jèze G, Bergot AS, Courau T, Churlaud G, Valdivia K, Strominger JL, Ruocco MG, Chaouat G, Klatzmann D: Self-specific memory regulatory T cells protect embryos at implantation in mice. J Immunol. 2013;191:2273-81. doi: 10.4049/jimmunol.1202413.

[56] Fujiwara H, Araki Y, Toshimori K: Is the zona pellucida an intrinsic source of signals activating maternal recognition of the developing mammalian embryo? J Reprod Immunol. 2009;81:1-8. doi: 10.1016/j.jri.2009.04.001.

[57] Wakuda K, Takakura K, Nakanishi K, Kita N, Shi H, Hirose M, Noda Y: Embryo-dependent induction of embryo receptivity in the mouse endometrium. J Reprod Fertil. 1999;115:315-24.

[58] Nance DM, Sanders VM: Autonomic innervation and regulation of the immune system (1987-2007). Brain Behav Immun. 2007;21:736-45.

[59] Panuncio AL, De La Peña S, Gualco G, Reissenweber N: Adrenergic innervation in reactive human lymph nodes. J Anat. 1999;194:143-6.

[60] Yuan XJ, Huang LB, Qiao HL, Deng ZP, Fa JJ: Uterine autonomic nerve innervation plays a crucial role in regulating rat uterine mast cell functions during embryo implantation. Prostaglandins Other Lipid Mediat. 2009;90:94-7.

[61] Okitsu O, Kiyokawa M, Oda T, Miyake K, Sato Y, Fujiwara H: Intrauterine administration of autologous peripheral blood mononuclear cells increases clinical pregnancy rates in frozen/thawed embryo transfer cycles of patients with repeated implantation failure. J Reprod Immunol. 2011;92:82-7. doi: 10.1016/j.jri.2011.07.001.

# 2

# Novel Cellular and Molecular Interactions During Limb Development, Revealed from Studies on the Split Hand Foot Congenital Malformation

Daniele Conte, Luisa Guerrini and Giorgio R. Merlo

### Abstract

The embryonic development of the limbs is widely used as a paradigm for the comprehension of the cellular processes and molecular mechanisms underlying organogenesis and pattern formation. The chick, mouse and (recently), zebrafish embryos are excellent models, for the ease of experimental manipulation and the availability of several mutant strains with limb malformation defects.

Knowledge on the molecular circuits that control cell expansion and position-dependent cell differentiation in the developing limb bud is rapidly expanding. Recently, a set of human congenital malformations known as split hand foot malformations (SHFM) together with the corresponding animal models have revealed novel molecular players and regulations, important for the function and maintenance of the apical ectodermal ridge, the structure that coordinates limb outgrowth with digit pattern.

In this chapter we illustrate the pathways centred on the master transcription factor p63, and discuss the mechanisms by which these pathways impact on the regulation of signalling molecule controlling growth and shape of the normal limb. Finally we indicate how the signalling networks are misregulated in SHFM, and point to emerging functions of the FGF8 and Wnt5a signalling molecules.

**Keywords:** Limb, Embryonic ectoderm, AER, SHFM, EEC, p63, Dlx5, Wnt5a, FGF8

# 1. Introduction

The limbs are projecting paired appendages of an animal body used especially for movement and grasping, for example, wings, arms, and legs. The development of the limb bud is often taken as a paradigm for a cellular and molecular comprehension of the common principles of organogenesis and pattern formation. Embryonic patterning implies that cells acquire positional information, usually by interpreting concentration gradient of signalling molecules. Accordingly, limb pattern is specified along three principal axes: anterior-posterior (A-P) (e.g., thumb to little finger), dorsal-ventral (D-V) (e.g., back of hand to palm) and proximal-distal (P-D) (e.g., shoulder to nails). Digit pattern across the A-P axis is a classic example of a signalling gradient that specifies positional values, linked to a gradient of Sonic-Hedgehog (SHH). D-V patterning is less studied and involves signals from dorsal and ventral ectoderm. The specification of P-D positional values has long been considered to involve a timing mechanism, under the control of ligands of the fibroblast growth factor (FGF) family. A concentration gradient of molecules can also give cells polarity information, recently shown to be critical for patterning and morphogenesis.

The limbs are not essential for life, thus a large number of mutant strains are available for studies on the genetic determinants of limb development, in normal and pathological conditions. Manipulation of chicken limb buds has been widely used in the past, mainly because of the ease of examination and manipulation, to postulate the first models of limb bud development leading to the identification of important regulatory genes and interactions. In addition to the chicken model, functional genetics has made great advances thanks to spontaneous and engineered loss- and gain-of-function mutant mouse strains, and recently with the advent of the zebrafish embryos as animal models.

In this chapter, we illustrate the pathways centred on the master transcription factor p63, and discuss the mechanisms by which these pathways impact on the regulation of signalling molecules controlling growth and patterning of the normal limb bud. Based on available knowledge, we propose how signalling networks are misregulated in the split hand foot malformation (SHFM) and related developmental conditions, and indicate emerging functions of the FGF8 and Wnt5a diffusible molecules.

### 1.1. Limb initiation

Around the embryonic age E8.0 in the mouse, limb buds are initiated as four lumps of mesenchymal cells covered by ectoderm, protruding from the main body axis at approximately the position of somites 6–11 (the forelimbs, FL) and somites 24–27 (the hindlimbs, HL). The limb buds are paired along the cephalo-caudal axis and develop at the same fixed locations on this body axis (Figure 1A). How are their positions defined?

It has been proposed that the position of several dorsal organs along the cephalo-caudal axis, their identity and timing of appearance depend on the expression of specific sets of *Hox* genes. The 39 vertebrate *Hox* genes code for homeodomain transcription factors, homologous with the genes of the Drosophila *HOM-C* complex, and are combinatorially expressed along the

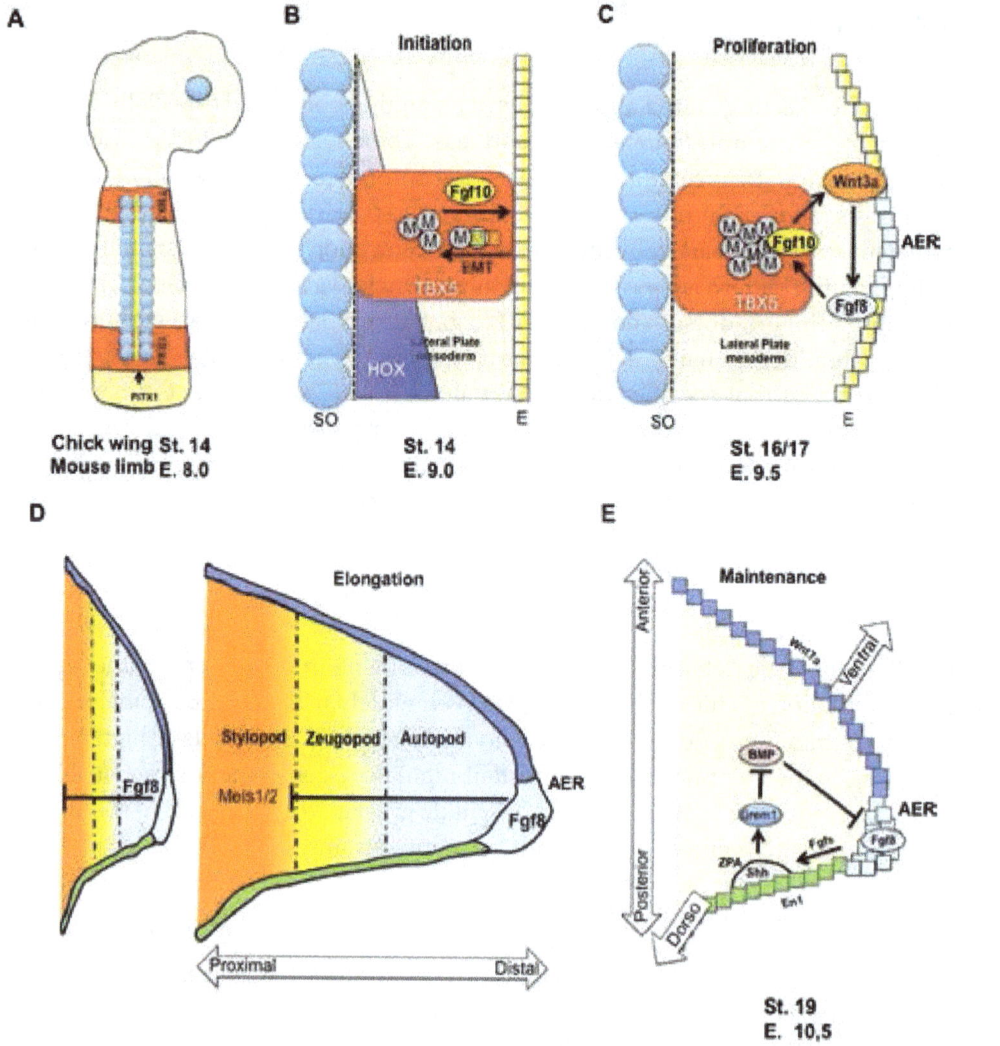


Conte et al.

**Figure 1.** Schematic representation of limb development with embryonic timeline for chick wing and mouse forelimb. A) Representation of the prospective limb territories in a stage 14/8 chick (Hamburger-Hamilton stages, HH))/mouse embryo. The forelimbs (FL) and hindlimbs (HL) derive from discrete regions of the lateral plate mesoderm (LPM). *Tbx5* (red) is expressed in the prospective FL, whereas *Tbx4* (red) is expressed in the prospective HL. In this stage, *Pitx1* (yellow) is expressed in a caudal domain that overlaps with *Tbx4*. The somites (blue) are numbered and serve as reference for the axial position of the FL and HL fields. B) Model of initiation of FL bud. Hox protein gradients establish the condition for the synthesis of retinoic acid (RA) in the LPM. RA causes induction of the transcription factors Tbx5 (or Tbx4 for the HL). *Tbx5*-expressing mesechymal cells express *FGF10* and induce the ectodermal cells of the surface (yellow square) to activate epithelial-mesenchymal transition (EMT). C) Newly generated mesenchymal cells express *FGF10* that induces the overlaying ectodermal cells to express *FGF8* giving rise to the apical ectodermal ridge (AER). Expression of *FGF8* by the AER induces the mesenchymal cells to express *FGF10,* thus establishing a positive feedback loop for the initial phases of limb outgrowth. D) Schematic representation of the progress zone (PZ) model. The AER maintains cells of the PZ in an unspecified state. For a detailed description of the proposed models of P-D patterning see the text. E) AER-derived FGF8 maintain the expression of *SHH* in the ZPA cells, which in turn gives feedback on the AER cells to maintain *FGFs* expression, via Grem1 and BMP inhibition. This signalling between the AER and ZPA contributes to co ordinate the patterning along the P-D and A-P axes.

main body axis. *Hox* genes are serially organized in four clusters (a, b, c, and d), each located on a different chromosome. Within each cluster, *Hox* genes are organized in a physical order collinear with the cephalo-caudal axis of the growing organism so that the genes lying at the 3′ end are expressed earlier and are localized in the most anterior domains. Moving toward the 5′ direction, each next gene is expressed in a progressively more posterior territory. Thus, each *Hox* gene has a specific anterior limit of expression, and each A-P embryonic territory expresses a specific combination of *Hox* genes, utilized as positional information.

A key signalling molecule for limb initiation is FGF10, a member of the FGF family of diffusible peptides. The *FGF10* mRNA is detected quite early in the presumptive limb mesenchyme and promotes AER induction (a key organizer and regulator of the P-D limb extension; see below) and initiation of ectopic limb development when applied exogenously [1]. Conversely, in *FGF10*-null mice, limb buds are initiated but the AER does not form, resulting in complete truncation of all four limbs [2 - 4].

The expression of *FGF10* coincides with the time when the trunk is only competent to form an ectopic limb, for example, the time at which the trunk mesenchyme becomes determined and can no longer be redirected to a limb fate (the HH stage 16–17 of the chick embryo) [5, 6]. The initial assumption was that limbs originate from a pre-existing mesenchymal population undergoing a localized regulation of proliferation. In fact, at the HH stage 17–18, there is a substantial decrease in proliferation of the flank mesoderm, while instead higher rates are maintained within the emerging limb buds.

The current model considers that, shortly after gastrulation, a re-epithelization of mesodermal cells occurs so that the entire embryo is essentially epithelial, including also the notochord, the somites, the intermediate mesoderm and the lateral plate mesoderm (LPM). At stage HH 13 in the chick, before limb initiation, the somatopleure displays epithelial rather than mesenchymal features. The LPM of the limb field starts out as an epithelium and ultimately generates limb-bud mesenchyme through a process termed epithelial-mesenchymal transition (EMT) [7] (Figure 1B). In embryos null for *FGF10* and *Tbx5* the proportion of mesenchymal cells compared to the proportion of epithelial cells was significantly lower than that of wild-type (WT). These mutants show hyperplasia of the somatopleure epithelium, in support of failure of these cells to undergo EMT. These new data show the time in which the trunk is competent to form an ectopic limb, is precisely the time at which the trunk mesenchyme is initially generated. The old experiments of ectopic application of FGF10 need to be re-interpreted, as induction of limb-bud formation from epithelial trunk somatopleure cells and not from mesenchymal cells of the same A-P level.

### 1.2. T-box genes and limb-type specification

The FL and HL of all vertebrate species are evidently different (e.g., wing vs. leg in the chick embryo, pectoral vs. pelvic fins in fish embryos, arms vs. legs in primates, etc.). The specification of limb-type identity and morphology is established before overt limb initiation. A large body of evidence indicates that two transcription factors of the T-box family participate in the early definition of limb-type identity: *Tbx5* for the presumptive territories of the mouse FL (wing of the chick, pectoral fins of fishes) and of *Tbx4* in the presumptive territory of the mouse

HL (leg of the chick, pelvic fins of fishes) (Figure 1A). These genes are expressed very early in the prospective limb mesoderm and, in addition to define limb-type identity, also appear to be necessary and sufficient for early limb induction [8 - 15].

However, although only expressed in FL and HL, respectively, *Tbx5* and *Tbx4* appear not to be the master directors of limb-bud identity/morphology design. Instead, the *Pitx1* gene, which codes for a paired-type homeodomain transcription factor and which is expressed in the HL bud, is the upstream regulator of *Tbx4*, and is directly implicated in HL specification. Multiple independent *cis*-regulatory elements of *Tbx4* expression have been identified, including the HL-specific enhancers [16]. Both may be targets of Pitx1 and other unknown upstream factors. Structural changes of these regulators might be some of the multiple factors responsible for the hind/lower limb morphology specification. However, limb-bud identity/morphology determination remains to a large extent unexplained.

### 1.3. Role of retinoic acid

A signalling molecule known to act upstream of *Tbx5* during forelimb/pectoral fin development is retinoic acid (RA) [17 - 21]. According to old observations, patterning along the proximal-distal axis of the vertebrate limb is controlled by opposing diffusible signals, in which RA functions as the proximal signal and FGF as the distal one [22, 23].

The mechanism through which RA controls limb development has been widely debated [21], but clear results have only been produced in recent years [17, 19, 22, 24 - 27]. Mouse and zebrafish embryos null for the gene *aldehyde dehydrogenase-1a2 (aldh1a2)* fail to synthesize RA and do not develop limbs/fins. These mutants fail to express *Tbx5*, and the exogenous application of RA can rescue both limb/fin development and *Tbx5* expression [18, 19, 25, 27, 28]. However, a recent paper shows that RA signalling is not required for P-D limb patterning, and instead provides genetic evidence that RA-FGF antagonism occur only along the trunk lateral plate mesoderm, prior to FL budding, to permit induction of *Tbx5* [29]. This study shows that RA controls limb development in a manner much different than that originally envisioned (see below).

### 1.4. Proximal-distal axis

The limb skeleton is laid down as five cartilage skeletal elements, not just the three referred to as stylopod (humerus/femur), zeugopod (radius-ulna/tibia-fibula), and autopod (digits); in fact two carpal regions between zeugopod and autopod are present, that initially have the same size as the other segments but then grow substantially less.

P-D extension and patterning is strictly linked to the signalling activity of the apical ectodermal ridge (AER), a morphologically distinct ectodermal thickening, extending along the entire A-P length, and lining the D-V border. The AER is present between E9 and E11 in the mouse embryo, consists of a pseudo-stratified epithelium in the chick and pluri-stratified epithelium in the mouse, and is a dynamic structure constantly undergoing morphogenetic changes [30 - 32].

The AER plays a fundamental role in promoting and regulating the outgrowth and patterning of the P-D limb axis. Experimental removal of the AER in chicken limb buds, causes a developmental arrest, and truncation of wing skeleton [33], meanwhile grafts of an AER to a recipient limb bud induces ectopic P-D outgrowth [34]. In 1993, Niswander identified FGFs as the relevant signals produced by the AER to induce P-D limb axis formation and extension. P-D extension and outgrowth is rescued by exogenous application of FGFs on AER removal [35]. This study provided the first molecular insights into how AER-FGF signalling controls in P–D extension and patterning. Four FGF ligands (4, -8, -9 and -17), are expressed by the AER cells with redundant functions during P–D patterning of mouse limb buds. Inactivation of the three FGFs expressed predominantly by the posterior AER (FGF4, -9, -17) does not alter limb-bud development [36]. In contrast, loss of *FGF8*, which is the first and only FGF ligand expressed by the entire AER from early stages onward, disrupts formation of the proximal-most limb skeletal element [37 - 40]. This early and transient disruption of P-D extension is rescued by the activation of FGF4 in the *FGF8*-deficient AER, which results in almost normal development of the more distal limb skeleton [41, 42]. Combined inactivation of both *FGF8* and *FGF4* causes a complete arrest of limb-bud development and limb agenesis [39, 42]. In addition, transient expression of *FGF8* and *FGF4* during initiation of limb-bud outgrowth is sufficient for specification of the entire PD axis, but the progressive proliferative expansion of such specified limb segments is disrupted [42].

Other AER-expressed FGFs, in particular *FGF9*, contribute to the proliferative expansion of the limb mesenchymal progenitors in a P-D sequential order, so that higher AER-expressed FGF levels are required for formation of more distal limb structures [36]. Taken together, this genetic analysis reveals an instructive role of AER-FGF signalling in the specification and proliferative expansion along the P–D axis.

The AER is first induced by the expression of *FGF10* in the prospective limb-bud mesenchyme. *FGF10* is expressed in the same territories as *Tbx4 and Tbx5* and interestingly, *FGF10* is a direct transcriptional target of these transcription factors. The expression of *FGF10* is essential to establish AER-expressed FGF signalling, which in turn is required to maintain *Ffg10* expression [1, 42]. The reciprocal induction of *FGF10-FGF8* requires the expression of *Wnt3a,* coding for a ligand of the Wnt family acting through the β-catenin pathway (described in the following sections). The activation of *Wnt3* expression couples *FGF8* and *FGF4* expression from cells of the AER with *FGF10* expression [43, 44]. Thus, in these early phases, a positive feedback loop between *FGF10* and *FGF8* is established in adjacent territories, and is required for reciprocal maintenance (Figure 1A-C).

### 1.5. Limb extension: The progress zone

Old experiments showed that removing the AER at progressively earlier stages resulted in truncations of the limb skeleton at progressively more proximal levels [33]. Thus, the acquisition of a P-D positional identity seemed to depend on the time that proliferating/unspecified cells spend near the AER (the progress zone, PZ) under the influence of AER signals. According to the model proposed by Summerbell and Wolpert [45] the mesenchymal progenitor cells leaving the PZ early would acquire proximal identities, whereas the same cells leaving the PZ later would acquire progressively more distal identities (Figure 1D).

The great merit of this model has been to introduce the notion of time as an important factor in morphogenetic signalling; however, as a result of extensive molecular and cellular analyses, the original PZ model has been largely abandoned. First, the loss of proximal but not distal skeletal elements in *FGF8*-deficient mouse limb buds [40] are difficult to reconcile. Second, fate mapping studies in chicken embryos provide good evidence for the presence of pools of progenitor cells with distinct P-D identities, specified very early and then expanded sequentially by proliferation [46]. Removal of the AER at progressively later stages simply eliminates the distal mesenchyme containing the specified but not yet expanded progenitor pools. These studies provide a straightforward alternative explanation for the loss of distal skeletal elements following AER removal [46]. These and other results led to the proposal of the early specification/expansion model as an alternative to the PZ model [42, 46]. This model proposes that AER-expressed FGF signalling controls survival and sequential proliferative expansion of a pool of progenitor/stem cells in P-D territories, in a dose- and time-dependent highly regulated fashion.

A third model has been proposed, in which P-D patterning is controlled by opposing diffusible signals, with RA functioning as a proximal signal and FGF acting as a distal signal [26]. Chick FL or HL ectopically exposed to RA or FGF8, or to antagonists of RAR or FGF receptor, display P-D fate changes that either expand or contract expression of proximal limb markers [23]. Further evidence has been recently provided, indicating that RA is needed for P–D patterning of both FL and HL [47, 48]. Using recombinant heterotopic chick limb transplantations they propose that the exposure to the activities of Wnt3a, FGF8 (distal molecule), and RA (proximal molecule) maintains the potential to form both proximal and distal structures. While these studies report the ability of RA treatment to reprogram distal limb mesenchyme to a proximal fate and to maintain early limb mesenchyme in a *Meis1*-expressing proximal fate alongside Wnt and FGF treatment [47], they do not address a requirement for endogenous RA in proximal limb mesenchyme. The ability of RA to increase *Meis1/2* (a proximal marker) could be a consequence of loss of FGF signalling, known to repress *Meis1/2* distally [36].

Recently, Cunningham and colleagues [29] provide convincing evidence that RA is not required for limb patterning and that RA-FGF antagonism does not occur along the limb P-D axis, as originally proposed [26]. They suggest that both the initial expression of *Meis1/2* in the LPM and later in the proximal limb bud do not require RA signalling, while the downregulation of *Meis1/2* expression in the distal limb requires AER-derived FGF8. They suggest that since *FGF8* expression in the AER appears after limb-bud formation [37], the proximal most limb domain is out of range of early AER-derived FGF signals, leading to maintenance of proximal *Meis1/2* expression and restricted distal *Meis1/2* expression (Figure 1D).

### 1.6. Anterior-posterior pattern

The mammalian limb bud is typically pentadactylous, for example, the autopodium gives rise to five skeletal elements. The digit organization, from anterior (pre-axial, the thumbs) to posterior (post-axial, the little finger) is referred to as the A-P pattern. It has long been recognized that the embryonic tissue mainly implicated in the regulation of the A-P pattern is the zone of polarizing activity (ZPA) (Figure 1E). In 1956, a region within the posterior-proximal limb mesenchyme was identified, that when grafted in the anterior margin of host chicken wing buds results in mirror image duplications of all digits [49, 50]. The ZPA acts as a signalling centre and specifies positional information in the limb-bud mesenchyme by secreting the diffusible molecule Sonic Hedgehog (SHH). Within the limb bud mesenchyme, SHH is present in a posterior (high) to anterior (low) gradient [51, 52]. Genetic studies indicate that the time spent expressing *SHH* provides cells with a kinetic memory relevant to specification of their A-P identities [53 - 56].

SHH signalling is translated into an intracellular, anterior (high) to posterior (low), gradient of the transcriptional repressor Gli3R within the limb mesenchyme [67]. Upon binding to the receptor Patched, SHH counteracts the conversion of Gli3 full-length into its cleaved repressor form. The Gli3R gradient is then required to establish the polarized expression of other genes involved in A-P patterning, and ultimately is translated into digit pattern, in ways not fully clarified [24, 57 - 61].

Further genetic studies in mouse and zebrafish embryos have implicated also HAND2 in the activation of *SHH* expression in both limb and fin buds [62]. Moreover, in the mouse embryo a mutual antagonistic interaction between Hand2 and Gli3, prior to *SHH* expression, establishes a A-P pre-pattern [60, 61, 63]. Finally, at later stages of development, the expression of the 5′ most members of the *Hoxd* gene cluster is activated within the posterior limb-bud mesenchyme. Cell biochemical studies have revealed a direct interaction of Hoxd proteins with the *cis*-regulatory limb-bud enhancer region of the *SHH* gene [64].

### 1.7. Hox genes and digit identity

An exhaustive illustration of this topic is beyond the scope of this chapter. Digit patterning has commonly been interpreted in the context of a gradient of expression of *SHH* preventing the processing of Gli3 to its repressor form (Gli3R) [65, 66].

Thus, a SHH gradient is translated into an inverse Gli3R gradient [24, 67]. However, between *Gli3* and *SHH;Gli3* null mutant mice display identical polydactylous limb phenotypes, indicating that an iterative series of (non-patterned) digits can form in the absence of SHH [24, 60], suggesting the existence of a SHH-independent prepatterning.

This observation, rather than supporting the SHH gradient model, is consistent with a Turing-type model of digit patterning [68 - 70]. According to this model, dynamic interactions between activator and inhibitor molecules produce periodic patterns of spots or stripes, serving as a molecular pre-pattern for chondrogenesis. Although the core molecules of a self-organizing mechanism remain poorly known, potential candidates for molecular modulators of the system include the *Hox* genes [70]. Distal *Hoxa* and *Hoxd* genes have a well-known impact on digit number, though their specific role remains unclear. *Hoxd* genes interact with the SHH-Gli3 pathway; these include the mutual transcriptional regulation between Hox genes and SHH and the binding of Hoxd12 to Gli3R, resulting in a blockage of Gli3R repressor activity [71 - 73]. In general, gain- and loss-of-function experiments suggest a positive relation between *Hox* genes and digit number [72, 74] that is also indicated by the ectopic anterior up-regulation of distal *Hoxd* genes in the Gli3-dependent polydactyly [24, 61]. Interestingly the disruption of various *Hox* genes combined with loss of *Gli3* results in polydactyly; more *Hox* genes are removed – more digits are formed [75]. Thus, losing *Hox* genes seemed to shorten the spacing between digits – the wavelength in Turing's mathematical language.

The Turing's model implies the activity of two diffusing and interacting molecules; however, *Hox* genes code for non-diffusible transcription factors, for example, they cannot directly participate. However, evidence that distal *Hox* genes are necessary for correct limb development is overwhelming. Indeed, in addition to a correct digit formation via a Turing-type regulation of SHH signalling, a second role of *Hox* genes in limb P-D patterning has been studied in depth. Caudal, late-expressed paralogs of the *Hox* gene clusters display a P-D as well as A-P gradient of expression within the limb mesenchyme [76, 77] suggesting a combinatorial role of these genes in patterning the limb skeletal elements. Experimental evidence leads to the conclusion that the paralogs 9–13 of the *Hox* gene clusters *-a* and *-d* specify individual limb segments [78]. Indeed *Hoxa11 -/-;Hoxd11 -/-* double mutant embryos lack radius and ulna [79] while *Hoxa13 -/-;Hoxd13 -/-* double mutants lack digits [80].

Finally, in spite of the major role played by posterior *Hox* genes, little is known about the cellular and/or molecular bases for the observed developmental defects. Attempts in this directions [81] show that malformation of the FL zeugopod in *Hoxa11/Hoxd11* double mutant mice results from multiple defects during the formation of the zeugopod, including reduced *FGF8* and *FGF10* expression, formation of smaller mesenchymal condensations, and failure to form normal growth plates at the proximal and distal ends of the zeugopod bones. As a consequence, growth and maturation of these bones is highly disorganized.

### 1.8. AER and ZPA interaction

The maintenance and propagation of *SHH* expression requires AER-derived FGF signalling as part of a positive epithelial-mesenchymal (E-M) feedback loop operating between the ZPA and the AER [82, 83] (Figure 1E). The BMP antagonist Gremlin1 (Grem1) was identified as a crucial mesenchymal component in this E-M feedback signalling system [59, 66, 84]. Grem1 is required to up-regulate AER-FGF signalling and to establish SHH/Grem1/FGF E-M feedback signalling. In *Grem1*-null limb buds, the establishment of this E-M feedback signalling loop is interrupted, and this in turn interferes with specification and expansion of the distal compartment (zeugopod and autopod) [59, 84].

### 1.9. Dorsal-ventral axis

Dorsal-ventral (D-V) patterning is mainly organized via signalling by Wnt7a, a diffusible molecule of the Wnt-family expressed in the dorsal ectoderm. Wnt7a is both necessary and sufficient to dorsalize the limb, indeed the loss of *Wnt7a* causes the dorsal side of limbs to acquire a ventral side identity, accompanied by missing posterior digits. Wnt7a is required to maintain expression of *SHH,* explaining the digit loss. Restoring the Wnt7a signal rescues both of these defects [85, 86].

Wnt7a induces the expression of *Lmx1,* coding for a Lim-family homeodomain-containing transcription factor. Lmx-1 is involved in dorsalization of the limb, which was shown by deleting *Lmx1* in mice: *Lmx1* null embryos produced ventral skin on both sides of their paws [87, 88]. There are other factors known to control the D-V patterning; on the ventral side the transcription factor-coding *Engrailed-1* gene, exclusively expressed in the ventral ectoderm, has been shown to repress the dorsalizing effect of Wnt7a in this territory [89] (Figure 1E).

## 2. Distal Limb Malformations in Human

Congenital limb malformations are relatively common, and are genetically and clinically heterogeneous, with a diverse spectrum in their epidemiology, aetiology and anatomy. They are often difficult to diagnose and categorize, because of their complex phenotypes and their association with other malformations and clinical symptoms. Many etiological factors have been suggested for limb anomalies, including inheritance of mutated genes, teratogenic drugs, environmental chemicals, ionizing radiation (atomic weapons, radioiodine and radiation therapy), infections, metabolic imbalance (e.g., maternal diabetes), or mechanical factors like amniotic band syndrome. With the advent of functional genetics, molecular pathways centred on disease genes are being unravelled.

A wide set of human congenital limb malformations can be attributed to defects in P-D development. In this chapter, we will attempt to link known disease-causing genes with their known or presumed function in the maintenance of the AER. We will focus on the genes for which more functional data are available: namely *Dlx5, FGF8, p63* and *Wnts*. These genes are co-expressed in the AER cells of the mouse limb [90] as well as in the fins of the zebrafish embryos [91, 92] and are known or proposed diseases-genes for the SHFM and EEC congenital limb malformations.

P-D defect refer to absence or hypoplasia of distal structure of the limb with more or less normal proximal structures. The spectrum of P-D limb reduction anomalies ranges from very mild disorders, such as syndactyly, to very severe forms, such as phocomelia or amelia. The most frequent congenital limb malformations are syndactylies, characterized by the fusion of the soft tissues of fingers and toes with or without bone fusion. Syndactylies are due to the lack of apoptosis in the interdigital mesenchyme and may also occur isolated or with other symptoms in a syndrome [93].

Polydactylies are distinguished by the appearance of supernumerary digits or parts of them, which may be present as a complete duplication of a whole limb or as a duplication of single digits [94]. Pre-axial polydactyly with extra digits located on the side of the hand or of the thumb or postaxial polydactyly where the extra digit is found on the side of the hand or foot of the fifth digit are common isolated limb malformation traits. On molecular level, many forms of polydactyly have been shown to be more or less directly linked to the SHH signal transduction pathway, which play a major role in A-P patterning of the limb [95, 96].

Brachydactylies are defined by shortened digits and are classified on an anatomic and genetic background into five groups from A to E [93]. Isolated brachydactylies are often inherited in an autosomal dominant manner and are characterized by a high degree of phenotypic variability. Type-B brachydactylies are associated to mutation in the *Ror2* gene, and *Ror2* mutations are also associated with the Robinow syndrome in which brachydactyly is a common feature [97 - 101].

A severe P-D arrest of the developing limb bud gives rise to phocomelia, characterized by undeveloped limbs [102]. Usually the upper limbs are not fully formed and sections of the "hands and arms may be missing". Short arm bones, fused fingers and missing thumbs will often occur. Legs and feet are also affected. Individuals with phocomelia will often lack thigh bones, and the hands or feet may be abnormally small or appear as stumps due to their close attachment to the body. Phocomelia is a known negative effect of the administration of thalidomide to pregnant women, in use in the late 1950s/early 1960s, to treat morning sickness, although the mechanism of action of this teratogen remains controversial [103, 104].

Failure of formation of limb buds gives rise to amelia, the complete absence of one or more limbs. The most severe form of amelia is the tetra-amelia, characterized by the absence of all four limbs, associated with craniofacial, pulmonary and urogenital defects. This autosomal recessive disorder has been linked to mutations of the *WNT3* gene (see the following section).

### 2.1. SHFM and EEC

SHFM, also known as ectrodactyly or lobster-claw malformation, is a congenital defect affecting predominantly the central rays of hands and/or feet. It may manifest either as an isolated trait or as part of syndromic conditions comprising other developmental disorders [105]. SHFM occurs with the incidence of about 1 in 18,000 live born infants and accounts for 8–17% of all limb malformations [106, 107]. SHFM is clinically heterogeneous, ranging from a relatively mild defect, such as hypoplasia of a single phalanx or syndactyly, to aplasia of one or more central digits (i.e., classical cleft, also known as lobster-claw anomaly).

Inter-individual and intra-familial variability of the SHFM is very high. Furthermore, variable expressivity of this feature can be so significant, that a different pattern of anomaly is seen in each limb of the same individual patient [93]. SHFM is mostly sporadic, although familial forms are known: in these cases an autosomal dominant transmission with reduced penetrance is the most common mode, but autosomal recessive and X-linked forms have been reported.

SHFM has been linked to (at least) six distinct loci [106] (Table 1). SHFM-I (MIM #183600) is the most frequent type and is linked to mutations and/or deletions/rearrangements of the *DLX5;DLX6* bigenic locus. Deletions, inversions and rearrangements affecting chromosome 7q21 have long been reported [108 - 112]. The smallest region of overlapping deletions encompasses several other genes in addition to *DLX5*, and *DLX6*: as *DYNC1I1, SLC25A13, DSS1*, but only *Dlx5* and *Dlx6* have been shown to be specifically expressed in the AER of the developing mouse limbs [113 - 115]. Recently, a point mutation in the DNA-binding domain of DLX5 (Q178P) has been reported in a SHFM-I family with a recessive transmission, co-segregating with the limb malformations [116]. In the mouse, the combined disruption of *Dlx5;Dlx6* leads to an ectrodactyly phenotype affecting the HLs [114, 115], fully confirming that the human orthologs *DLX5* (and presumably *DLX6)* are the disease genes for this malformation. Interestingly, SHFM type-V (MIM #606708) is linked to deletions of a region on chromosome 2 encompassing the *HOXD* gene cluster, near *DLX1* and *DLX2* [117 - 119]. Although no clear evidence for the involvement of *DLX1* and *DLX2* in this malformation is available, it is tempting to imagine that similar to *DLX5*, misregulated expression of *DLX1/2* in the human embryonic limb bud could be the molecular mechanism leading to SHFM type-V.

SHFM type-III (MIM# 600095) is associated with duplications/rearrangements around the *DACTYLIN* (*FBXW4*) locus on chromosome 10q and the synthetic one in mice [120, 121]. The genomic lesion involves the *DACTYLIN, LBX1, βTRCP* and other more distant genes, but none of these is directly disrupted by the rearrangement and no point mutation has been reported. Interestingly, the *FGF8* locus is located in the proximity of the rearrangement breakpoints [122], and considering its importance for P-D limb development, it represents a valid candidate SHFM type-III disease gene.

Mutations of p63 are associated to SHFM type-IV (MIM #605289), a condition in which ectrodactyly appears as an isolated non-syndromic disorder linked to mutations or chromosomal anomalies in the DBD or in the C-terminal domain of p63$\alpha$ [123 - 125]. The $\alpha$ tail of p63 contains a sumoylation site, inactivated by *p63* mutations found in SHFM-IV (E639X). Sumoylation can modulate p63 half-life [126] and naturally occurring mutated p63 proteins often display altered stability, suggesting that the final effect of the mutations could be the persistence of the mutated protein and consequent misexpression of p63 targets [125, 127, 128]. p63 mutations also cause the ectodermal dysplasia-ectrodactyly-cleft lip/palate syndrome type-III (EEC-3) syndrome (MIM #604292) [129] in which ectrodactyly is a common feature.

SHFM type-VI (MIM #225300) is the only autosomal recessive form of this malformation, and is due to homozygous point mutations of the *WNT10B* gene [130 - 133]. Finally, the X-linked SHFM type-II form (MIM #313350) has been mapped to chromosome Xq26.3 [134] but no disease gene has yet been identified.

| SHFM locus | Chromosome/gene affected | Case reported | Inheritancepattern | Limb phenotypes | Additional phenotypes | References |
|---|---|---|---|---|---|---|
| **SHFM-I** | Rearrangements 7q21.3-q22.1*DLX5* mutation | 1 family | Autosomal dominant Autosomal recessive | SHFM | EEC, mental retardation, sensorineural deafness | Crackower et al. (1996) Marinoni et al. (1995) Shamseldin et al. (2012) |
| **SHFM-II** | Xq26 | 1 family | X-linked recessive | SHFM, syndactyly, metacarpalhypo plasia, phalangeal hypoplasia | | Faiyaz ul Haque et al. (2005) |

| SHFM locus | Chromosome/gene affected | Case reported | Inheritancepattern | Limb phenotypes | Additional phenotypes | References |
|---|---|---|---|---|---|---|
| **SHFM-III** | Duplication 10q24 | 20% | Autosomal dominant | SHFM, triphalangeal and/ orduplicated thumbs | | de Mollerat et al. (2003) |
| **SHFM-IV** | *TP63* mutations | 10% non syndromic93% EEC syndromes | Autosomal dominant | SHFM | EEC, ADULT, LADD, CHARGE,VATE R/mental retardation | van Bokhoven et al. (2001) Ianakiev et al. (2000) |
| **SHFM-V** | Deletion 2q31 | | Autosomal dominant | SHFM | Mental retardation, ectodermal and craniofacialfindi ngs, orofacial clefting | Goodman et al. (2002) Del Campo et al. (1999) |
| **SHFM-VI** | *WNT10B* mutation | 3 family1 sporadic case | Autosomal recessive | SHFM, tibial aplasia/ hypoplasia | | Ugur and Tolun (2008) Blattner et al. (2012) Khan et al. (2012) |

SHFM – Split Hand/Foot Malformation, EEC – Ectrodactyly-Ectodermal dysplasia-Cleft lip/palate, ADULT – Acro-Dermato-Ungual-Lacrimal-Tooth syndrome, LADD – Lacrimo-Auriculo-Dento-Digital syndrome,

CHARGE syndrome (Coloboma of the eye, Heart defects, atresia of the nasal choanae, Retardation of growth and/or development, Genital and/or urinary abnormalities, Ear abnormalities and deafness), VATER association - vertebral anomalies, anal atresia, cardiovascular anomalies, tracheoesophageal fistula, renal and/or radial anomalies, limb defects.

**Table 1.** Genetic alterations and SHFM-related phenotypes

## 2.2. p63-Dlx5;Dlx6 Regulation

SHFM type-IV and EEC are caused by mutations in the *p63* gene, which codes for a highly conserved transcription factor related to the *p53* and *p73* tumour-suppressor genes [129, 135 - 137]. A common feature of these disorders is ectodermal dysplasia, consisting in abnormal maturation and stratification of the skin and abnormal development of hairs, teeth, nails, exocrine glands and cornea. The other two consistent features of *p63*-linked disorders are cleft lip/palate and ectrodactyly.

p63 is expressed in the basal or progenitor layers of many epithelial tissues [138, 139], and is able to promote the epithelial stratification program typical of the mammalian skin, as well as to control proliferation and exit from the cell cycle of epidermal stem cells. For these activities p63 has been proposed as a master regulator of epidermal stem cell maintenance, proliferation and stratification [140]. The *TP63* gene is translated into ten protein isoforms [141]: the trans-activating (TA) isoforms, closely resembling p53, and the delta-N (ΔN) isoforms, devoid of the TA-domain-1 (TA1). Although the TA isoforms were initially thought to be the ones to possess transcriptional regulatory functions, it has well been established that the ΔN isoforms can activate transcription of a distinct set of target genes via a second TA-domain-2 (TA2) [142]. Five TA and ΔN isoforms are generated by two transcripts which are subjected to alternative splicing, thus the final protein products differ at the carboxyl termini ($\alpha$, $\beta$, $\gamma$, $\delta$ and $\varepsilon$). In addition to TA1 or TA2 domain, the p63 proteins contain a DNA-binding domain (DBD) and an oligomerization domain (OD). The $\alpha$-isoforms (either TA or ΔN) also contain a sterile alpha motif (SAM) domain, a protein-protein interaction module found in developmentally relevant proteins [143, 144]. Recent studies have identified a transcriptional inhibitory (TI) domain located between the SAM domain and the C-terminus of p63$\alpha$; this domain is believed to be responsible for the lower transcriptional activity of TAp63$\alpha$ compared to the -$\beta$ and the -$\gamma$ isoforms [145]. ΔNp63$\alpha$ is the most expressed isoform in the embryonic ectoderm.

Attempts to establish genotype–phenotype correlations are hampered by the variable clinical expressivity observed within families: SHFM type-IV and the EEC syndromes are due to mutations in the DNA-binding domain of p63 [129]. In these cases, all p63 isoforms are affected by the mutations. DBD mutants usually act as dominant-negative effectors and render the WT protein unable to bind DNA [129], explaining the dominant transmission of EEC. In contrast, the Hay Wells or ankyloblepharon-ectodermal dysplasia-cleft palate syndrome (AEC, MIM #106260) manifests with normal limbs but severe skin defects, and is typically associated with heterozygous missense mutations in the SAM domain of p63. The acro-dermato-ungual lacrimal tooth (ADULT, MIM #103285) syndrome is associated with a specific gain-of-function mutation R298Q/G in exon 8, affecting the DNA-binding domain of p63. Finally, both limb-mammary syndrome (LMS, MIM #603543), very similar to ADULT and EEC syndromes, and Rapp-Hodgkin syndrome (RHS, MIM #129400), resembling AEC, are due to p63 mutations. *p63* mutations causing EEC are usually not found in AEC, LMS and SHFM [146 - 148].

Mice null for *p63* have been generated by two groups independently [136, 137]; at birth these mice show severe defects affecting their skin, limb and craniofacial skeleton, teeth, hair, and mammary glands. Specifically, the skin appears thin, mostly single layered and translucent, unable to prevent water loss. The HLs fail to form altogether, while the FLs are severely truncated and lack most of their distal skeletal elements. The altered phenotypes observed in these mutant mice are a direct consequence of altered cellular properties affecting the same tissues and organs as in EEC patients [90, 136, 137, 149, 150]. While in the null embryos the *p63* protein is missing altogether (i.e., both the TA and ΔN isoforms), in EEC, AEC, LMS, and SHFM-IV patients the mutated p63 protein coexists with half of the normal dose of the wild-type protein. To better model the disease, the group of Dr. A. Mills (CSHL, USA) has generated mice bearing the *R279H* mutation (found in EEC patients). Homozygous embryos and newborn animals show a global phenotype similar, but not identical, to that of *p63-/-* [90], consisting in the absence of the HL, severely truncated FL, a thin translucent skin and cranio-facial and palatal defects. The HL defects in both the *p63* null and in the *p63-R279H* homozygous embryos are evident as early as E9.5, and are accompanied by loss of AER stratification and *FGF8* expression [90, 136, 137]. Interestingly, mild limb defects are observed in heterozygous p63-R279H mice, the mouse model closer to EEC.

Mouse models of the AEC syndrome have also been generated. Compared to EEC patients, AEC patients suffer of extreme skin fragility but have normal limbs. The AEC-mutant p63 proteins appear to act in a dominant-negative fashion. Mice were generated in which either ΔNp63a is down regulated in the skin, as a way to mimic the dominant negative action of mutant p63 in the AEC patients, or an AEC-mutant p63 was introduced [151 - 153]. These mice show severe skin erosion resembling the AEC phenotype, characterized by suprabasal epidermal proliferation, delayed terminal differentiation and altered basement membrane.

p63 mutations cause limb congenital phenotypes due to their impact on the AER Animal models show p63 is essential for epidermal stratification [90, 139, 154 - 156]. Considering that the AER is one of the earliest attempt of the embryonic (non-neural) ectoderm to organize into a multilayered epithelial tissue [157], it is not surprising that in *p63* null or *p63 R279H* homozygous mice the AER is thinner and poorly stratified. Failure to maintain AER stratification and FGF8 expression is a common feature of various ectrodactyly phenotypes [90, 157 - 159].

p63 is expected to control AER functions via transcriptional regulation of AER-restricted target genes [122, 154 - 156], indeed failure of AER stratification has also been associated with loss of expression of key morphogens for limb development, such as *FGF8* and *Dlx5;Dlx6* [122]. *Dlx* genes are the vertebrate homologs of Drosophila *Dll*, a homeodomain transcription factors required for the specification of distal limb elements in the fly embryo. In *Dll* hypomorphic mutant flies, a variable set of phenotypes is observed depending on the mutation, ranging from fusion of the distal segments (weak mutants) to complete loss of distal and medial leg segments (severe mutants) [160, 161]. In mice *Dlx* genes have a prominent role in specifying the mandible and maxillary skeletal structures [162, 163], as well as controlling normal limb development [114, 115]. Point mutations of *DLX5* have been found to co-segregate in familiar cases of SHFM [116] and the combined deletion of *Dlx5* and *Dlx6* leads to ectrodactyly of the HLs, that is, a true mouse model of SHFM type-I. There is evidence that until E11.5 the AER appears and functions normally, including a normal morphology and normal expression of AER markers (*FGF4, FGF8, Msx2*). On the contrary, at E11.5-E12 the expression of AER markers indicate that the central wedge of the AER fails to function. At about the same time the first signs of dysmorphology are visible. The expression of *FGF8* and other markers declines in the central sector of the limb bud, accompanied by loss of stratification in the same territory [158], while the expression of *SHH, Hand2* and *Tbx4* in the mutant limbs is unchanged. Considering the expression pattern of *Dlx* genes in the limb, the *Dlx5;Dlx6* null defect can be summarized as a cell-autonomous failure of the central AER to maintain and express morphogenetic molecules.

*p63* and Dlx proteins are co-expressed in the AER cells [90] as well as in the fins of the zebrafish embryos [91, 92]. In homozygous *p63* null and *p63EEC* (R279H) mutant limbs, the expression of four *Dlx* genes is strongly reduced. Functionally, when the *p63+/EEC* (heterozygous) mutation is combined with an incomplete loss of *Dlx5* and *Dlx6* alleles, severe limb phenotypes are observed, not present in mice with either mutation alone [90]. Together, there is a clear evidence for p63-Dlx regulatory cascade that is functional for distal limb development.

In vitro, ΔNp63$\alpha$ induces transcription from the *Dlx5* and *Dlx6* promoters, an activity abolished by EEC and SHFM-IV mutations, but not by AEC-associated mutations. ChIP analysis shows that p63 occupies the *Dlx5* and *Dlx6* promoters. This regulation takes place both at the proximal promoter level [90] and via a conserved *cis*-acting genomic element, located 250 kb centromeric to DLX5, an element that is specifically deleted in few SHFM patients [164]. Recent studies have identified a tissue-specific enhancer located within the coding exons 15 and 17 of the *Dync1/1* gene (near the *Dlx5;Dlx6* locus). This genomic element is characterized by an enhancer-type chromatin signature and physically interacts with a *DLX5/6* promoter region 900 kb distal to *DYNC1/1*, specifically in the limb [165, 166]. Using copy number variation (CNV) analyses in SHFM patients, combined with whole genome sequencing to map deletion and translocation breakpoints, a recent study shows that the *DYNC1I1* enhancers are also critical for limb development in humans [167]. An additional enhancer was identified in an intron of the *Slc25a13* locus, close to *Dlx5;Dlx6*, and was shown to drive *Dlx* gene expression in the otic vesicle, forebrain, branchial arch and limbs of the developing embryo [165, 166]. It is plausible that the SHFM phenotype linked with mutations in these enhancers is caused by an altered regulation of Dlx5/6 transcription.

### 2.3. Downstream of Dlx5;Dlx6

Sp8 is a transcription factor of the Sp1 zinc-finger family [168, 169], homologous to the Drosophila *D-Sp1* gene that has been implicated in appendage development [170]. In the developing limbs *Sp8* shows restricted expression in the ectoderm, including the AER cells [168]. Mouse embryos null for *Sp8* show severe developmental defects affecting the distal portion of the limbs, associated with a strongly reduced expression of *FGF8* [168, 169, 171], *Sp8* is co-expressed with *Dlx* genes in the murine AER and forebrain [172] and appears in the top 1% of a list of conserved/co-expressed genes in microarray data [173]. Furthermore, conserved Dlx5 DNA-binding sites are predicted near the *Sp8* locus, thus *Sp8* is a likely direct *Dlx5* transcriptional target. A Dlx5-Sp8 transcriptional cascade could be upstream of *FGF8* expression, which in turn maintains p63 protein stability.

A number of observations suggest that p63 and Dlx proteins may regulate *FGF8* expression by acting directly on the genomic region corresponding to the SHFM type-III critical region [120, 121]: indeed p63-binding sites are present within the region, as demonstrated by ChIP-seq screening [164], and several predicted *Dlx5* binding sites cluster around the *FGF8* locus, in genomic regions conserved across mammalian species [158] (unpublished data).

Considering that the AER of *Dac* heterozygous embryos shows reduced *FGF8* expression and defective cell layering [159], and considering that rearrangements/duplications around *Dactylin* do not disrupt or interrupt the gene, and since *Dactylin* is ubiquitously expressed in mouse tissues, the role of *Dactylin* as disease-gene is doubtful [122]. In alternative, *FGF8* and components of the NFkB pathway might be the disease-genes. It is tempting to speculate that the complex duplication rearrangement modifies the position/organization of *cis*-acting control elements, which in turn affect expression of *FGF8* and components of the NFkB pathway. Thus SHFM type-III could be a genome-misorganization type of genetic disease.

In further support of this, genome-wide CNV analyses on a Chinese family with SHFM type-III revealed a micro-duplication on chromosome 10q24 co-segregating with the SHFM phenotype [174]. This novel duplication contains two discontinuous DNA fragments: the minimal centromeric duplicated segment involves *LBX1, POLL* and a disrupted *BTRC;* the telomeric duplication encompasses *DPCD* and part of *FBXW4.* No coding and splice-site mutations of candidate genes in the region were found. Interestingly, the second duplicated fragment comprises Dlx5 and p63 DNA binding sites [164].

Another pathway that links p63 and Dlx5 in the regulation of the *FGF8* locus implicates the gene *IKKα,* a direct transcriptional target of p63 relevant for ectoderm development and limb morphogenesis [175 - 177]. Interestingly, while mutations of *p63* and loss of *Dlx5;6* lead to a reduced *FGF8* expression in the AER, in *IKKα* mutant embryos the AER shows an increased *FGF8* expression [178], which nevertheless results in distal limb truncations and severe malformations.

From the above considerations, it appears that numerous players in the p63-Dlx5 cascade may contribute to regulate *FGF8* expression in the AER. The possibility that the *FGF8* locus is a common target of the p63 and the Dlx5 networks during limb development is in agreement with the well-known functions of FGF8 to sustain epithelial mesenchymal signalling and assure the timely generation of mesenchymal progenitors [36].

### 2.4. Post-translational p63 protein regulations

Several biochemical observations indicate that the ΔN- and TAp63 proteins are tightly regulated at post-translational level, via protein modification (phosphorylation, sumoylation and ubiquitination) and protein-protein interactions [126, 158, 179, 180]. Such modifications modulate the stability of the p63 protein, regulate its transcriptional activity and ultimately modulate its ability to orchestrate the timing of exit from the cell cycle and the dynamic of stratification of mammalian ectoderm [156, 181, 182].

Among the interacting or modifying proteins, MDM2 and p53 have been previously recognized [179, 180]. Recently we have shown that the peptidyl-prolyl *cis/trans* isomerase NIMA-interacting-1, Pin1, is a regulator of ΔNp63α protein stability, inducing its proteasome-mediated degradation [158] resulting in diminished transcription of two p63 targets [183] (Figure 2).

Another modification is acetylation, catalyzed by histone acetyl-transferase on lysine residues, and known to finely regulate p53 and p73 stability and transcriptional activity [184 - 189]. p73 is acetylated by p300 on lysine residues in the DBD and Oligomerization Domain [190] enhancing p73 ability to bind and activate proapototic target genes [191]. The p73-p300 interaction requires the prolyl-isomerase Pin1, which induces conformational changes following phosphorylation by the tyrosine kinase c-Abl [192]. Acetylation of p53 correlates with its stabilization and activation by antagonizing the activity of the MDM2 ubiquitin-ligase. It is interesting to note that a naturally occurring p63 mutation found in SHFM type-IV patients

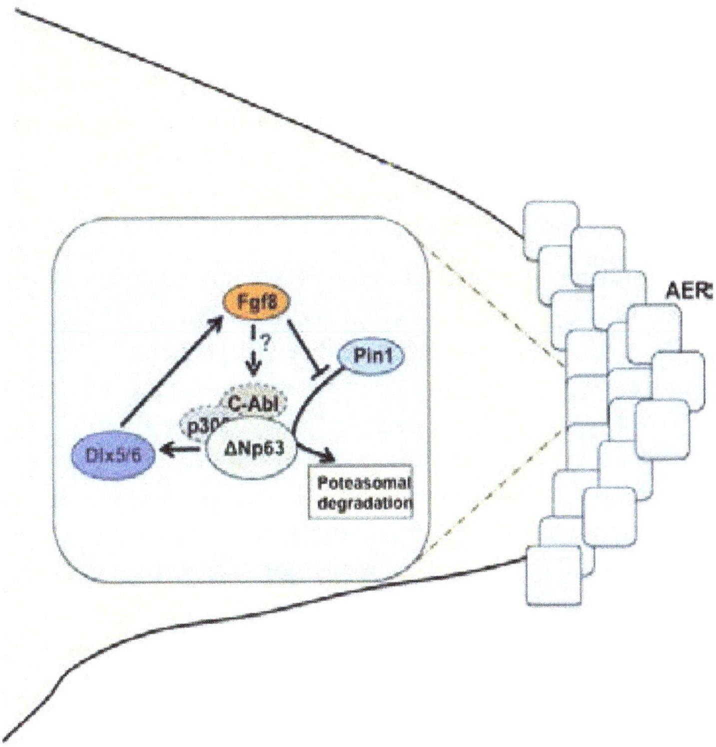


Conte et al.

**Figure 2.** Schematic representation of the molecules and their interactions that regulate the stability of ΔNp63 during the AER stratification. p63 regulates its own stability via to the expression of *FGF8*; this pathway includes the *Dlx5/ Dlx6* disease genes. Fgf8 stabilizes p63 by counteracting the activity of Pin1 to induce proteasome-mediated degradation of ΔNp63$\alpha$. Novel results indicate that FGF8 activates a signalling cascade leading to activation of c-Abl that promotes phosphorylation of ΔNp63$\alpha$ on tyrosine residues. This phosphorylation event is required for the interaction of ΔNp63$\alpha$ with the p300 acetyl-transferase, which modulated ΔNp63$\alpha$ stabilization and transcriptional activity. Although only shown in vitro, we speculate that regulation may also occur in the AER cells (dotted line).

changes lysine 193 into glutamic acid (K193E) [125, 146, 147, 193]. Our unpublished data show that ΔNp63$\alpha$ is acetylated by p300 on the K193 residue, and that the K193E mutation prevents this modification (Guerrini and Restelli, unpublished) (Figure 2).

## 2.5. Emerging roles of FGF8

Expression of *FGF8* is strongly reduced in the AER of the *p63* null, *R279H p63* mutant, and *Dlx5;Dlx6* mutant embryos [90, 115] as well as several other mouse strains with distal limb defects. The AER of these mutants appears poorly stratified. Thus, loss of AER stratification and reduced *FGF8* expression are a common theme during the onset of this specific class of malformations. The link between *FGF8* expression and AER stratification is not totally clear. When *FGFR2* gene is deleted in the AER cells, via conditional genetics, the AER loses stratification as well as Fgf*8* expression. In this case, the AER cells cannot respond to (AER-derived?) FGFs [194] and it can be concluded that AER-expressed FGFs are needed for AER maintenance, apparently in an autocrine fashion.

An emerging role of FGF8 is the control of p63 stability in the AER cells. The AER of *Dlx5/Dlx6* null mice shows poor stratification as well as reduced *FGF8* expression, similar to what is seen in *p63* mutant mice. We have documented that *Dlx5;Dlx6* are transcriptional targets of p63, and that in turn *FGF8* is a target of Dlx5. As already said, ΔNp63α protein stability is negatively regulated by the interaction with Pin1, via proteasome-mediated degradation. Recently we have shown that FGF8 counteracts Pin1-ΔNp63α interaction, thus indicating that FGF8 participates in a feedback loop which involves the p63-Dlx5 cascade [158] (Figure 2).

p63 stability might also be regulated by another post-translational modification, namely acetylation by the p300 histone acetylase. c-Abl is a key regulator of the p53 family members and is known to be activated by treatment with FGF2 [192, 195 - 198]. Recently we have collected new data showing that FGF8 is able to stabilize ΔNp63α also via a novel pathway that requires the c-Abl tyrosine kinase and the protein acetylation by p300 (Guerrini and Restelli, unpublished). Thus, Dlx5, p63, Pin1, p300 and FGF8 participate in a time- and location-restricted regulatory loop that seems to be able to self-maintain and whose normal functioning is necessary for AER stratification, hence for normal extension and patterning of the limb buds. These results shed new light on the general molecular mechanisms at the basis of the SHFM and EEC limb malformations (Figure 2).

In an interesting set of experiments using cultured embryonic limbs, it was recently shown that the FGF/MAPK pathway establishes a high-distal to low-proximal gradient that controls the migration velocity of mesenchymal cells [199]. These cell movements enable continuous rearrangement of the cells at the distal tip of the limb bud. The effect of FGF/MAPK signalling emanating from the AER is different than the effect induced by Wnt5a in the limb bud. While Wnt5a induces directional movement of cells, FGF8 acts to induce rapid, yet disorganized, movements. Ultimately, the activity of both Wnt5a and FGF results in distal elongation (Figure 3). These observations suggest that FGF8 acts by inducing random movements, but with a higher velocity as cells move close to the source. A study proposes that the FGF pathway drives tail-bud elongation in the chick embryo by promoting random cell movements [200]. According to these authors FGF creates a gradient of cell motility and that the tail bud elongates by mass action of random cell movement at the posterior end of the embryo. Although this data indicate a similar mode of FGF action, cells in the limb bud additionally undergo oriented processes of cell division and directional movements under the influence of Wnt5a. This study indicates that it is the combined action of non-canonical WNT and FGF that integrates orientation and movement, consequently driving limb-bud elongation and thereby establishing a progenitor field of the proper dimensions for the subsequent patterning and morphogenesis of limb anatomy.

### 2.6. Wnt signalling and limb development

Wnt molecules are the vertebrate homologs of the Drosophila *wingless* gene, required for wing development. Wnt molecules are involved in all aspects of embryonic development, from patterning to morphogenesis and cell-tissue interactions [201 - 203].

Several members of the Wnt family of ligands are expressed in the ectoderm and mesenchyme of the developing limbs. At early stages, *Wnt8c* and *Wnt2b* are transiently expressed in the

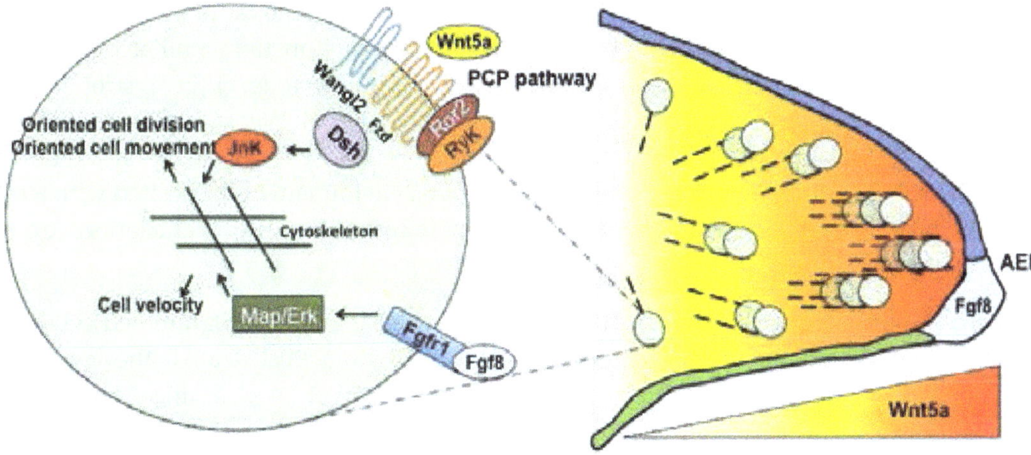


Conte et al.

**Figure 3.** Schematic representation of the mesenchymal cells orientation and organization in the early limb bud. These cellular events are regulated by the combined activities of the WNT and FGF pathways. Wnt5A/Jnk/PCP pathway is necessary for the proper orientation of cell movements and cell division. In contrast, the FGF/MAPK signaling pathway, emanating from the AER establishes a gradient of cell velocity. The combination of oriented cell divisions and movements drives the P-D extension of the limb bud necessary for subsequent morphogenesis.

LPM and participate in the initiation of HL and FL outgrowth, respectively [43]. At later stages, *Wnt3/Wnt3a* and *Wnt5a* are expressed by the AER cells while *Wnt7a* is expressed in the dorsal ectoderm.

Wnt ligands signal through the Frizzled (Fz) seven-pass trans-membrane receptors. In the "canonical" pathway, binding of Wnt ligands to Fz receptors represses the axin/glycogen synthase kinase-3β (GSK3β) complex, which in the absence of the ligand promotes the degradation of β-catenin via the ubiquitin pathway (reviewed in reference [204]). In Wnt-activated cells, cytoplasmic β-catenin accumulates and translocates to the nucleus where, in conjunction with T cell-specific factor/lymphoid enhancer binding factor-1 (Tcf/Lef1) transcription factors, activates transcription of target genes.

A role of "canonical" Wnt signalling in limb development has long been recognized [205]. In the chick limb bud, the Wnt/β-catenin pathway is essential for the induction and maintenance of the AER. Indeed, ectopic expression of Wnts in the interflank region prior to limb outgrowth induces ectopic *FGF10* expression and limb formation. FGF10 subsequently induces *Wnt3a* expression in the AER, which in turn switches on the expression of Fgf8, again via the β-catenin pathway, and promotes AER formation [43, 44, 206].

In the chick embryo *Wnt3a* mediates the Wnt/β-catenin signalling required for establishment of the AER. In the mouse, old data indicate that mouse embryos lacking the Wnt/β-catenin pathway component *LRP6*, or simultaneously lacking *Lef1* and *Tcf1*, exhibit defective AER formation and limb defects, indicating that his pathway is indeed essential for AER formation [207, 208]. However, *Wnt3a* is not expressed in the limb ectoderm of the mouse embryo, and *Wnt3a* null embryos do not show limb defects [209, 210]. Instead, the closely related *Wnt3* gene is expressed in the limb ectoderm [210] and the conditional removal of *Wnt3* in the limb ectoderm leads to severe distal limb truncations and AER malfunction. Similar results were obtained by the conditional removal of β-catenin in the limb ectoderm [211], strongly suggesting that the murine *Wnt3* is functionally homologous to chick *Wnt3a,* and that a pre-AER active Wnt3/β-catenin pathway in the embryonic ectoderm is essential for AER formation and maintenance. Notably, homozygous mutations of *WNT3* in human are associated with a rare autosomal recessive congenital disorder known as tetra-amelia [212] characterized by the absence of all four limbs.

Wnt signalling has been implicated in removing "excess" tissue by programmed cell death and sculpting the limb shape. Indeed, the ability of BMP4 to induce cell death in the developing limb appears to be mediated by Dkk1 [213]. Loss of function of Dkk1 in mice results in the downregulation of *Msx1,* a component of the cell death pathway, in the anterior and posterior necrotic zones and the interdigital mesenchyme, whilst gain of Dkk1 function in chicks causes excessive cell death via activation of the c-jun pathway [213, 214]. The decrease in cell death in the mouse mutants contributes to the polydactyly and fusion of digits that occur in *Dkk1* mutant mice [214]. In addition, Fz2, –3 and –4, and Dkk2, and –3, are expressed in the interdigit mesenchyme, suggesting that a fine balance of Wnt signalling controls cell death/survival in this region [215, 216].

### 2.7. Emerging role of Wnt5a and non-canonical signalling

Wnt ligands can also activate two other branches of "non-canonical" pathways; one of these is known as the planar cell polarity (PCP) pathway, involves Fz receptors and dishevelled (Dvl), which interact with a distinct set of "PCP proteins" such as Van Gogh (Vang) and Prickle [217]. The PCP pathway recruits the small GTPases Rho and Cdc42 and the c-Jun N-terminal kinase (JNK) [218 - 220]. Initially identified in Drosophila, PCP establishes cellular polarity in the plane of an epithelium, perpendicular to the apical-basal orientation [217]. Studies in vertebrate model systems, including Xenopus and zebrafish, indicate that the PCP pathway also regulates a morphogenetic process known as convergent extension (CE). CE was first demonstrated in gastrulating *Xenopus* embryos in which mesodermal cells underwent medio-laterally oriented intercalation, leading to concomitant tissue lengthening and narrowing [221]. Imaging experiments in zebrafish indicate that, in addition to polarized cell intercalation, the PCP pathway also regulates directional cell migration and oriented cell division underlying CE [222 - 225]. A second branch of "non-canonical" Wnt transduction pathways leads to the release of intracellular Ca2+ and the activation of protein kinase C (PKC) and Ca2+/Calmodulin-dependent Kinase-II (CamKII) [226 - 229]. The choice of the pathway being activated by a Wnt ligand appears to depend mostly on the receptor profile and on the intracellular signalling molecules available in a given cell type, and little on the Wnt ligand itself.

A role of "non-canonical" Wnt signalling during limb development has been recognized, although the cellular and molecular mechanisms are not fully clarified. The vertebrate *Wnt5a* gene, the homolog to Drosophila *Dwnt-5* gene essential for limb and appendage development, is considered the typical non-canonical Wnt, involved in the establishment of PCP [230 - 232]. Wnt5a together with Wnt11 mediates the activation of PCP during the CE in frogs and zebrafish [223, 233, 234], and during mouse limb development *Wnt5a* is expressed in a gradient from the AER to the proximal mesechymal cells, is regulated by FGF signalling from the AER and has been shown to inhibit β-catenin degradation [235, 236].

In addition to the PCP pathway, Wnt5a has been shown to activate at least two other non-canonical pathways. The first is known as the Wnt–Ca2+ pathway, in which Wnt5a stimulation induces Ca2+ release and subsequent activation of the Ca2+-sensitive kinases protein kinase C and Ca2+/calmodulin-dependent kinase [226, 227, 237, 238]. Over-expression of the core PCP proteins, Dvl and Pk, can also activate the Wnt–Ca2+ cascade in zebrafish and *Xenopus*, suggesting that the Wnt–Ca2+ and PCP pathways either overlap substantially or are components of the same signalling network [229, 239, 240]. Second, in mammalian cells Wnt5a has been shown to antagonize the canonical Wnt pathway by either promoting GSK3β-independent β-catenin degradation [236] or by inhibiting β-catenin-dependent transcription [241].

Wnt5a can signal through different Fz receptors and co-receptors, but also via non-conventional tyrosine-kinase like receptors (Ror2 and Ryk) and can activate both the canonical and the non-canonical Wnt pathways [241, 242]. Activation of the canonical pathway entails the Lrp5 and Lrp6 co-receptors, which through cytoplasmic Dvl promote stabilization of β-catenin, its nuclear translocation and the activation of gene transcription [243, 244]. However, the distinct phenotypes observed between *Wnt3, β-catenin, Lrp5/Lrp6* and *Wnt5a* mutant mice [245] argues that during limb development Wnt5a does not signal through the β-catenin pathway [246].

In human, missense mutations in *WNT5A* have been documented in an autosomal dominant form of RRS (MIM #180700) [247 - 249] implying that a disruption of Wnt5a signalling may underlie both RRS and BDB1. Homozygous *ROR2* mutations have been linked to the autosomal recessive form of Robinow syndrome (or COVESDEM syndrome) (MIM #268310), while heterozygous *ROR2* mutations lead to type brachydactyly (MIM #113000) [250] and autosomal Dominant Brachydactyly type-B (BDB1, MIM #113000). BDB1 is the most severe form of brachydactyly and is characterized by loss of nails and varying number of phalanges [100, 251]. In contrast, RRS patients display broader skeletal dysplasia including mesomelic limb shortening and dwarfism, and may or may not display brachydactyly [97, 98, 101].

In mice, the disruption of *Wnt5a* results in short metacarpal elements, absence of phalanges and truncations of proximal elements [236, 252, 253]. The remaining limb skeletal elements are significantly shortened and the severity of the phenotype follows a gradient, with distal bones more affected than proximal ones, reminiscent of mesomelic limb shortening in RRS patients. Interestingly, the AER appears normally stratified and expresses *FGF8* [252]. Strong evidence of the involvement of the Wnt5-dependent pathways in limb development is derived from phenotypes of mice with loss of Wnt5a receptors. In addition to Fz receptors, Wnt5a binds to both Ryk and Ror2 receptors and regulates PCP by promoting Vangl2 stability during limb extension [242, 254]. Ryk and Ror2 are single-pass tyrosine-kinase type of receptors [241, 255]. Ror2 (an orphan tyrosine kinase receptor) activates JNK [256] and in Xenopus has been shown to interact with Wnt11 and Fz7 to regulate CE, suggesting that it may be part of the PCP pathway [257]. Upon binding with Wnt5a, Ror2 inhibits the canonical Wnt signalling. Furthermore, Ror2 also plays an important role in chondrogenesis. *Ror2* is selectively expressed in chondrocytes of cartilage anlagen, and is thus probably important in their initial growth and patterning. Mice mutant for *Ror2* and double mutants for *Ror1;Ror2* exhibit phenotypes that correspond to human RRS malformation, and bear similarities with the *Wnt5a* mutant mice [258, 259]. *Ryk* is another unconventional Wnt5a receptor, consisting in a single trans-membrane pass, catalytically-inactive, tyrosine kinase molecule. Ryk mutant mice show limb truncation similar to those of *Wnt5a* null embryos [260]. Finally, disruption of PCP signalling as Vangl2 in mice causes limb morphogenesis and skeletal defects and may underlie the Robinow syndrome and brachydactyly type B [261]. Together, these observations indicate that Wnt5a, Ryk and Ror2 molecules produce similar phenotypes when lost, for example, the disruption of components of the Wnt non-canonical pathway causes similar limb developmental defects.

### 2.8. Wnt5a controls aspects of PCP and CE in limb development

Recent data [199] shed light on the cellular functions of Wnt5a during limb development. Inspired by the CE process and the PCP pathway, first described in lower organisms, the authors examined the proliferative expansion and migration of mesenchymal cells of the mouse limb bud; in particular, they examined the orientation of cell division and movements in response to Wnt5a. The combination of oriented cell divisions and movements drives the P-D elongation of the limb bud necessary to set the stage for subsequent morphogenesis. They show that Wnt5a via the JNK PCP pathway is needed for the proper orientation of mesenchymal cell movements and cell division reminiscent of CE in *Xenopus* and zebrafish [222 - 225] (Figure 3).

Although these recent studies implicate Wnt5a in the oriented migration and cell division of the mesenchymal cells, little is known about the ectoderm cells, and in particular the AER cells, in which *Wnt5a* is expressed. It is conceivable that the AER cells might be the prime (autocrine) cellular target of Wnt5a, and that the acquisition of a correct planar orientation is a requisite for correct AER formation. Wnt5a and Dlx5 have an overlapping expression pattern, and the phenotype of *Wnt5a* null mice, although not identical, is quite similar to that of *Dlx5/Dlx6* mutant. One possibility is that a deregulation of *Wnt5a* expression, secondary to the disruption of *Dlx5;Dlx6* may underlie ectrodactyly of the *Dlx5;Dlx6* mutant embryos (Figure 4). In support of this, we have evidence that *Dlx* genes promote neuronal differentiation via *Wnt5a*, and that Dlx2 and Dlx5 physically occupy conserved genomic elements near the *Wnt5a* locus and activate its transcription [262]. This interaction and regulation is likely to occur also in the AER cells, a possibility that remains to be investigated.

### 2.9. Quantitative and dynamic gene expression in limb development

An emerging theme in developmental biology is the importance of gene dosage and dynamic gene expression for correct morphogenesis [56]. Several *Dlx* (*1, 2, 3, 5* and *6*) and *FGF* (*4, 8, 9* and *17*) genes are co-expressed in the AER, and their expression is dynamically regulated, both with respect to time (embryonic age) and location (territory of expression). In addition, there is evidence that *Dlx* and *FGF* genes are functionally redundant, at least in part. For example, no limb phenotype is observed in mice null for only one *Dlx* gene, while ectrodactyly is

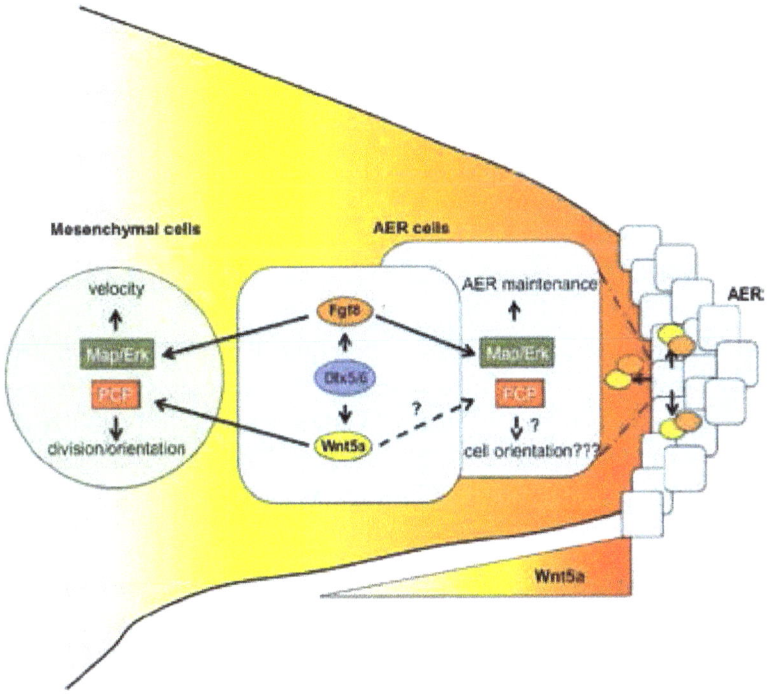


Conte et al.

**Figure 4.** Proposed model of regulation of the AER cell orientation. Dlx5 is known to regulate the transcription of both *FGF8* and *Wnt5a*. In turn, FGF8 is required for AER maintenance and stratification, via p63, while the function of Wnt5a for AER maintenance is still poorly known. Recent data of the regulation of orientation and velocity of mesenchymal cells by, respectively, the Wnt5a/PCP and the FGF8-MAP-Erk pathways open the possibility that Wnt5a may regulate the orientation/motility of the AER cell and assure a correct stratification (dotted line).

observed in *Dlx2;Dlx5* null mice [161] and the ectrodactyly of *Dlx5;Dlx6* null mice is fully rescued by the re-expression of *Dlx5* alone [115]. Likewise, an increased severity of craniofacial phenotypes correlates with progressive loss of *Dlx* gene [263, 264]. All these are indications of gene-dosage effects between functionally redundant genes.

We propose that the portion of the p63 network that (direct or indirect) regulates *FGF8* expression is exerted in a quantitative and dynamic mode. To support this, we should consider that although *p63* null and *p63EEC* homozygous mice show severe limb truncation or absence, the heterozygous mice appear to be normal. When heterozygous EEC mice are bred with heterozygous *Dlx5;Dlx6* ones (the latter have normal limbs), anomalies are clearly observed [90].

A gene-dosage effect combined with the co-expression of functionally redundant genes implies the existence of a threshold level to be maintained to assure AER stratification and signalling functions. Indeed, we have noted that the expression of *Dlx2* and *Dlx5* is lower in the central portion of the AER, compared to the anterior or posterior segments [122]. Thus, the central AER might be more sensitive to reduced *Dlx* expression due to intrinsic lower expression. On the same line, there is evidence that certain amount of AER-derived pan-FGF is required to induce and maintain the underlying mesenchymal progenitors [36, 56, 157]. In fact, in the *Dlx5; Dlx6* mutant limbs, the reduction of *FGF8* expression is restricted to the central AER, the region where epithelial-mesenchymal signalling is primarily defective and the region where morphogenesis fails [114, 115]. Thus, the entire p63-Dlx-FGF cascade is sensitive to gene dosage and position of expression.

## 3. Concluding remarks

p63 is a master regulator of ectodermal cell proliferation, differentiation and stratification, and has a key role in the establishment of a positive loop that maintains *FGF8* expression. In turn, our recent data reveal a novel role of FGF8 to (directly and indirectly) stabilize the p63 proteins and modulate their transcriptional activity. Thus, in the biology and development of the ectoderm, p63 post-translational modifications are as important as *p63* gene expression and may reveal novel targets to be used in p63 modulation.

We illustrate that the p63-Dlx5 transcriptional regulation is at the centre of a pathway relevant for the SHFM malformation. The stability of p63 and the activation of the pathway appear to be under the regulation of FGF8, which in turn is regulated by the pathway. In addition to decipher this positive regulatory loop, these data support a model to attempt to explain the SHFM-III pathogenesis in terms of genome positional effects on the *FGF8* locus.

FGF8 and Wnt5a provide instructions for mesoderm cells as to which direction and orientation to take, at the basis of AER formation and proper migration of mesenchymal cells. This instruction adopts molecules of the PCP pathway, most likely inducing convergent extension. While this has been recently demonstrated for the mesenchymal cells, the possibility that a Wnt5a-dependent PCP pathway is also functional for the organization and stratification of the AER cells remains to be addressed. Notably, data from the human malformation diseases and the corresponding animal models clearly suggest so.

The study of animal models of EEC and SHFM diseases has provided much of this knowledge, and will continue to do so. The big hope is that, once the pathways will be elucidated, we might be able to exploit diffusible molecules and attempt to correct the limb malformation defects. Preliminary attempts are being conducted on whole-organ cultured limbs.

## Nomenclature

A-P, anterior-posterior

D-V, dorsal-ventral

P-D, proximal-distal

SHH, sonic hedgehog

FGF, fibroblast growth factor

FL, forelimb

HL, hindlimb

ZPA, zone of polarizing activity

AER, apical ectodermal ridge

PZ, progress zone

KO, knock-out

PCP, planar cell polarity

CE, convergent extension

LPM, lateral plate mesoderm

## Author details

Daniele Conte[1], Luisa Guerrini[2] and Giorgio R. Merlo[1*]

*Address all correspondence to: giorgioroberto.merlo@unito.it

1 Department of Molecular Biotechnology and Health Sciences, Università degli Studi di Torino, Italy

2 Department of Biosciences, Università degli Studi di Milano, Italy

## References

[1] Ohuchi, H., *et al.* (1997) The mesenchymal factor, FGF10, initiates and maintains the outgrowth of the chick limb bud through interaction with FGF8, an apical ectodermal factor. *Development* 124, 2235–2244

[2] Xu, X., *et al.* (1998) Fibroblast growth factor receptor 2 (FGFR2)-mediated reciprocal regulation loop between FGF8 and FGF10 is essential for limb induction. *Development* 125, 753–765

[3] Min, H., *et al.* (1998) Fgf-10 is required for both limb and lung development and exhibits striking functional similarity to Drosophila branchless. *Genes Dev* 12, 3156–3161

[4] Sekine, K., *et al.* (1999) FGF10 is essential for limb and lung formation. *Nat Genet* 21, 138–141

[5] Ohuchi, H., *et al.* (1995) An additional limb can be induced from the flank of the chick embryo by FGF4. *Biochem Biophys Res Commun* 209, 809–816

[6] Vogel, A., *et al.* (1996) Involvement of FGF-8 in initiation, outgrowth and patterning of the vertebrate limb. *Development* 122, 1737–1750

[7] Gros, J., and Tabin, C.J. (2014) Vertebrate limb bud formation is initiated by localized epithelial-to-mesenchymal transition. *Science* 343, 1253–1256

[8] Agarwal, P., *et al.* (2003) Tbx5 is essential for forelimb bud initiation following patterning of the limb field in the mouse embryo. *Development* 130, 623–633

[9] Ahn, D.G., *et al.* (2002) T-box gene tbx5 is essential for formation of the pectoral limb bud. *Nature* 417, 754–758

[10] Begemann, G., *et al.* (2002) Cloning of zebrafish T-box genes tbx15 and tbx18 and their expression during embryonic development. *Mech Dev* 114, 137–141

[11] Garrity, D.M., *et al.* (2002) The heartstrings mutation in zebrafish causes heart/fin Tbx5 deficiency syndrome. *Development* 129, 4635–4645

[12] Minguillon, C., *et al.* (2005) Tbx5 and Tbx4 are not sufficient to determine limb-specific morphologies but have common roles in initiating limb outgrowth. *Dev Cell* 8, 75–84

[13] Rallis, C., *et al.* (2003) Tbx5 is required for forelimb bud formation and continued outgrowth. *Development* 130, 2741–2751

[14] Saito, D., *et al.* (2002) Specification and determination of limb identity: evidence for inhibitory regulation of Tbx gene expression. *Development* 129, 211–220

[15] Takeuchi, J.K., *et al.* (2003) Tbx5 and Tbx4 trigger limb initiation through activation of the Wnt/Fgf signaling cascade. *Development* 130, 2729–2739

[16] Menke, J. (2008) Contrast-enhanced magnetic resonance angiography in peripheral arterial disease: improving image quality by automated image registration. *Magn Reson Med* 60, 224–229

[17] Mic, F.A., *et al.* (2004) Retinoic acid synthesis controlled by Raldh2 is required early for limb bud initiation and then later as a proximodistal signal during apical ectodermal ridge formation. *J Biol Chem* 279, 26698–26706

[18] Begemann, G., and Meyer, A. (2001) Hindbrain patterning revisited: timing and effects of retinoic acid signalling. *Bioessays* 23, 981–986

[19] Gibert, Y., *et al.* (2006) Induction and prepatterning of the zebrafish pectoral fin bud requires axial retinoic acid signaling. *Development* 133, 2649–2659

[20] Maden, M. (1982) Vitamin A and pattern formation in the regenerating limb. *Nature* 295, 672–675

[21] Tickle, C., *et al.* (1982) Local application of retinoic acid to the limb bond mimics the action of the polarizing region. *Nature* 296, 564–566

[22] Mercader, N., *et al.* (2006) Prdm1 acts downstream of a sequential RA, Wnt and Fgf signaling cascade during zebrafish forelimb induction. *Development* 133, 2805–2815

[23] Mercader, N., *et al.* (2000) Opposing RA and FGF signals control proximodistal vertebrate limb development through regulation of Meis genes. *Development* 127, 3961–3970

[24] Litingtung, Y., *et al.* (2002) SHH and Gli3 are dispensable for limb skeleton formation but regulate digit number and identity. *Nature* 418, 979–983

[25] Grandel, H., *et al.* (2002) Retinoic acid signalling in the zebrafish embryo is necessary during pre-segmentation stages to pattern the anterior-posterior axis of the CNS and to induce a pectoral fin bud. *Development* 129, 2851–2865

[26] Tabin, C., and Wolpert, L. (2007) Rethinking the proximodistal axis of the vertebrate limb in the molecular era. *Genes Dev* 21, 1433–1442

[27] Zhao, X., *et al.* (2009) Retinoic acid promotes limb induction through effects on body axis extension but is unnecessary for limb patterning. *Curr Biol* 19, 1050–1057

[28] Niederreither, K., *et al.* (1999) Embryonic retinoic acid synthesis is essential for early mouse post-implantation development. *Nat Genet* 21, 444–448

[29] Cunningham, T.J., *et al.* (2013) Antagonism between retinoic acid and fibroblast growth factor signaling during limb development. *Cell Rep* 3, 1503–1511

[30] Bell, S.M., *et al.* (1998) The loss of ventral ectoderm identity correlates with the inability to form an AER in the legless hindlimb bud. *Mech Dev* 74, 41–50

[31] Todt, W.L., and Fallon, J.F. (1986) Development of the apical ectodermal ridge in the chick leg bud and a comparison with the wing bud. *Anat Rec* 215, 288–304

[32] Todt, W.L., and Fallon, J.F. (1987) Posterior apical ectodermal ridge removal in the chick wing bud triggers a series of events resulting in defective anterior pattern formation. *Development* 101, 501–515

[33] Saunders, J.W., Jr. (1948) The proximo-distal sequence of origin of the parts of the chick wing and the role of the ectoderm. *J Exp Zool* 108, 363–403

[34] Fallon, J.F., *et al.* (1986) Apical ectodermal ridge maintenance *in ovo* and *in vitro*. *Prog Clin Biol Res* 226, 103–113

[35] Niswander, L., *et al.* (1993) FGF-4 replaces the apical ectodermal ridge and directs outgrowth and patterning of the limb. *Cell* 75, 579–587

[36] Mariani, F.V., *et al.* (2008) Genetic evidence that FGFs have an instructive role in limb proximal-distal patterning. *Nature* 453, 401–405

[37] Crossley, P.H., *et al.* (1996) Roles for FGF8 in the induction, initiation, and maintenance of chick limb development. *Cell* 84, 127–136

[38] Moon, A.M., and Capecchi, M.R. (2000) Fgf8 is required for outgrowth and patterning of the limbs. *Nat Genet* 26, 455–459

[39] Boulet, A.M., *et al.* (2004) The roles of FGF4 and Fgf8 in limb bud initiation and outgrowth. *Dev Biol* 273, 361–372

[40] Lewandoski, M., *et al.* (2000) Fgf8 signalling from the AER is essential for normal limb development. *Nat Genet* 26, 460–463

[41] Lu, P., *et al.* (2006) Increasing FGF4 expression in the mouse limb bud causes polysyndactyly and rescues the skeletal defects that result from loss of Fgf8 function. *Development* 133, 33–42

[42] Sun, X., *et al.* (2002) Functions of FGF signalling from the apical ectodermal ridge in limb development. *Nature* 418, 501–508

[43] Kawakami, Y., *et al.* (2001) WNT signals control FGF-dependent limb initiation and AER induction in the chick embryo. *Cell* 104, 891–900

[44] McQueeney, K., *et al.* (2002) Beta-catenin-dependent Wnt signaling in apical ectodermal ridge induction and FGF8 expression in normal and limbless mutant chick limbs. *Dev Growth Differ* 44, 315–325

[45] Summerbell, D., *et al.* (1973) Positional information in chick limb morphogenesis. *Nature* 244, 492–496

[46] Dudley, A.T., *et al.* (2002) A re-examination of proximodistal patterning during vertebrate limb development. *Nature* 418, 539–544

[47] Cooper, K.L., *et al.* (2011) Initiation of proximal-distal patterning in the vertebrate limb by signals and growth. *Science* 332, 1083–1086

[48] Rosello-Diez, A., *et al.* (2011) Diffusible signals, not autonomous mechanisms, determine the main proximodistal limb subdivision. *Science* 332, 1086–1088

[49] Tickle, C., *et al.* (1975) Positional signalling and specification of digits in chick limb morphogenesis. *Nature* 254, 199–202

[50] Zwilling, E. (1956) Genetic mechanism in limb development. *Cold Spring Harb Symp Quant Biol* 21, 349–354

[51] Riddle, R.D., *et al.* (1993) Sonic hedgehog mediates the polarizing activity of the ZPA. *Cell* 75, 1401–1416

[52] Wolpert, L. (1969) Positional information and the spatial pattern of cellular differentiation. *J Theor Biol* 25, 1–47

[53] Harfe, B.D., *et al.* (2004) Evidence for an expansion-based temporal SHH gradient in specifying vertebrate digit identities. *Cell* 118, 517–528

[54] Scherz, P.J., *et al.* (2007) Extended exposure to Sonic hedgehog is required for patterning the posterior digits of the vertebrate limb. *Dev Biol* 308, 343–354

[55] Zeller, R. (2004) It takes time to make a pinky: unexpected insights into how SHH patterns vertebrate digits. *Sci STKE* 2004, pe53

[56] Zeller, R. (2010) The temporal dynamics of vertebrate limb development, teratogenesis and evolution. *Curr Opin Genet Dev* 20, 384–390

[57] Panman, L., *et al.* (2006) Differential regulation of gene expression in the digit forming area of the mouse limb bud by SHH and gremlin 1/FGF-mediated epithelial-mesenchymal signalling. *Development* 133, 3419–3428

[58] Robert, B., and Lallemand, Y. (2006) Anteroposterior patterning in the limb and digit specification: contribution of mouse genetics. *Dev Dyn* 235, 2337–2352

[59] Michos, O., *et al.* (2004) Gremlin-mediated BMP antagonism induces the epithelial-mesenchymal feedback signaling controlling metanephric kidney and limb organogenesis. *Development* 131, 3401–3410

[60] te Welscher, P., *et al.* (2002) Mutual genetic antagonism involving GLI3 and dHAND prepatterns the vertebrate limb bud mesenchyme prior to SHH signaling. *Genes Dev* 16, 421–426

[61] te Welscher, P., *et al.* (2002) Progression of vertebrate limb development through SHH-mediated counteraction of GLI3. *Science* 298, 827–830

[62] Cohn, M.J., *et al.* (2002) Branching, segmentation and the metapterygial axis: pattern versus process in the vertebrate limb. *Bioessays* 24, 460–465

[63] Ros, M.A., *et al.* (1996) The limb field mesoderm determines initial limb bud anteroposterior asymmetry and budding independent of sonic hedgehog or apical ectodermal gene expressions. *Development* 122, 2319–2330

[64] Capellini, T.D., *et al.* (2006) Pbx1/Pbx2 requirement for distal limb patterning is mediated by the hierarchical control of Hox gene spatial distribution and SHH expression. *Development* 133, 2263–2273

[65] Bastida, M.F., *et al.* (2009) A BMP-SHH negative-feedback loop restricts SHH expression during limb development. *Development* 136, 3779–3789

[66] Zeller, R., *et al.* (2009) Vertebrate limb bud development: moving towards integrative analysis of organogenesis. *Nat Rev Genet* 10, 845–858

[67] Wang, B., *et al.* (2000) Hedgehog-regulated processing of Gli3 produces an anterior/posterior repressor gradient in the developing vertebrate limb. *Cell* 100, 423–434

[68] Kondo, S., and Miura, T. (2010) Reaction-diffusion model as a framework for understanding biological pattern formation. *Science* 329, 1616–1620

[69] Turing, A.M. (1990) The chemical basis of morphogenesis. 1953. *Bull Math Biol* 52, 153–197; discussion 119–152

[70] Miura, T., *et al.* (2006) Mixed-mode pattern in Doublefoot mutant mouse limb--Turing reaction-diffusion model on a growing domain during limb development. *J Theor Biol* 240, 562–573

[71] Kmita, M., *et al.* (2005) Early developmental arrest of mammalian limbs lacking HoxA/HoxD gene function. *Nature* 435, 1113–1116

[72] Zakany, J., *et al.* (2004) A dual role for Hox genes in limb anterior-posterior asymmetry. *Science* 304, 1669–1672

[73] Chen, Y., *et al.* (2004) Direct interaction with Hoxd proteins reverses Gli3-repressor function to promote digit formation downstream of SHH. *Development* 131, 2339–2347

[74] Kmita, M., *et al.* (2002) Serial deletions and duplications suggest a mechanism for the collinearity of Hoxd genes in limbs. *Nature* 420, 145–150

[75] Sheth, R., *et al.* (2012) Hox genes regulate digit patterning by controlling the wavelength of a Turing-type mechanism. *Science* 338, 1476–1480

[76] Beauchemin, M., *et al.* (1998) Graded expression of Emx-2 in the adult newt limb and its corresponding regeneration blastema. *J Mol Biol* 279, 501–511

[77] Geraudie, J., and Ferretti, P. (1998) Gene expression during amphibian limb regeneration. *Int Rev Cytol* 180, 1–50

[78] Shubin, N., *et al.* (1997) Fossils, genes and the evolution of animal limbs. *Nature* 388, 639–648

[79] Davis, A.P., *et al.* (1995) Absence of radius and ulna in mice lacking hoxa-11 and hoxd-11. *Nature* 375, 791–795

[80] Fromental-Ramain, C., *et al.* (1996) Hoxa-13 and Hoxd-13 play a crucial role in the patterning of the limb autopod. *Development* 122, 2997–3011

[81] Boulet, A.M., and Capecchi, M.R. (2004) Multiple roles of Hoxa11 and Hoxd11 in the formation of the mammalian forelimb zeugopod. *Development* 131, 299–309

[82] Laufer, E., *et al.* (1994) Sonic hedgehog and Fgf-4 act through a signaling cascade and feedback loop to integrate growth and patterning of the developing limb bud. *Cell* 79, 993–1003

[83] Niswander, L., *et al.* (1994) Function of FGF-4 in limb development. *Mol Reprod Dev* 39, 83–88; discussion 88–89

[84] Khokha, M.K., *et al.* (2003) Gremlin is the BMP antagonist required for maintenance of SHH and Fgf signals during limb patterning. *Nat Genet* 34, 303–307

[85] Parr, B.A., *et al.* (1998) The classical mouse mutant postaxial hemimelia results from a mutation in the Wnt 7a gene. *Dev Biol* 202, 228–234

[86] Parr, B.A., and McMahon, A.P. (1995) Dorsalizing signal Wnt-7a required for normal polarity of D-V and A-P axes of mouse limb. *Nature* 374, 350–353

[87] Chen, H., *et al.* (1998) Limb and kidney defects in Lmx1b mutant mice suggest an involvement of LMX1B in human nail patella syndrome. *Nat Genet* 19, 51–55

[88] Riddle, R.D., *et al.* (1995) Induction of the LIM homeobox gene Lmx1 by WNT7a establishes dorsoventral pattern in the vertebrate limb. *Cell* 83, 631–640

[89] Loomis, C.A., *et al.* (1998) Analysis of the genetic pathway leading to formation of ectopic apical ectodermal ridges in mouse Engrailed-1 mutant limbs. *Development* 125, 1137–1148

[90] Lo Iacono, N., *et al.* (2008) Regulation of Dlx5 and Dlx6 gene expression by p63 is involved in EEC and SHFM congenital limb defects. *Development* 135, 1377–1388

[91] Bakkers, J., *et al.* (2002) Zebrafish DeltaNp63 is a direct target of Bmp signaling and encodes a transcriptional repressor blocking neural specification in the ventral ectoderm. *Dev Cell* 2, 617–627

[92] Lee, H., and Kimelman, D. (2002) A dominant-negative form of p63 is required for epidermal proliferation in zebrafish. *Dev Cell* 2, 607–616

[93] Temtamy, S.A., and McKusick, V.A. (1978) The genetics of hand malformations. *Birth Defects Orig Artic Ser* 14, i–xviii, 1–619

[94] Schwabe, G.C., and Mundlos, S. (2004) Genetics of congenital hand anomalies. *Handchir Mikrochir Plast Chir* 36, 85–97

[95] Lettice, L.A., *et al.* (2003) A long-range SHH enhancer regulates expression in the developing limb and fin and is associated with preaxial polydactyly. *Hum Mol Genet* 12, 1725–1735

[96] Tsukurov, O., *et al.* (1994) A complex bilateral polysyndactyly disease locus maps to chromosome 7q36. *Nat Genet* 6, 282–286

[97] Afzal, A.R., and Jeffery, S. (2003) One gene, two phenotypes: ROR2 mutations in autosomal recessive Robinow syndrome and autosomal dominant brachydactyly type B. *Hum Mutat* 22, 1–11

[98] Afzal, A.R., *et al.* (2000) Recessive Robinow syndrome, allelic to dominant brachydactyly type B, is caused by mutation of ROR2. *Nat Genet* 25, 419–422

[99] Ho, H.Y., *et al.* (2012) Wnt5a-Ror-Dishevelled signaling constitutes a core developmental pathway that controls tissue morphogenesis. *Proc Natl Acad Sci U S A* 109, 4044–4051

[100] Schwabe, G.C., *et al.* (2000) Distinct mutations in the receptor tyrosine kinase gene ROR2 cause brachydactyly type B. *Am J Hum Genet* 67, 822–831

[101] Schwarzer, W., *et al.* (2009) A gradient of ROR2 protein stability and membrane localization confers brachydactyly type B or Robinow syndrome phenotypes. *Hum Mol Genet* 18, 4013–4021

[102] Newman, C.G. (1986) The thalidomide syndrome: risks of exposure and spectrum of malformations. *Clin Perinatol* 13, 555–573

[103] Ito, T., and Handa, H. (2012) Deciphering the mystery of thalidomide teratogenicity. *Congenit Anom (Kyoto)* 52, 1–7

[104] Therapontos, C., *et al.* (2009) Thalidomide induces limb defects by preventing angiogenic outgrowth during early limb formation. *Proc Natl Acad Sci U S A* 106, 8573–8578

[105] Duijf, P.H., *et al.* (2003) Pathogenesis of split-hand/split-foot malformation. *Hum Mol Genet* 12 Spec No 1, R51–60

[106] Gurrieri, F., and Everman, D.B. (2013) Clinical, genetic, and molecular aspects of split-hand/foot malformation: an update. *Am J Med Genet A* 161A, 2860–2872

[107] Sowinska-Seidler, A., *et al.* (2014) Split-hand/foot malformation – molecular cause and implications in genetic counseling. *J Appl Genet* 55, 105–115

[108] Crackower, M.A., *et al.* (1996) Characterization of the split hand/split foot malformation locus SHFM1 at 7q21.3-q22.1 and analysis of a candidate gene for its expression during limb development. *Hum Mol Genet* 5, 571–579

[109] Del Porto, G., *et al.* (1983) [Interstitial deletion of the long arm of chromosome 7 and its clinical correlations]. *Pathologica* 75 Suppl, 268–271

[110] Marinoni, J.C., *et al.* (1995) Split foot and developmental retardation associated with a deletion of three microsatellite markers in 7q21.2-q22.1. *Clin Genet* 47, 90–95

[111] Scherer, S.W., *et al.* (2003) Human chromosome 7: DNA sequence and biology. *Science* 300, 767–772

[112] Scherer, S.W., *et al.* (1994) Fine mapping of the autosomal dominant split hand/split foot locus on chromosome 7, band q21.3-q22.1. *Am J Hum Genet* 55, 12–20

[113] Acampora, D., *et al.* (1999) Craniofacial, vestibular and bone defects in mice lacking the Distal-less-related gene Dlx5. *Development* 126, 3795–3809

[114] Merlo, G.R., *et al.* (2002) Mouse model of split hand/foot malformation type I. *Genesis* 33, 97–101

[115] Robledo, R.F., *et al.* (2002) The Dlx5 and Dlx6 homeobox genes are essential for craniofacial, axial, and appendicular skeletal development. *Genes Dev* 16, 1089–1101

[116] Shamseldin, H.E., *et al.* (2012) Identification of a novel DLX5 mutation in a family with autosomal recessive split hand and foot malformation. *J Med Genet* 49, 16–20

[117] Del Campo, M., *et al.* (1999) Monodactylous limbs and abnormal genitalia are associated with hemizygosity for the human 2q31 region that includes the HOXD cluster. *Am J Hum Genet* 65, 104–110

[118] Goodman, F.R., *et al.* (2002) A 117-kb microdeletion removing HOXD9-HOXD13 and EVX2 causes synpolydactyly. *Am J Hum Genet* 70, 547–555

[119] Goodman, F.R. (2002) Limb malformations and the human HOX genes. *Am J Med Genet* 112, 256–265

[120] Sidow, A., *et al.* (1999) A novel member of the F-box/WD40 gene family, encoding dactylin, is disrupted in the mouse dactylaplasia mutant. *Nat Genet* 23, 104–107

[121] de Mollerat, X.J., *et al.* (2003) A genomic rearrangement resulting in a tandem duplication is associated with split hand-split foot malformation 3 (SHFM3) at 10q24. *Hum Mol Genet* 12, 1959–1971

[122] Guerrini, L., *et al.* (2011) A symphony of regulations centered on p63 to control development of ectoderm-derived structures. *J Biomed Biotechnol* 2011, 864–904

[123] van Bokhoven, H., *et al.* (2001) p63 Gene mutations in eec syndrome, limb-mammary syndrome, and isolated split hand-split foot malformation suggest a genotype-phenotype correlation. *Am J Hum Genet* 69, 481–492

[124] Elliott, A.M., *et al.* (2006) Clinical and epidemiological findings in patients with central ray deficiency: split hand foot malformation (SHFM) in Manitoba, Canada. *Am J Med Genet A* 140, 1428–1439

[125] Rinne, T., *et al.* (2007) p63-associated disorders. *Cell Cycle* 6, 262–268

[126] Ghioni, P., *et al.* (2005) The protein stability and transcriptional activity of p63alpha are regulated by SUMO-1 conjugation. *Cell Cycle* 4, 183–190

[127] Elliott, A.M., *et al.* (2005) Split hand foot malformation (SHFM). *Clin Genet* 68, 501–505

[128] van Bokhoven, H., and Brunner, H.G. (2002) Splitting p63. *Am J Hum Genet* 71, 1–13

[129] Celli, J., *et al.* (1999) Heterozygous germline mutations in the p53 homolog p63 are the cause of EEC syndrome. *Cell* 99, 143–153

[130] Aziz, A., *et al.* (2013) Novel homozygous mutations in the WNT10B gene underlying autosomal recessive split hand/foot malformation in three consanguineous families. *Gene* 534, 7

[131] Blattner, A., *et al.* (2012) Homozygous nonsense mutation in WNT10B and sporadic split-hand/foot malformation (SHFM) with autosomal recessive inheritance. *Am J Med Genet A* 152A, 2053–2056

[132] Khan, S., *et al.* (2012) A novel homozygous missense mutation in WNT10B in familial split-hand/foot malformation. *Clin Genet* 82, 48–55

[133] Ugur, S.A., and Tolun, A. (2008) Homozygous WNT10b mutation and complex inheritance in Split-Hand/Foot Malformation. *Hum Mol Genet* 17, 2644–2653

[134] Faiyaz-Ul-Haque, M., *et al.* (2005) Fine mapping of the X-linked split-hand/split-foot malformation (SHFM2) locus to a 5.1-Mb region on Xq26.3 and analysis of candidate genes. *Clin Genet* 67, 93–97

[135] Berdon-Zapata, V., *et al.* (2004) p63 gene analysis in Mexican patients with syndromic and non-syndromic ectrodactyly. *J Orthop Res* 22, 1–5

[136] Yang, A., *et al.* (1999) p63 is essential for regenerative proliferation in limb, craniofacial and epithelial development. *Nature* 398, 714–718

[137] Mills, A.A., *et al.* (1999) p63 is a p53 homologue required for limb and epidermal morphogenesis. *Nature* 398, 708–713

[138] Senoo, M., *et al.* (2007) p63 Is essential for the proliferative potential of stem cells in stratified epithelia. *Cell* 129, 523–536

[139] Candi, E., *et al.* (2008) p63 in epithelial development. *Cell Mol Life Sci* 65, 3126–3133

[140] Romano, R.A., *et al.* (2012) DeltaNp63 knockout mice reveal its indispensable role as a master regulator of epithelial development and differentiation. *Development* 139, 772–782

[141] Mangiulli, M., *et al.* (2009) Identification and functional characterization of two new transcriptional variants of the human p63 gene. *Nucleic Acids Res* 37, 6092–6104

[142] Ghioni, P., *et al.* (2002) Complex transcriptional effects of p63 isoforms: identification of novel activation and repression domains. *Mol Cell Biol* 22, 8659–8668

[143] Thanos, C.D., and Bowie, J.U. (1999) p53 Family members p63 and p73 are SAM domain-containing proteins. *Protein Sci* 8, 1708–1710

[144] Yang, A., *et al.* (2006) Relationships between p63 binding, DNA sequence, transcription activity, and biological function in human cells. *Mol Cell* 24, 593–602

[145] Serber, Z., *et al.* (2002) A C-terminal inhibitory domain controls the activity of p63 by an intramolecular mechanism. *Mol Cell Biol* 22, 8601–8611

[146] Brunner, H.G., *et al.* (2002) P63 gene mutations and human developmental syndromes. *Am J Med Genet* 112, 284–290

[147] Brunner, H.G., *et al.* (2002) The p63 gene in EEC and other syndromes. *J Med Genet* 39, 377–381

[148] van Bokhoven, H., and McKeon, F. (2002) Mutations in the p53 homolog p63: allele-specific developmental syndromes in humans. *Trends Mol Med* 8, 133–139

[149] Lopardo, T., *et al.* (2008) Claudin-1 is a p63 target gene with a crucial role in epithelial development. *PLoS One* 3, e2715

[150] Radoja, N., *et al.* (2007) Homeobox gene Dlx3 is regulated by p63 during ectoderm development: relevance in the pathogenesis of ectodermal dysplasias. *Development* 134, 13–18

[151] Clements, S.E., *et al.* (2012) Mutations in AEC syndrome skin reveal a role for p63 in basement membrane adhesion, skin barrier integrity and hair follicle biology. *Br J Dermatol* 167, 134–144

[152] Ferone, G., *et al.* (2013) p63 control of desmosome gene expression and adhesion is compromised in AEC syndrome. *Hum Mol Genet* 22, 531–543

[153] Ferone, G., *et al.* (2012) Mutant p63 causes defective expansion of ectodermal progenitor cells and impaired FGF signalling in AEC syndrome. *EMBO Mol Med* 4, 192–205

[154] Koster, M.I., *et al.* (2004) p63 is the molecular switch for initiation of an epithelial stratification program. *Genes Dev* 18, 126–131

[155] Koster, M.I., and Roop, D.R. (2004) p63 and epithelial appendage development. *Differentiation* 72, 364–370

[156] Koster, M.I., and Roop, D.R. (2007) Mechanisms regulating epithelial stratification. *Annu Rev Cell Dev Biol* 23, 93–113

[157] Fernandez-Teran, M., and Ros, M.A. (2008) The Apical Ectodermal Ridge: morphological aspects and signaling pathways. *Int J Dev Biol* 52, 857–871

[158] Restelli, M., *et al.* (2014) DLX5, FGF8 and the Pin1 isomerase control $\Delta Np63\alpha$ protein stability during limb development: a regulatory loop at the basis of the SHFM and EEC congenital malformations. *Hum Mol Genet* 23, 3830–3842

[159] Crackower, M.A., *et al.* (1998) Defect in the maintenance of the apical ectodermal ridge in the Dactylaplasia mouse. *Dev Biol* 201, 78–89

[160] Panganiban, G. (2000) Distal-less function during Drosophila appendage and sense organ development. *Dev Dyn* 218, 554–562

[161] Panganiban, G., and Rubenstein, J.L. (2002) Developmental functions of the Distal-less/Dlx homeobox genes. *Development* 129, 4371–4386

[162] Beverdam, A., *et al.* (2002) Jaw transformation with gain of symmetry after Dlx5/Dlx6 inactivation: mirror of the past? *Genesis* 34, 221–227

[163] Depew, M.J., *et al.* (2002) Specification of jaw subdivisions by Dlx genes. *Science* 298, 381–385

[164] Kouwenhoven, E.N., *et al.* (2010) Genome-wide profiling of p63 DNA-binding sites identifies an element that regulates gene expression during limb development in the 7q21 SHFM1 locus. *PLoS Genet* 6, e1001065

[165] Birnbaum, R.Y., *et al.* (2012) Functional characterization of tissue-specific enhancers in the DLX5/6 locus. *Hum Mol Genet* 21, 4930–4938

[166] Birnbaum, R.Y., *et al.* (2012) Coding exons function as tissue-specific enhancers of nearby genes. *Genome Res* 22, 1059–1068

[167] Lango Allen, H., *et al.* (2014) Next generation sequencing of chromosomal rearrangements in patients with split-hand/split-foot malformation provides evidence for DYNC1I1 exonic enhancers of DLX5/6 expression in humans. *J Med Genet* 51, 264–267

[168] Bell, S.M., *et al.* (2003) Sp8 is crucial for limb outgrowth and neuropore closure. *Proc Natl Acad Sci U S A* 100, 12195–12200

[169] Treichel, D., *et al.* (2003) mBtd is required to maintain signaling during murine limb development. *Genes Dev* 17, 2630–2635

[170] Schock, F., *et al.* (1999) Common and diverged functions of the Drosophila gene pair D-Sp1 and buttonhead. *Mech Dev* 89, 125–132

[171] Kawakami, Y., *et al.* (2004) Sp8 and Sp9, two closely related buttonhead-like transcription factors, regulate Fgf8 expression and limb outgrowth in vertebrate embryos. *Development* 131, 4763–4774

[172] Waclaw, R.R., *et al.* (2006) The zinc finger transcription factor Sp8 regulates the generation and diversity of olfactory bulb interneurons. *Neuron* 49, 503–516

[173] Ala, U., *et al.* (2008) Prediction of human disease genes by human-mouse conserved coexpression analysis. *PLoS Comput Biol* 4, e1000043

[174] Dai, L., *et al.* (2013) Discontinuous microduplications at chromosome 10q24.31 identified in a Chinese family with split hand and foot malformation. *BMC Med Genet* 14, 45

[175] Candi, E., *et al.* (2006) Differential roles of p63 isoforms in epidermal development: selective genetic complementation in p63 null mice. *Cell Death Differ* 13, 1037–1047

[176] Marinari, B., *et al.* (2008) The tumor suppressor activity of IKKalpha in stratified epithelia is exerted in part via the TGF-beta antiproliferative pathway. *Proc Natl Acad Sci U S A* 105, 17091–17096

[177] Marinari, B., *et al.* (2009) IKKalpha is a p63 transcriptional target involved in the pathogenesis of ectodermal dysplasias. *J Invest Dermatol* 129, 60–69

[178] Sil, A.K., *et al.* (2004) IkappaB kinase-alpha acts in the epidermis to control skeletal and craniofacial morphogenesis. *Nature* 428, 660–664

[179] Galli, F., *et al.* (2010) MDM2 and Fbw7 cooperate to induce p63 protein degradation following DNA damage and cell differentiation. *J Cell Sci* 123, 2423–2433

[180] Ratovitski, E.A., *et al.* (2001) p53 associates with and targets Delta Np63 into a protein degradation pathway. *Proc Natl Acad Sci U S A* 98, 1817–1822

[181] Moretti, F., *et al.* (2010) A regulatory feedback loop involving p63 and IRF6 links the pathogenesis of 2 genetically different human ectodermal dysplasias. *J Clin Invest* 120, 1570–1577

[182] Browne, G., *et al.* (2011) Differential altered stability and transcriptional activity of DeltaNp63 mutants in distinct ectodermal dysplasias. *J Cell Sci* 124, 2200–2207

[183] Girardini, J.E., *et al.* (2011) A Pin1/mutant p53 axis promotes aggressiveness in breast cancer. *Cancer Cell* 20, 79–91

[184] Brooks, C.L., and Gu, W. (2003) Ubiquitination, phosphorylation and acetylation: the molecular basis for p53 regulation. *Curr Opin Cell Biol* 15, 164–171

[185] Gu, B., and Zhu, W.G. (2012) Surf the post-translational modification network of p53 regulation. *Int J Biol Sci* 8, 672–684

[186] Luo, J., *et al.* (2004) Acetylation of p53 augments its site-specific DNA binding both *in vitro* and *in vivo*. *Proc Natl Acad Sci U S A* 101, 2259–2264

[187] Marmorstein, R., and Roth, S.Y. (2001) Histone acetyltransferases: function, structure, and catalysis. *Curr Opin Genet Dev* 11, 155–161

[188] Meek, D.W., and Anderson, C.W. (2009) Posttranslational modification of p53: cooperative integrators of function. *Cold Spring Harb Perspect Biol* 1, a000950

[189] Tang, Y., *et al.* (2008) Acetylation is indispensable for p53 activation. *Cell* 133, 612–626

[190] Zeng, X., *et al.* (2000) The N-terminal domain of p73 interacts with the CH1 domain of p300/CREB binding protein and mediates transcriptional activation and apoptosis. *Mol Cell Biol* 20, 1299–1310

[191] Costanzo, A., *et al.* (2002) DNA damage-dependent acetylation of p73 dictates the selective activation of apoptotic target genes. *Mol Cell* 9, 175–186

[192] Mantovani, F., *et al.* (2004) Pin1 links the activities of c-Abl and p300 in regulating p73 function. *Mol Cell* 14, 625–636

[193] Ianakiev, P., *et al.* (2000) Split-hand/split-foot malformation is caused by mutations in the p63 gene on 3q27. *Am J Hum Genet* 67, 59–66

[194] Lu, P., *et al.* (2008) The apical ectodermal ridge is a timer for generating distal limb progenitors. *Development* 135, 1395–1405

[195] Agami, R., *et al.* (1999) Interaction of c-Abl and p73alpha and their collaboration to induce apoptosis. *Nature* 399, 809–813

[196] Levav-Cohen, Y., *et al.* (2005) C-Abl as a modulator of p53. *Biochem Biophys Res Commun* 331, 737–749

[197] Sanchez-Prieto, R., *et al.* (2002) Regulation of p73 by c-Abl through the p38 MAP kinase pathway. *Oncogene* 21, 974–979

[198] Yan, W., *et al.* (2008) Distinct angiogenic mediators are required for basic fibroblast growth factor- and vascular endothelial growth factor-induced angiogenesis: the role of cytoplasmic tyrosine kinase c-Abl in tumor angiogenesis. *Mol Biol Cell* 19, 2278–2288

[199] Gros, J., *et al.* (2010) WNT5A/JNK and FGF/MAPK pathways regulate the cellular events shaping the vertebrate limb bud. *Curr Biol* 20, 1993–2002

[200] Benazeraf, B., *et al.* (2010) A random cell motility gradient downstream of FGF controls elongation of an amniote embryo. *Nature* 466, 248–252

[201] Pandur, P., *et al.* (2002) Increasingly complex: new players enter the Wnt signaling network. *Bioessays* 24, 881–884

[202] Huelsken, J., and Behrens, J. (2002) The Wnt signalling pathway. *J Cell Sci* 115, 3977–3978

[203] Hendriks, B., and Reichmann, E. (2002) Wnt signaling: a complex issue. *Biol Res* 35, 277–286

[204] Clevers, H., and Nusse, R. (2012) Wnt/beta-catenin signaling and disease. *Cell* 149, 1192–1205

[205] Church, V.L., and Francis-West, P. (2002) Wnt signalling during limb development. *Int J Dev Biol* 46, 927–936

[206] Kengaku, M., *et al.* (1997) Expression of Wnt and Frizzled genes during chick limb bud development. *Cold Spring Harb Symp Quant Biol* 62, 421–429

[207] Galceran, J., *et al.* (1999) Wnt3a-/--like phenotype and limb deficiency in Lef1(-/-)Tcf1(-/-) mice. *Genes Dev* 13, 709–717

[208] Pinson, K.I., *et al.* (2000) An LDL-receptor-related protein mediates Wnt signalling in mice. *Nature* 407, 535–538

[209] Takada, S., *et al.* (1994) Wnt-3a regulates somite and tailbud formation in the mouse embryo. *Genes Dev* 8, 174–189

[210] Roelink, H., and Nusse, R. (1991) Expression of two members of the Wnt family during mouse development--restricted temporal and spatial patterns in the developing neural tube. *Genes Dev* 5, 381–388

[211] Barrow, J.R., *et al.* (2003) Ectodermal Wnt3/beta-catenin signaling is required for the establishment and maintenance of the apical ectodermal ridge. *Genes Dev* 17, 394–409

[212] Niemann, S., *et al.* (2004) Homozygous WNT3 mutation causes tetra-amelia in a large consanguineous family. *Am J Hum Genet* 74, 558–563

[213] Grotewold, L., and Ruther, U. (2002) The Wnt antagonist Dickkopf-1 is regulated by Bmp signaling and c-Jun and modulates programmed cell death. *EMBO J* 21, 966–975

[214] Mukhopadhyay, M., *et al.* (2001) Dickkopf1 is required for embryonic head induction and limb morphogenesis in the mouse. *Dev Cell* 1, 423–434

[215] Monaghan, A.P., *et al.* (1999) Dickkopf genes are co-ordinately expressed in mesodermal lineages. *Mech Dev* 87, 45–56

[216] Nohno, T., *et al.* (1999) Differential expression of the frizzled family involved in Wnt signaling during chick limb development. *Cell Mol Biol (Noisy-le-grand)* 45, 653–659

[217] Zallen, J.A. (2007) Planar polarity and tissue morphogenesis. *Cell* 129, 1051–1063

[218] Boutros, M., *et al.* (1998) Dishevelled activates JNK and discriminates between JNK pathways in planar polarity and wingless signaling. *Cell* 94, 109–118

[219] Li, L., *et al.* (1999) Dishevelled proteins lead to two signaling pathways. Regulation of LEF-1 and c-Jun N-terminal kinase in mammalian cells. *J Biol Chem* 274, 129–134

[220] McEwen, D.G., and Peifer, M. (2000) Wnt signaling: Moving in a new direction. *Curr Biol* 10, R562–564

[221] Keller, R. (2002) Shaping the vertebrate body plan by polarized embryonic cell movements. *Science* 298, 1950–1954

[222] Gong, Y., *et al.* (2004) Planar cell polarity signalling controls cell division orientation during zebrafish gastrulation. *Nature* 430, 689–693

[223] Heisenberg, C.P., *et al.* (2000) Silberblick/Wnt11 mediates convergent extension movements during zebrafish gastrulation. *Nature* 405, 76–81

[224] Jessen, J.R., *et al.* (2002) Zebrafish trilobite identifies new roles for Strabismus in gastrulation and neuronal movements. *Nat Cell Biol* 4, 610–615

[225] Yin, C., *et al.* (2008) Cooperation of polarized cell intercalations drives convergence and extension of presomitic mesoderm during zebrafish gastrulation. *J Cell Biol* 180, 221–232

[226] Kuhl, M., *et al.* (2000) The Wnt/Ca2+ pathway: a new vertebrate Wnt signaling pathway takes shape. *Trends Genet* 16, 279–283

[227] Kuhl, M., *et al.* (2000) Ca(2+)/calmodulin-dependent protein kinase II is stimulated by Wnt and Frizzled homologs and promotes ventral cell fates in Xenopus. *J Biol Chem* 275, 12701–12711

[228] Sheldahl, L.C., *et al.* (1999) Protein kinase C is differentially stimulated by Wnt and Frizzled homologs in a G-protein-dependent manner. *Curr Biol* 9, 695–698

[229] Sheldahl, L.C., *et al.* (2003) Dishevelled activates Ca2+ flux, PKC, and CamKII in vertebrate embryos. *J Cell Biol* 161, 769–777

[230] Eisenberg, L.M., *et al.* (1992) Cloning and characterization of a novel Drosophila Wnt gene, Dwnt-5, a putative downstream target of the homeobox gene distal-less. *Dev Biol* 154, 73–83

[231] Rao, T.P., and Kuhl, M. (2010) An updated overview on Wnt signaling pathways: a prelude for more. *Circ Res* 106, 1798–1806

[232] van Amerongen, R., and Nusse, R. (2009) Towards an integrated view of Wnt signaling in development. *Development* 136, 3205–3214

[233] Kilian, B., *et al.* (2003) The role of Ppt/Wnt5 in regulating cell shape and movement during zebrafish gastrulation. *Mech Dev* 120, 467–476

[234] Wallingford, J.B., *et al.* (2001) Regulation of convergent extension in Xenopus by Wnt5a and Frizzled-8 is independent of the canonical Wnt pathway. *Int J Dev Biol* 45, 225–227

[235] Kawakami, Y., *et al.* (1999) Involvement of Wnt-5a in chondrogenic pattern formation in the chick limb bud. *Dev Growth Differ* 41, 29–40

[236] Topol, L., *et al.* (2003) Wnt-5a inhibits the canonical Wnt pathway by promoting GSK-3-independent beta-catenin degradation. *J Cell Biol* 162, 899–908

[237] Slusarski, D.C., *et al.* (1997) Modulation of embryonic intracellular Ca2+ signaling by Wnt-5A. *Dev Biol* 182, 114–120

[238] Slusarski, D.C., *et al.* (1997) Interaction of Wnt and a Frizzled homologue triggers G-protein-linked phosphatidylinositol signalling. *Nature* 390, 410–413

[239] Veeman, M.T., *et al.* (2003) A second canon. Functions and mechanisms of beta-catenin-independent Wnt signaling. *Dev Cell* 5, 367–377

[240] Westfall, T.A., *et al.* (2003) Wnt-5/pipetail functions in vertebrate axis formation as a negative regulator of Wnt/beta-catenin activity. *J Cell Biol* 162, 889–898

[241] Mikels, A.J., and Nusse, R. (2006) Purified Wnt5a protein activates or inhibits beta-catenin-TCF signaling depending on receptor context. *PLoS Biol* 4, e115

[242] Andre, P., *et al.* (2012) The Wnt coreceptor Ryk regulates Wnt/planar cell polarity by modulating the degradation of the core planar cell polarity component Vangl2. *J Biol Chem* 287, 44518–44525

[243] Logan, C.Y., and Nusse, R. (2004) The Wnt signaling pathway in development and disease. *Annu Rev Cell Dev Biol* 20, 781–810

[244] Sokol, S.Y., and Wharton, K.A., Jr. (2007) WNTers in La Jolla. *Development* 134, 3393–3399

[245] Zylstra, C.R., *et al.* (2008) Gene targeting approaches in mice: assessing the roles of LRP5 and LRP6 in osteoblasts. *J Musculoskelet Neuronal Interact* 8, 291–293

[246] Yang, Y. (2003) Wnts and wing: Wnt signaling in vertebrate limb development and musculoskeletal morphogenesis. *Birth Defects Res C Embryo Today* 69, 305–317

[247] Patton, M.A., and Afzal, A.R. (2002) Robinow syndrome. *J Med Genet* 39, 305–310

[248] Person, A.D., *et al.* (2010) WNT5A mutations in patients with autosomal dominant Robinow syndrome. *Dev Dyn* 239, 327–337

[249] Roifman, M., *et al.* (2015) De novo WNT5A-associated autosomal dominant Robinow syndrome suggests specificity of genotype and phenotype. *Clin Genet* 87, 34–41

[250] Jeffery, A. (2003) Insulin resistance. *Nurs Stand* 17, 47–53; quiz 54–45

[251] Oldridge, M., *et al.* (2000) Dominant mutations in ROR2, encoding an orphan receptor tyrosine kinase, cause brachydactyly type B. *Nat Genet* 24, 275–278

[252] Yamaguchi, T.P., *et al.* (1999) A Wnt5a pathway underlies outgrowth of multiple structures in the vertebrate embryo. *Development* 126, 1211–1223

[253] Yang, Y., *et al.* (2003) Wnt5a and Wnt5b exhibit distinct activities in coordinating chondrocyte proliferation and differentiation. *Development* 130, 1003–1015

[254] Gao, B., *et al.* (2011) Wnt signaling gradients establish planar cell polarity by inducing Vangl2 phosphorylation through Ror2. *Dev Cell* 20, 163–176

[255] Mikels, A., *et al.* (2009) Ror2 receptor requires tyrosine kinase activity to mediate Wnt5A signaling. *J Biol Chem* 284, 30167–30176

[256] Oishi, I., *et al.* (2003) The receptor tyrosine kinase Ror2 is involved in non-canonical Wnt5a/JNK signalling pathway. *Genes Cells* 8, 645–654

[257] Hikasa, H., *et al.* (2002) The Xenopus receptor tyrosine kinase Xror2 modulates morphogenetic movements of the axial mesoderm and neuroectoderm via Wnt signaling. *Development* 129, 5227–5239

[258] Nomi, M., *et al.* (2001) Loss of mRor1 enhances the heart and skeletal abnormalities in mRor2-deficient mice: redundant and pleiotropic functions of mRor1 and mRor2 receptor tyrosine kinases. *Mol Cell Biol* 21, 8329–8335

[259] Schwabe, G.C., *et al.* (2004) Ror2 knockout mouse as a model for the developmental pathology of autosomal recessive Robinow syndrome. Dev Dyn 229, 400–410

[260] Halford, M.M., et al. (2000) Ryk-deficient mice exhibit craniofacial defects associated with perturbed Eph receptor crosstalk. Nat Genet 25, 414–418

[261] Wang, B., et al. (2011) Disruption of PCP signaling causes limb morphogenesis and skeletal defects and may underlie Robinow syndrome and brachydactyly type B. Hum Mol Genet 20, 271–285

[262] Paina, S., et al. (2011) Wnt5a is a transcriptional target of dlx homeogenes and promotes differentiation of interneuron progenitors in vitro and in vivo. J Neurosci 31, 2675–2687

[263] Depew, M.J., et al. (2005) Reassessing the Dlx code: the genetic regulation of branchial arch skeletal pattern and development. J Anat 207, 501–561

[264] Vieux-Rochas, M., et al. (2010) Spatio-temporal dynamics of gene expression of the Edn1-Dlx5/6 pathway during development of the lower jaw. Genesis 48, 262–373

# 3

# Reactive Oxygen Species (ROS) and Male Fertility

Simona Tafuri, Francesca Ciani, Eugenio Luigi Iorio,
Luigi Esposito and Natascia Cocchia

**Abstract**

Oxidative energy production is inevitably associated with the generation of reactive oxygen species (ROS), excessive concentrations of which can lead to cellular pathology. A free radical may be defined as any molecule that has one or more unpaired electrons. The superoxide anion, the hydroxyl radical, and the hypochlorite radical are some of the highest reactive radicals of oxygen. Owing to their high reactivity and to their capability of initiating an uncontrolled cascade of chain reactions, ROS produce extensive protein damage and cytoskeletal modifications and inhibit cellular mechanisms. Aerobic organisms are equipped with a powerful battery of mechanisms that protect them from the adverse effects of lipid peroxidation (LPO) and other manifestations of oxygen toxicity. Defective sperm function frequently causes male infertility, due to abnormal flagella movement, failure to recognize the zona, and inhibition of sperm-oocyte fusion. ROS are fundamental mediators of physiological sperm function, such as signal transduction mechanisms that have an effect on fertility. ROS can have positive effects on sperm and the concentration functions depending on the nature and the concentration of the ROS involved. They are necessary in regulating the hyperactivation and the ability of the spermatozoa to undergo acrosome reaction. An increased amount of superoxide anion ($O_2^-$) is one of the first steps required by the spermatozoa for induction and development of hyperactivation and capacitation. Numerous studies have shown that oxidative stress plays an important role in the pathophysiology of infertility and assisted fertility. The paternal genome is of primary importance in the normal embryo and fetal development. ROS-induced sperm damage during sperm translation, such as signal transduction through the seminiferous tubules and epididymis, is one of the most important mechanisms leading to sperm DNA damage. Male germ cells are extremely vulnerable to oxidative stress as the sperm membrane is rich in unsaturated fatty acids and lacks the capacity for DNA repair. Spermatozoa are particularly susceptible to ROS-induced damage because their plasma membranes contain large quantities of polyunsaturated fatty acids (PUFA) and their cytoplasm contains low concentrations of the scavenging enzymes. Many clinical and research institutes are investigating the usefulness of antioxidant supplementation and their role in prevention of the infertility problems. Incubation under oxygen in vitro was detrimental to human spermatozoa, decreasing motility and viability. Since then, many reports have associated ROS with impaired sperm function, including decreased motility, abnormal morphology, and decreased sperm-egg penetration. Increasing knowledge of the mechanisms whereby ROS and endogenous antioxidant systems influence reproductive processes can assist to optimize the application of exogenous antioxidants to fertility treatment.

**Keywords:** ROS, Fertility, Oxidative stress

# 1. Introduction

## 1.1. Mammalian testis and reproduction

The primary sex organs of the male reproductive system are the two testes in which sperm is produced [1, 2]; the testis contains seminiferous tubules that consist of germinal epithelium and peritubular tissue [2, 3]. The epithelium contains two basic cell types, the somatic and germinal cells [4]. At different developmental stages, germ cells, including spermatogonial stem cells and differentiated cells formed during and following meiosis, are primary and secondary spermatocytes and spermatids, respectively.

These cells are located within invaginations of somatic Sertoli cells, with which maintain an intimate and cooperative relationship [3, 4]. Sertoli cells form the blood-testis barrier and are implicated in phagocytosis, secretion of testicular fluid for sperm transport, production of endocrine and paracrine substances that regulate spermatogenesis, and secretion of androgen-binding protein [5].

The development of the testis is a paradigm for the development of other organs, incorporating mechanisms for determining organ shape, size, internal architecture, vascularization, and interaction with other tissues physically, hormonally, and neurally. In the testis's development, several cells are bipotential, since the genital ridges must be able to differentiate into testes or ovaries depending on signals received; the differentiation of these cell lineages does not proceed independently, but it follows from differentiation of Sertoli cells, which then orchestrate the behavior of all other cell types [6]. Finally, the testis is built from a combination of innate precursors and immigrant cells such as germ cells.

Testosterone-secreting Leydig cells are found in the intertubular tissue surrounding the capillaries and have an important role in the spermatogenesis and the differentiation of sexual organs and secondary male sex characteristics. The Leydig cell is a polyhedral epithelioid cell with a single ovoid nucleus that contains one to three nucleoli and abundant dark-staining peripheral heterochromatin. The acidophilic cytoplasm contains many membrane-bound lipid droplets and a large amount of smooth endoplasmic reticulum. Testicular Leydig cells are the principal source of androgens in the male.

Spermatogenesis occurs in the seminiferous tubules, and it is a dynamic and metabolically active biological process during which haploid spermatozoa are produced through a gradual transformation of germ cells. These cells migrate from the basal compartment toward the luminal regions of the tubules, passing the blood-testis barrier.

The secretion of luteinizing hormone (LH) and follicle-stimulating hormone (FSH) from the pituitary, under the influence of gonadotropin-releasing hormone (GnRH) released by the hypothalamus, affects the male reproductive function. LH stimulates Leydig cells to produce testosterone, which exerts a negative feedback on GnRH and gonadotropin secretion. FSH stimulates Sertoli cell proliferation, a necessary step for the maturation of germ cells, given that the number of Sertoli cells largely determines the number of germ cells that can be correctly nurtured in the testis. During spermatogenesis, FSH and testosterone act in synergy [7, 8].

The early development of gonads has a higher energy requirement than ovaries [9]. The presence of many mitochondria in male germ cells highlights their importance in testicular metabolism [10, 11]. The germ cells's survival in the adult testis is dependent from carbohydrate metabolism, including glycolysis and mitochondrial oxidative phosphorylation. During spermatogenesis, many changes in the energy metabolism of germ cells are involved, mainly due to the blood-testis barrier and changes to the surrounding medium.

The spermatogonia, mature sperm, and the somatic Sertoli cells show high glycolytic activity, whereas spermatocytes and spermatids produce adenosine triphosphate (ATP) by mitochondrial oxidative phosphorylation [12, 13]. During spermatogenesis, three types of mitochondria are identified: the mitochondria in Sertoli cells, spermatogonia, and preleptotene and leptotene spermatocytes; the intermediate form in zygotene spermatocytes; and the condensed form in pachytene spermatocytes, secondary spermatocytes, and early spermatids [7]. The physiological death of germ cells via apoptosis occurs in the spermatogenic process and can be increased by hormone deprivation, heat, and toxin exposure [3]. Therefore, mitochondria play a central and important role in Leydig cell steroidogenesis.

### 1.2. ROS and male fertility

Oxygen is essential for animal life. Most of the body's energy is produced by the enzymatically controlled reaction of oxygen with hydrogen in oxidative phosphorylation occurring in the mitochondria during oxidative respiration. In controlled reaction steps, hydrogen is provided in the form of reducing equivalent and the energy produced is conserved in the form of high-energy phosphates. A four-electron reduction of molecular oxygen to water involving cytochrome oxidase occurs in the mitochondria. During this stepwise, enzymatic reduction of oxygen, free radicals are formed [14].

Free radicals were first described more than a century ago [15]; more than 30 years later, it was showed that all oxidation reactions involving organic molecules would be mediated by free radicals [16]. Then, free radicals were found in biological systems and were involved in many pathological processes and aging [17-19]. Subsequently, their signaling function was evaluated, and then it was found that they were regulated by hormones like insulin and were regulators of metabolic pathways [20-22].

They are short-lived reactive chemical intermediates, which contain one or more electrons with unpaired spin. Free radicals are highly reactive and oxide lipids in membranes, carbohydrates and amino acids in proteins, and damage nucleic acids. Free radicals are active participants in different processes, and they cannot be considered only damaging agents, but real players in many normal functions of living organisms. They are normal by-products in various metabolic and physiological processes, whereas excessive production of them results in the oxidative stress.

The dioxygen molecule ($O_2$) is a biradical, because it contains two electrons with the same spin in an external antibonding molecular orbital. Molecular oxygen can be reduced via a four-electron mechanism with acceptance of four protons yielding two water molecules. In this case, the free biradical is simply converted to a non-radical species due to acceptance of the four electrons and four protons. However, there is another way to reduce molecular oxygen; this is one-electron successive reduction. Receiving one electron, $O_2$ is converted to the superoxide anion radical ($O_2^{\cdot -}$), containing one unpaired electron in an external antibonding orbital. Accepting a second electron and two protons converts the superoxide anion radical into hydrogen peroxide ($H_2O_2$); $H_2O_2$ has a non-radical nature and is chemically more active than molecular oxygen but less active than $O_2^{\cdot -}$.

The formation of the most reactive of oxygen species, the hydroxyl radical ($HO^{\cdot}$), results from the further reduction of $H_2O_2$ leading to its dismutation. Finally, acceptance of a fourth (final) electron and one more proton $HO^{\cdot}$ forms a water molecule. Since $O_2^{\cdot -}$, $H_2O_2$, and $HO^{\cdot}$ are chemically more reactive than molecular oxygen, they are collectively called ROS, but only $O_2^{\cdot -}$ and $HO^{\cdot}$ are actually free radicals, whereas $H_2O_2$ is not. Therefore, in biological research, the term "free radicals" is frequently replaced by "reactive oxygen species" (ROS), which is a more general term and includes both free radical and non-radical species.

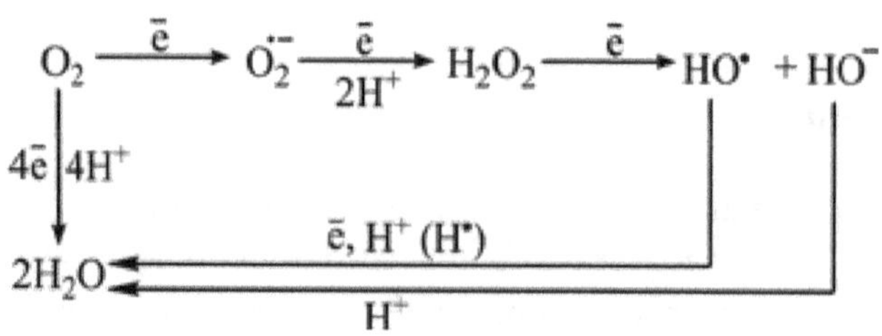

ROS formation and redox signaling play a role in physiology and in a variety of pathologies, including inflammatory, infectious, and degenerative disorders, either in humans or in animals [23-25]. ROS are involved in a variety of pathophysiological conditions of the testis, and oxidative stress is known to inhibit ovarian and testicular steroidogenesis. The disruption of redox signaling and control and imbalance in favor of prooxidant species define oxidative stress [26, 27].

Oxidative stress is a state in which an oxidant-generating system overcomes an antioxidant defense system, a process that is involved in many diseases including male factor infertility and/or subfertility. ROS are products of normal cellular metabolism and are formed during the normal enzymatic reactions of intercellular and intracellular signaling [28]. ROS overproduction can be induced through physiological or pathological mechanisms, including ROS generation by leukocytes as a cytotoxic mechanism of host defense, during hypoxic states leading to high levels of ROS, as well as by drugs with oxidizing effects on cells. Then, when mitochondria become a target of elevated levels of ROS, the process of oxidative phosphorylation might be affected because of a possible damage of proteins and membrane lipids. Lipids are present in the sperm plasma membrane in the form of polyunsaturated fatty acids (PUFAs) that contain more than two carbon-carbon double bonds. ROS attacks PUFA in the cell membrane, leading to a cascade of chemical reactions called lipid peroxidation.

[1] $O_2^{-\bullet} + O_2^{-\bullet} + 2H^+ = H_2O_2 + O_2$

[2] $O_2^{-\bullet} + H_2O_2 \overset{Fe^{2+}}{=} O_2 + OH^\bullet + OH^-$

[3] $-CH_2- + OH^\bullet = -\dot{C}H- + H_2O$

[4] $R^\bullet + O_2 = ROO^\bullet$

[5] $ROO^\bullet + -CH_2- = ROOH + -\dot{C}H-$

At low concentrations, ROS are metabolic intermediates in the metabolism of prostanoids, in gene regulation and cellular growth and in signal transduction [29, 30]. At high concentrations, ROS exert bionegative effects and damage all major classes of biomolecules.

During reproduction, ROS are involved in many important mechanisms of sperm physiology. An increase in ROS generation at the beginning of capacitation is followed by an increase in tyrosine phosphorylation [31]. The motility was associated with the generation of superoxide anion and a phosphorylation of tyrosine residues.

Furthermore, the acrosome reaction was associated with an extracellular superoxide anion of spermatozoa [32]. In the male genital tract, ROS are generated by spermatozoa and leukocytes including neutrophils and macrophages. In the semen, sperm cells are one of the major cellular sources of ROS. The male germ cells produced a small amount of ROS from the earliest stages of the development [33]. They are involved in the sperm chromatin condensation, regulating the number of germ cells by induction of apoptosis or proliferation of spermatogonia [34]. In the mature sperm, ROS play an important role in the capacitation, acrosome reaction and sperm motility, and they can also function as signaling molecules. There are at least two mechanisms of their production: the membrane nicotinamide adenine dinucleotide phosphate

(NADPH) oxidase, an enzyme complex that is contained in the cell membrane, and the mitochondria.

Furthermore, many studies have demonstrated that low and physiological levels of ROS play an important role in processes such as capacitation, hyperactivation, acrosome reaction, and sperm-oocyte fusion in order to ensure appropriate fertilization, whereas high levels of ROS cause sperm pathologies such as ATP depletion and loss of sperm motility and viability [35]. When the ROS overcomes the antioxidant defense systems and disrupts the intricate balance between ROS and antioxidants, pathological defects occur that causes significant damage to biomolecules such as lipids, proteins, nucleic acids, and carbohydrates [36]. The ROS found in the seminal plasma originates from various endogenous and exogenous sources; there are many endogenous sources of ROS in the seminal plasma such as peroxidase-positive leukocytes including polymorphonuclear leukocytes and macrophages [37]. Most of these peroxidase-positive leukocytes derive from the prostate and seminal vesicles; if these sources of ROS are triggered by many intracellular or extracellular stimuli, as inflammation or infection, they can increase ROS and the NADPH production via the hexose monophosphate shunt [38, 39]. An increase in proinflammatory cytokines, such as interleukin (IL)-8, and a decrease in the antioxidant superoxide dismutase (SOD) can result in a respiratory burst, production of high levels of ROS, and oxidative stress. Between exogenous sources of ROS, there are toxins, phthalates, and others [40]. Infections lead to an excessive ROS production, resulting in an oxidative burst from neutrophils/macrophages as a first-line defense mechanism. When there is an infection, an imbalance of prooxidants and antioxidants favors the oxidative stress that damages the sperm functions such as motility and fertilization. In the testis and epididymis infections, the ROS produced are very detrimental to the spermatozoa because of the long contact time and the loss of antioxidant protection.

During the final phase of the ejaculation, only high numbers of ROS-producing leukocytes are harmful to sperm functions. An infection which involves ROS in the epididymis, prostate gland, and/or seminal vesicles could indirectly damage sperm functions [41].

In 1943, a paper was published showing the effect of high oxygen tensions on motility and prevention of this phenomenon by adding catalase, which suggested the involvement of oxygen overload in motility of spermatozoa [42]. Indeed, ROS generation was dependent on the oxygen tension; higher oxygen tensions increased ROS generation, mainly from leukocytes, whereas low oxygen tensions improved the survival rate and penetration capacity [43].

Oxidative stress has been considered a main cause to male infertility, but studies have showed that low and verified concentrations of ROS play a pivotal role in sperm physiological processes such as capacitation, hyperactivation, acrosome reactions, and signaling processes to provide a suitable fertilization, but an increase in oxidative stress leads to male infertility by the induction of peroxidative damage to the sperm plasma membrane, DNA damage, and apoptosis. ROS must be maintained at appropriate levels to ensure appropriate physiological function while preventing pathological damage to the spermatozoa. ROS is thought to influence fertility by affecting sperm membranes and sperm DNA. They reduce sperm motility and its ability to fuse with the oocyte and compromise paternal genomic contribution to the embryo; in fact, sperm are vulnerable to oxidative stress-induced damage due to the high portion of PUFA and also due to the low concentrations of scavenging enzymes in their cytoplasm, both contributing to the defective sperm function observed in a high percentage of infertility.

There are many agents that cause an increase in testicular oxidative stress, such as environmental toxins or conditions such as varicocele, orchitis, cryptorchidism, and aging, all of which leads to an increase in germ cell apoptosis and hypospermatogenesis. ROS-induced DNA damage may also potentiate germ cell apoptosis, leading to a decrease in sperm count and thus to the decline of semen quality, both of which are associated with male infertility [39]. Large amounts of pathogenic mutant mtDNA accumulate in the testis; the resulting mitochondrial respiratory dysfunction in spermatogenic cells leads to a decrease in energy production that ultimately induces meiotic arrest and abnormalities in sperm morphology, stressing the importance of mitochondrial respiratory function in mammalian spermatogenesis [44].

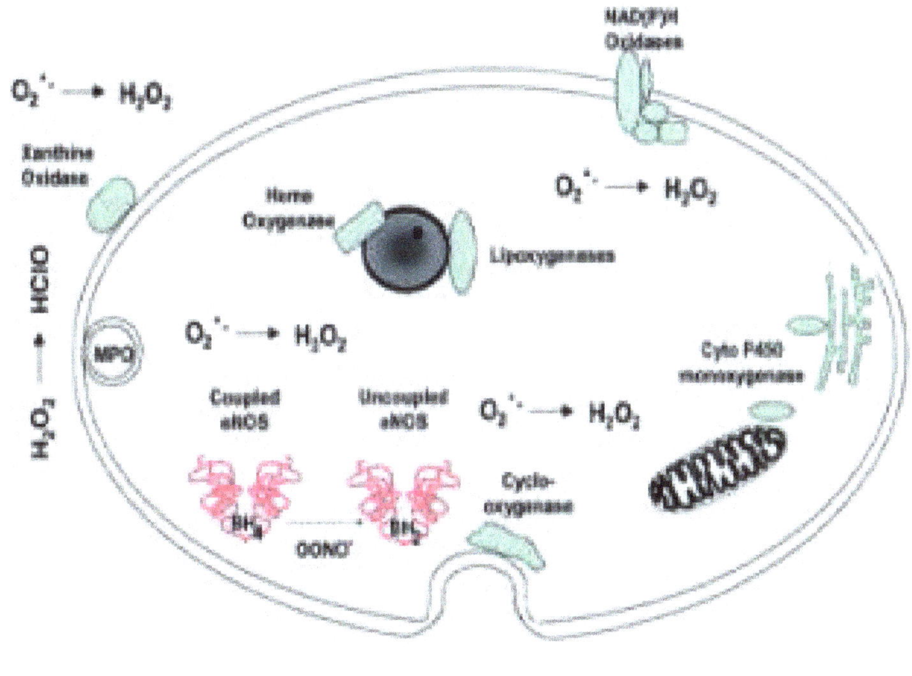


## 2. Apoptosis and oxidative stress

Oxidative stress is implicated between causes of male infertility. ROS production and its effects on semen quality have been widely clarified. Oxygen is essential to sustain life, and physiological levels of ROS are necessary to maintain normal cell functions. However, products of oxygen such as ROS can be detrimental to cell function and survival [45].

ROS are detrimental to sperm survival and function due to its adverse effects on sperm membrane and genetic material. High frequency of single- and double-stranded DNA breaks due to oxidative stress activates apoptosis by inducing cytochrome c and caspases 9 and 3 [46]. Disruption of inner and outer mitochondrial membranes results in release of cytochrome c, a protein which activates caspases and induces apoptosis. Mitochondrial exposure to ROS results in the release of apoptosis-inducing factor, which directly interacts with the DNA and leads to DNA fragmentation [46]. Seminal oxidative stress, sperm DNA damage, and apoptosis constitute a unified pathogenic molecular mechanism in infertility. Therefore, apoptosis in semen could be a useful indicator of semen quality.

## 3. Antioxidants in male fertility

Antioxidants are substances, enzymatic and nonenzymatic, which serve to eliminate ROS. Enzymatic oxidants, or natural oxidants, include glutathione reductase (GSH), superoxide dismutase (SOD), and catalase, while some non-enzymatic oxidants include vitamins (C, E, and B), carotenoids, carnitines, cysteines, pentoxifylline, metals, taurine, and albumin [47]. Glutathione reductase and peroxidase are the principal reducing agents in the body and behave as antioxidant scavengers in the epididymis and testes [48]. Their action on sperm membranes confers protection on to the lipid components, preserving the sperm viability and motility [49]. Preceding in vitro studies have demonstrated that GSH reduces lipid peroxidation and improves the sperm membrane characteristics [50]. The main antioxidant enzyme system in the semen includes SOD, catalase, and glutathione peroxidase.

SODs are metalloenzymes that catalyze the dismutation reactions of the superoxide anion and are present in intracellular and extracellular forms; two of the intracellular forms are copper-zinc SOD, which is localized in the cytoplasm and contains copper and zinc (Cu, ZnSOD, SOD1) in the active site, and manganese SOD, which is located primarily in the mitochondrial matrix and contains manganese in the active site (MnSOD, SOD2). The extracellular form of SOD (EC-SOD, SOD3) acts in the extracellular space and it is related to the surface polysaccharides though it may also be present in a free form [51]. SOD presents high activity in the seminal plasma with 75% of its activity connected to the activity of SOD1 and the remaining 25% to SOD3; these isoenzymes are maybe derived from the prostate [52]. SOD and catalase protect sperm from superoxide anions catalyzing the conversion of superoxide into oxygen and $H_2O_2$, thereby preventing lipid peroxidation and enhancing motility [53].

$$\cdot O_{2^-} + \cdot O_{2^-} \times + 2H^+ \rightarrow H_2O_2 + O_2$$

SOD and catalase assist in removing ROS that has the potential to damage sperm. Catalase catalyzes the conversion of $H_2O_2$ to $O_2$ and $H_2O$ and presents a heme group with a central iron atom. It acts mainly in the endoplasmic reticulum, peroxisomes, mitochondria, and cytosol in many cell types [54]. Catalase was found in the human and rat sperm cells and in the seminal plasma; the prostate seems to be its source [55]. The sperm cell capacitation induced by nitric oxide is activated by catalase [56].

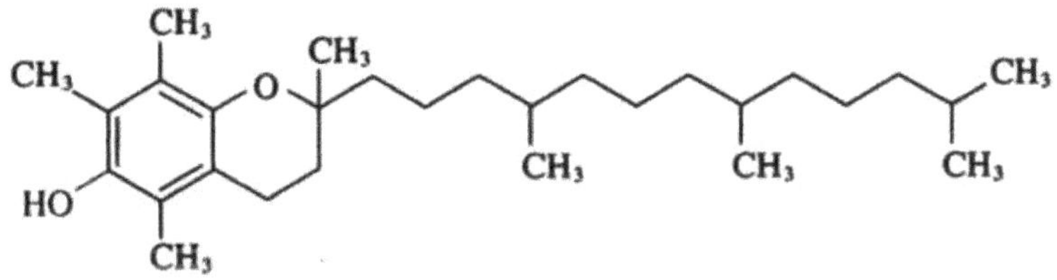

$$2H_2O_2 \quad O_2 + 2H_2O$$

Glutathione peroxidase (GPX), another antioxidant enzyme in the semen, catalyzes the reduction of $H_2O_2$ and organic peroxides [51]. GPX contains selenium in the form of selenocysteine in its active site. It is located in the sperm in the mitochondrial matrix [52] but has also been found to have a nuclear form that preserves sperm DNA from oxidative damage and enters in the process of chromatin condensation. It was found in the seminal plasma; therefore, it could originate from the prostate [57, 58].

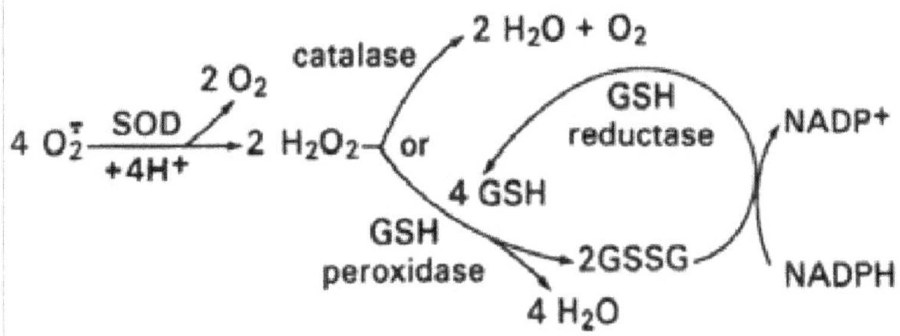


Between nonenzymatic antioxidants, there are vitamin E which encompass a group of potent, lipid-soluble, chain-breaking antioxidants. Structural analyses have revealed that molecules having vitamin E antioxidant activity include four tocopherols (α, β, γ, δ) and four tocotrienols (α, β, γ, δ). Vitamin E (α-tocopherol), a chain-breaking antioxidant in the sperm's cell membrane, neutralizes $H_2O_2$ and quenches free radicals, therefore stopping chain reactions that develop lipid peroxides and protecting the membrane from the oxidative damage [48]. Vitamin E improves the activity of other scavenging oxidants and helps to keep motility and morphology of the sperm [54]. It preserves the spermatogenesis in male rats and fails to conserve zygotes in female rats. Selenium deficiency can induce male infertility and could thus support an antioxidant function of vitamin E in the reproductive system. Therefore, vitamin E and selenium can act in synergy in membrane protection from oxidative stress. Vitamin E is known to readily reduce alkyl peroxy radicals of unsaturated lipids, thereby generating hydroperoxides that are reduced by the selenoperoxidases, in particular by phospholipid-hydroperoxide glutathione peroxidase.

Vitamin C or L-ascorbic acid, or ascorbate (the anion of ascorbic acid), is an essential nutrient for humans and many animals. Vitamin C is a major chain-breaking antioxidant and is present in the extracellular fluid. It neutralizes hydroxyl, superoxide, and hydrogen peroxide radicals

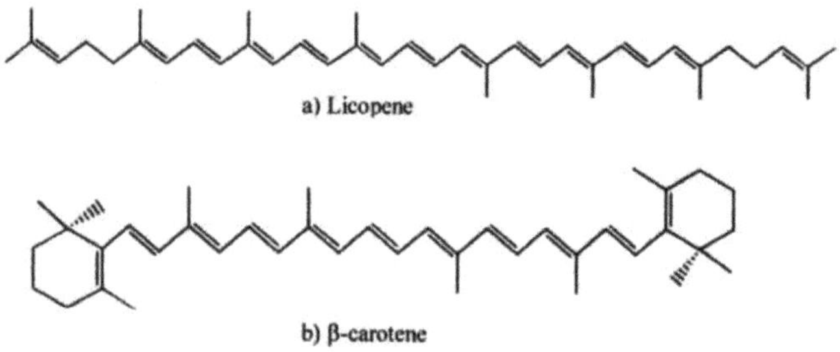


and prevents sperm agglutination [53]. It also helps to recycle vitamin E. It plays a significant role in removing oxidative stress in the seminal plasma. It reacts with $OH^-$, $O_2^-$, and $H_2O_2$ in the extracellular fluid, thus protecting sperm viability and motility [59].

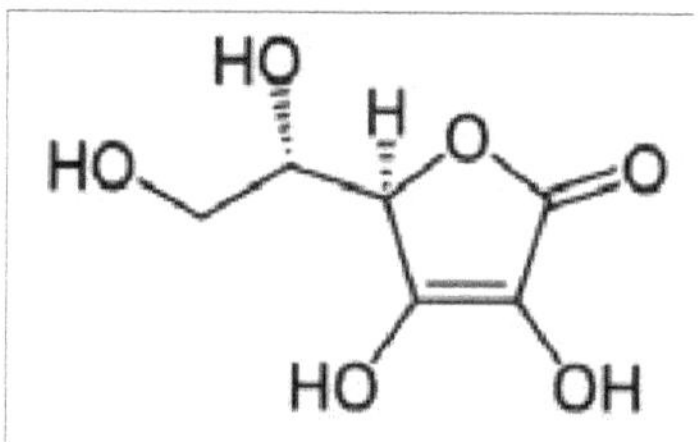


Carnitine, a water-soluble antioxidant, participates in sperm motility and prevents lipid oxidation; it protects the sperm DNA and membranes from oxidative damage and maintains sperm viability and motility [60].

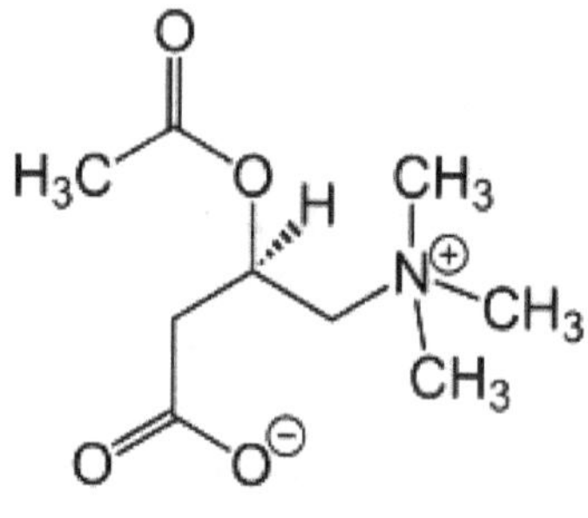


Carotenoids are a family of pigmented compounds that are synthesized by plants and microorganisms, but not animals. They are present as micro-components in fruits and vegetables and are responsible for their yellow, orange, and red colors. Carotenoids are thought to be responsible for the beneficial properties of fruits and vegetables in preventing diseases including cardiovascular diseases, cancer, and other chronic diseases. Carotenoids (β-carotene and lycopene) are very efficient singlet molecular oxygen quenchers; they prevent peroxidation in the seminal plasma [59].

Cysteines, precursors of intracellular GSH, increase the amount of GSH synthesized that prevents oxidative damage to the cell membrane and DNA. There are a few other minor antioxidants that contribute to relieving oxidative stress, such as albumin, taurine/hypotaurine, inositol, and some metals. Albumin, a plasma protein, interacts with peroxyl radicals and inhibits the chain reactions that generate ROS production and preserve motility and viability of sperm.

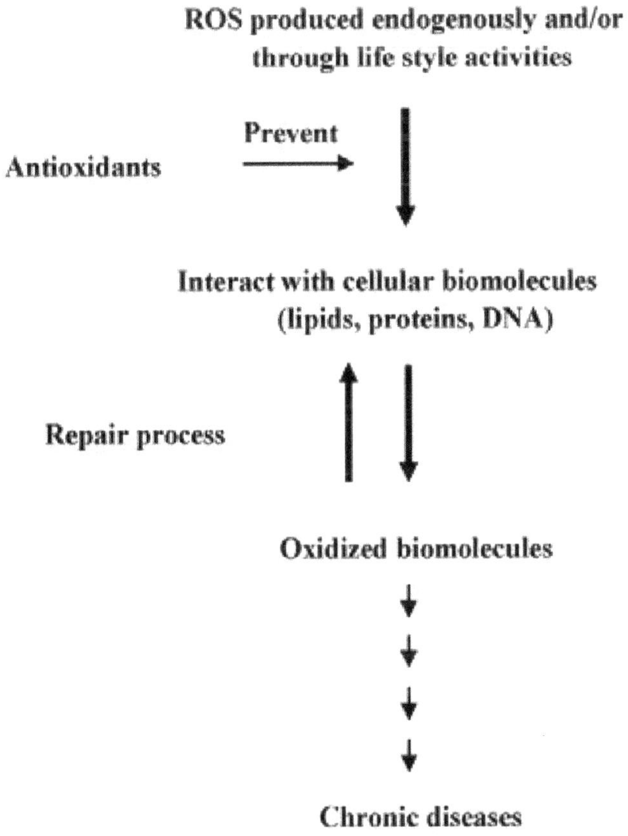


Taurine, a non-enzymatic antioxidant, scavenges ROS; inositol enhances GSH activity and preserves normal sperm morphology.

Selenium is an important component in the regular development and maturation of the testes and contributes to the protection of sperm DNA and cell membranes, particularly when used as an adjunct to vitamin E. The specific role of selenium in spermatogenesis appears to be related to phospholipid hydroperoxide glutathione peroxidase, which is expressed depending on the developmental state of spermatids.

Zinc acts as a chelator and binds ROS; manganese enhances sperm motility and viability [61, 62]. Chrome, another essential micronutrient, is a component of enzymes involved in carbohydrate metabolism. Its supplementation reduces fat deposition in rats, preventing obesity, the initial phase of inflammation, and oxidative stress [63]. Although seminal plasma contains a range of protective antioxidants such as SOD, catalase, and glutathione peroxidase, these defenses are less abundant in the sperm and seem to be impaired in cases of male infertility [64].

## 4. Measurement of ROS

Oxidative stress results from an imbalance between ROS production and the intracellular and extracellular antioxidants that scavenge ROS. There are many direct assays that measure the oxidation of the sperm cell membrane. The most used assay measures malondialdehyde (MDA), one of the final products of sperm cell membrane lipid peroxidation [65, 66]. Increased levels of MDA correlate with decreased sperm parameters.

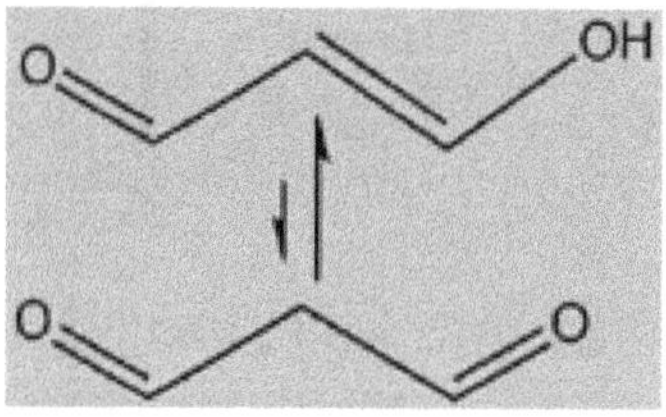

Quantification of sperm DNA damage has also been used as assay for intracellular ROS-induced oxidant injury by measuring a specific product of oxidant-induced DNA damage, 8-oxo-7, 8, -dihydro 2′ deoxyguanoside (8-OHdG), used as a specific marker of oxidative injury to sperm DNA [67].

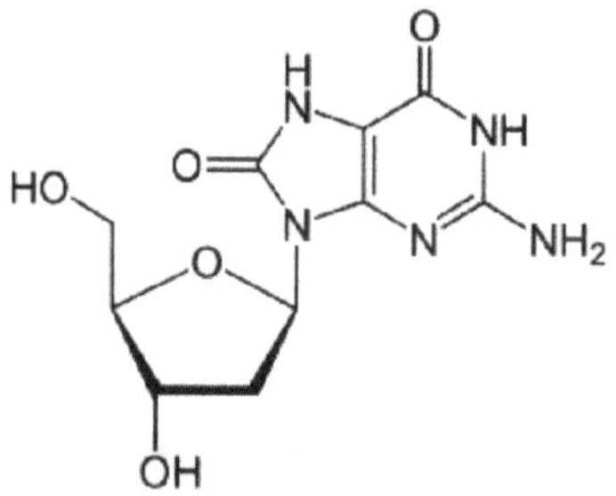

The most used method for measurement of seminal ROS is the indirect chemiluminescence assay. Luminol (5-amino-2, 3, dihydro 1, 4, phthalazinedione), or lucigen, can be used for quantification of redox activities of spermatozoa [68]. Lucigen measures only extracellular superoxide radicals, while luminol is used to measure extracellular and intracellular levels of ROS.

The nitroblue tetrazolium assay requires a light microscope and allows differentiation of spermatic and leukocytic ROS without the steps required in chemiluminescence assays. Nitroblue tetrazolium interacts with superoxide radicals in the sperm and leukocytes by changing to diformazan, a blue pigment. The concentration of diformazan correlates with the concentration of intracellular ROS [68].

The antioxidant levels of the semen can also be determined by chemiluminescence assay or by a colorimetric assay. Antioxidant levels are measured through the addition of a known concentration of ROS to the semen, leading to the development of the chemiluminescence signal or a color change. This assay allows the antioxidants in the semen to scavenge the known ROS and then the measurement of residual ROS level. The intensity of the signal produced is inversely correlated with the total antioxidant capacity of the sample [69].

Another method for measuring oxidative stress can be carried through the measurement of lipid peroxidation in the whole sperm by a commercially assay kit (LP Sperm Test, Diacron International, Grosseto, Italy). The assay is based on the ability of peroxides to promote the oxidation of $Fe^{2+}$ to $Fe^{3+}$; the product of peroxidation ($Fe^{3+}$) binds to the thiocyanate, developing a colored complex measured photometrically [70].

## 5. ROS In Vitro Fertilization (IVF) or artificial insemination

New studies are underway to find new methods for supporting longer storage of cooled animal semen. All aerobic organisms require oxygen for life; although it is an essential element, oxygen is responsible for ROS production. It is known that high concentrations of ROS cause sperm pathology. Low concentrations of ROS play an important role in sperm physiology, while higher concentrations are detrimental. A study showed the influence of ROS on capacitation and the acrosome reaction in frozen-thawed bull spermatozoa; they concluded that ROS is required in the capacitation process and that hydrogen peroxide may participate as an inducer of the acrosome reaction [71, 72].

ROS act as second messengers and are involved in the sperm capacitation, acrosome reaction, and oocyte fertilization. They regulate the increase of cyclic adenosine monophosphate (cAMP), protein kinase A (PKA) activation, and phosphorylation of PKA substrates (arginine-X-X-(serine/threonine) motif), phosphorylation of extracellular signal-regulated kinase (ERK) and mitogen-activated protein kinase kinase (MEK) proteins and threonine-glutamate-tyrosine motif, and tyrosine phosphorylation of fibrous sheath proteins [73]. When ROS increase, the endogenous antioxidant defenses of gametes decrease and oxidative stress is induced [74]. High concentrations of ROS induce changes in sperm cell functions, altering fluidity and integrity of sperm membranes due to lipid peroxidation. Furthermore, ROS can damage DNA in the sperm nucleus, deplete ATP in mitochondria, and cause loss of sperm motility, viability, and capacity for fertilization [75]. Oxidative stress may be a cause of male infertility and contribute to DNA fragmentation in spermatozoa. There are few studies on the effects of antioxidant addition to extenders during cooling and/or freezing mammalian spermatozoa. Spermatozoa are subjected to peroxidative damage due to an excess of ROS because of the high presence of polyunsaturated fatty acids in membrane phospholipids. The antioxidant systems control the balance between production and neutralization of ROS and protect spermatozoa against peroxidative damage [76]. Recent studies moreover show a physiological SOD activity in human seminal plasma [77, 78]. SOD is an important antioxidant defense in all cells exposed to oxygen. Their use as additives in semen extenders has had controversial effects [79, 80]. SOD is responsible for $H_2O_2$ and $O_2$ production, by dismutation of superoxide radicals. The addition of SOD to semen improves the quality of semen and reduces ERK activation [81, 82]. The addition of SOD to the semen extender could prolong storage of stallion semen, allowing longer distance shipments and a more precise timing of insemination, increasing the high rates of fertility. Furthermore, the antioxidant addition might also bring benefits to spermatozoa in the female reproductive tract [83]. ROS are responsible for the deterioration in quality of semen stored at 5°C, and the addition of SOD to the semen extender improves the quality of cold-stored semen.

Another work evaluated the effect of SOD supplementation in ovary transport media during 4°C storage of cat ovaries at different time intervals on the occurrence of ovarian apoptosis and on the ability to undergo in vitro oocyte development. The authors by immunohistochemical analysis, reverse transcriptase polymerase chain reaction (RT-PCR) analysis, and viability test analysis have demonstrated that SOD supplementation in transport media of domestic cat ovaries reduces cellular apoptosis and enhances COC survival and in vitro embryo production (IVEP) [84].

## 6. Conclusion

Oxidative stress has been extensively studied for about four decades. Substantial progress has been achieved to date from descriptive characterization of this process to delineation of molecular mechanisms underlining adaptive responses and targeted manipulations of expected responses. Oxygen toxicity is an inherent challenge to aerobic life, including spermatozoa, the cells responsible for propagation of the species. The oxidative damage to sperm membranes, proteins, and DNA is connected with changes in signal transduction mechanisms that affect fertility.

Spermatozoa and oocytes possess an inherent but limited capacity to generate ROS to aid in the fertilization process. Although a variety of defense mechanisms including antioxidant enzymes, vitamins, and biomolecules are available, a balance of the benefits and risks from ROS and antioxidants appears to be necessary for the survival and function of spermatozoa.

The antioxidants $\alpha$-tocopherol (Vitamin A), ascorbic acid (Vitamin C), and retinoids (Vitamin A) are all potent scavengers of reactive oxygen species. Many studies have investigated the role of these and other antioxidants in improving sperm parameters.

The origin and the etiologies of increased ROS in males with suboptimal sperm quality are increasingly clear, presenting many pathways for a potential therapy. However, well-designed randomized controlled trials will be required to evaluate the potential of antioxidant systems. Furthermore, prooxidative and antioxidative properties of therapeutics are currently receiving more attention as part of anti-infectious therapies too.

ROS production might be beneficial or harmful for living organisms; this also applies in spermatozoa, which require low levels of ROS to show their full capacity in fertilizing. Conversely, oxidative stress is damaging for spermatozoa and many other cellular types; an excess of ROS has been associated with many diseases including diabetes, cancer, atherosclerosis, and Parkinson disease.

Oxidative stress might also be a consequence of unhealthy lifestyles such as smoking, alcohol abuse, or exposure to chemical or electromagnetic pollution. ROS are important contributors to the regulation of sperm function in both a positive and a negative sense. Thus, these cells generate low levels of ROS in order to promote capacitation and the functional evolution of sperm behaviors needed for fertilization, including hyperactivation and the presentation of zona recognition molecules on their surface. If fertilization does not occur, the continued generation of ROS activates the intrinsic apoptotic cascade.

Future progress in the field needs identification of the most crucial cellular targets for ROS action as well as discovery of the underlying mechanisms and consequences of the interaction between ROS and cellular components.

The mechanisms responsible for removing ROS and their regulation would be the second hot topic for ongoing studies of ROS metabolism.

In recent years, it was discovered that ROS and ROS-regulated pathways are actively involved in modification of diverse cellular processes starting from core metabolism and hormonal signaling through to complicated processes such as fertilization and development. The latter along with some biotechnological avenues would also extend ROS-related studies in practical directions. Therefore, much remains to be learned about the effects of ROS on biological systems, the adaptive strategies that overcome ROS attack, and the natural use of ROS in the signaling and regulation of metabolism.

## Author details

Simona Tafuri[1], Francesca Ciani[1*], Eugenio Luigi Iorio[2], Luigi Esposito[1] and Natascia Cocchia[1]

*Address all correspondence to: ciani@unina.it

1 Department of Veterinary Medicine and Animal Productions - University of Naples Federico II, Naples, Italy

2 International Observatory of Oxidative Stress, Salerno, Italy

## References

[1] Shauf C., Moffett D., Moffett S. Reproduction and its endocrine control. In Allen D. (ed.) Human physiology. Times Mirror/Mosby College Publishing, St Louis, 1990; 646–661.

[2] Junqueira L., Carneiro J. The male reproductive system. In Foltin J., Lebowitz H., Boyle P. (eds.) Basic histology. McGraw Hill Companies, New York, 2003; 431–447.

[3] Holstein A., Schulze W., Davidoff M. Understanding spermatogenesis is a prerequisite for treatment. Reproductive Biology and Endocrinology 2003; 1; 107.

[4] Hess R. Spermatogenesis. In Knobil E., Neill J. (eds.) Encyclopedia of reproduction. Academic Press, San Diego, 1999; 539–545.

[5] De Kreteser D., Kerr J.B. The cytology of the testis. In Knobil E., Neill J. (eds.) The physiology of reproduction. Raven Press Ltd., New York, 1994; 1212–1241.

[6] Burgoyne P.S., Thornhill A.R., Boudrean S.K., Darling S.M., Bishop C.E., Evans E.P. The genetic basis of XX–XY differences present before gonadal sex differentiation in the mouse. Philosophical Transactions of the Royal Society of London. Series B, Biological Sciences 1995; 350; 253–260.

[7] Holdcraft R., Braun R. Hormonal regulation of spermatogenesis. International Journal of Andrology 2004; 27; 335–342.

[8] Maclachlan R., Wreford N., O'Donnell L., De Kretser D., Robertson D. The endocrine regulation of spermatogenesis: Independent roles for testosterone and FSH. Journal of Endocrinology 1996; 148; 1–9.

[9] Matoba S., Hiramatsu R., Kanai-Azuma M., Tsunekawa N., Harikae K., Kawakami H., Kurohmaru M., Kanai Y. Establishment of testis-specific SOX9 activation requires high glucose metabolism in mouse sex differentiation. Developmental Biology 2008; 324; 76–87.

[10] Meinhardt A., Wilhelm B., Seitz J. Expression of mitochondrial marker proteins during spermatogenesis. Human Reproduction Update 1999; 5; 108–119.

[11] Amaral S., Amaral A., Ramalho-Santos J. Aging and male reproductive function: A mitochondrial perspective. Frontiers in Bioscience 2013; 5; 181–197.

[12] Robinson R., Fritz I. Metabolism of glucose by Sertoli cells in culture. Biology of Reproduction 1981; 24; 1032–1041.

[13] Grootegoed J., Jansen R., Van der Molen H. The role of glucose, pyruvate and lactate in ATP production by rat spermatocytes and spermatids. Biochimica et Biophysica Acta 1984; 767; 248–256.

[14] Fridovich I. The biology of oxygen radicals. Science 1978; 201(4359); 875–880.

[15] Gomberg M. An instance of trivalent carbon: Triphenylmethyl. Journal of the American Chemical Society 1900; 22; 757–771.

[16] Michaelis L. Free radicals as intermediate steps of oxidation–reduction. Cold Spring Harbor Symposia on Quantitative Biology 1939; 7; 33–49.

[17] Commoner B., Townsend J., Pake G.E. Free radicals in biological materials. Nature 1954; 174; 689–691.

[18] Gerschman R., Gilbert D.L., Nye S.W., Dwyer P., Fenn W.O. Oxygen poisoning and X-irradiation: A mechanism in common. Science 1954; 119; 623–626.

[19] Harman D. Origin and evolution of the free radical theory of aging: A brief personal history, 1954–2009. Biogerontology 2009; 10; 773–781.

[20] Christman M.F., Morgan R.W., Jacobson F.S., Ames B.N. Positive control of a regulon for defenses against oxidative stress and some heat-shock proteins in Salmonella typhimurium. Cell 1985; 41; 753–762.

[21] Spagnoli A., Spadoni G.L., Sesti G., Del Principe D., Germani D., Boscherini B. Effect of insulin on hydrogen peroxide production by human polymorphonuclear leukocytes. Studies with monoclonal anti-insulin receptor antibodies, and an agonist and an inhibitor of protein kinase C. Hormone Research 1995; 43; 286–293.

[22] Shaikhali I., Heiber T., Seidel E., Ströher H., Hiltscher S., Birkmann K.J., Dietz M., Baier M. The redox-sensitive transcription factor Rap2.4a controls nuclear expression of 2-Cys peroxiredoxin A and other chloroplast antioxidant enzymes. BMC Plant Biology 2008; 8-48.

[23] Bildik A., Kargin F., Seyrek K., Pasa S., Ozensoy S. Oxidative stress and non-enzymatic antioxidative status in dogs with visceral Leishmaniasis. Research in Veterinary Science 2004; 77(1); 63–66.

[24] Kumaraguruparan R., Kabalimoorthy J., Nagini S. Correlation of tissue lipid peroxidation and antioxidants with clinical stage and menopausal status in patients with adenocarcinoma of the breast. Clinical Biochemistry 2005; 38(2); 154–158.

[25] Vajdovich P., Kriska T., Mézes M., Szabó P.R., Balogh N., Bánfi A., Arany-Tóth A., Gaál T., Jakus redox status of dogs with non-Hodgkin lymphomas. An ESR study. J. Cancer Letters 2005; 224(2); 339–346.

[26] Cadenas E., Sies H. Oxidative stress: Excited oxygen species and enzyme activity. Advances in Enzyme Regulation 1985; 23; 217–237.

[27] Jones DP. Disruption of mitochondrial redox circuitry in oxidative stress. Chemico Biological Interaction 2006; 163(1–2); 38–53.

[28] Agarwal A., Prabakaran S., Allamaneni S. What an andrologist/urologist should know about free radicals and why. Urology 2006; 67; 2–8.

[29] Lands WE. Interactions of lipid hydroperoxides with eicosanoid biosynthesis. Free Radical Biology and Medicine 1985; 1(2); 97–101.

[30] Joseph JA., Cutler RC. The role of oxidative stress in signal transduction changes and cell loss in senescence. Annals of the New York Academy of Sciences 1994; 738; 37–43.

[31] de Lamirande E., Gagnon C. Paradoxical effect of reagents for sulfhydryl and disulfide groups on human sperm capacitation and superoxide production. Free Radical Biology and Medicine 1998; 25(7); 803–817.

[32] de Lamirande E., Tsai C., Harakat A., Gagnon C. Involvement of reactive oxygen species in human sperm arcosome reaction induced by A23187, lysophosphatidylcholine, and biological fluid ultrafiltrates. Journal of Andrololology 1998; 19(5); 585–594.

[33] Fisher H.M., Aitken R.J. Comparative analysis of the ability of precursor germ cells and epididymal spermatozoa to generate reactive oxygen metabolites. Journal of Experimental Zoology 1997; 277; 390–400.

[34] Aitken R.J. The Amoroso lecture. The human spermatozoon – A cell in crisis? Journal of Reproduction and Fertility 1999; 115; 1–7.

[35] Saleh R.A., Agarwal A. Oxidative stress and male infertility: From research bench to clinical practice. Journal of Andrololology 2002; 23; 737–752.

[36] Agarwal A., Prabakaran S.A. Mechanism, measurement, and prevention of oxidative stress in male reproductive physiology. Indian Journal of Experimental Biology 2005; 43; 963–974.

[37] Saleh R.A., Agarwal A., Nada E.A., El-Tonsy M.H., Sharma R.K., Meyer A. Negative effects of increased sperm DNA damage in relation to seminal oxidative stress in men with idiopathic and male factor infertility. Fertility and Sterility 2003; 79; 1597–1605.

[38] Lavranos G., Balla M., Tzortzopoulou A., Syriou V., Angelopoulou R. Investigating ROS sources in male infertility: A common end for numerous pathways. Reproductive Toxicology 2012; 34; 298–307.

[39] Agarwal A., Saleh R.A., Bedaiwy M.A. Role of reactive oxygen species in the pathophysiology of human reproduction. Fertility and Sterility 2003; 79; 829–843.

[40] Pant N., Shukla M., Kumar Patel D., Shukla Y., Mathur N., Kumar Gupta Y. Correlation of phthalate exposures with semen quality. Toxicology and Applied Pharmacology 2008; 231; 112–116.

[41] Ochsendorf F.R. Infections in the male genital tract and reactive oxygen species. Human Reproduction Update 1999; 5; 399–420.

[42] MacLeod J. The role of oxygen in the metabolism and motility of human spermatozoa. American Journal of Physiology 1943; 138; 512–518.

[43] Whittington K., Ford WC. The effect of incubation periods under 95% oxygen on the stimulated acrosome reaction and motility of human spermatozoa. Molecular Human Reproduction 1998; 4(11); 1053–1057.

[44] Nakada K., Sato A., Yoshida K., Morita T., Tanaka H., Inoue S., Yonekawa H., Hayashi J. Mitochondria-related male infertility. Proceedings of the National Academy of Sciences USA 2006; 103; 15148–15153.

[45] Griveau J.F., Renard P., Le Lannou D. Superoxide anion production by human spermatozoa as a part of the ionophore induced acrosome reaction process. International Journal of Andrology 1995; 18; 67–74.

[46] Aitken R.J., Koppers A.J. Apoptosis and DNA damage in human spermatozoa. Asian Journal of Androlology 2011; 13; 36–42.

[47] Bansal A.K., Bilaspuri G.S. Impacts of oxidative stress and antioxidants on semen functions. Veterinary Medicine International 2010; doi: 10.4061/2011/686137.

[48] Mora-Esteves C., Shin D. Nutrient supplementation: Improving male fertility fourfold. Seminars in Reproductive Medicine 2013; 31, 293–300.

[49] Lanzafame F.M., La Vignera S., Vicari E., Calogero A.E. Oxidative stress and medical antioxidant treatment in male infertility. Reproductive Biomedicine Online 2009; 19; 638–659.

[50] Griveau J.F., Le Lannou D. Effects of antioxidants on human sperm preparation techniques. International Journal of Andrology 1994; 17; 225–231.

[51] Galecka E., Jacewicz R., Mrowicka M., Florkowski A., Galecki P. Antioxidative enzymes – Structure, properties, functions. Polski Merkuriusz Lekarski 2008; 25; 266–268.

[52] Peeker R., Abramsson L., Marklund S.L. Superoxide dismutase isoenzymes in human seminal plasma and spermatozoa. Molecular Human Reproduction 1997; 3; 1061–1066.

[53] Agarwal A., Nallella K.P., Allamaneni S.S., Said T.M. Role of antioxidants in treatment of male infertility: An overview of the literature. Reproductive Biomedicine Online 2004; 8; 616–627.

[54] Scibior D., Czeczot H. Catalase: Structure, properties, functions. Postepy higieny i medycyny doświadczalne Online 2006; 60; 170–180.

[55] Fraczek M., Kurpisz M. The redox system in human semen and peroxidative damage of spermatozoa. Postepy higieny i medycyny doświadczalne Online 2005; 59: 523–534.

[56] de Lamirande E., Leclerc P., Gagnon C. Capacitation as a regulatory event that primes spermatozoa for the acrosome reaction and fertilization. Molecular Human Reproduction 1997; 3; 175–194.

[57] Pfeifer H., Conrad M., Roethlein D., Kyriakopoulos A., Brielmeier M., Bronkamm G.W. Identification of a specific sperm nuclei selenoenzyme necessary for protamine thiol cross-linking during sperm maturation. FASEB Journal 2001; 15; 1236–1238.

[58] Yeung C.H., Cooper T.G., De Geyter M., De Geyter C., Rolf C., Kamischke A., Nieschlag E. Studies on the origin of redox enzymes in seminal plasma and their relationship with results of in vitro fertilization. Molecular Human Reproduction 1998; 4; 835–839.

[59] Lampiao F. Free radicals generation in an in vitro fertilization setting and how to minimize them. The World Journal of Obstetrics and Gynecology 2012; 1; 29–34.

[60] Sharma R.K., Agarwal A. Role of reactive oxygen species in male infertility. Urology 1996; 48; 835–850.

[61] Sies H. Strategies of antioxidant defense. European Journal of Biochemistry 1993; 215, 213–219.

[62] Lombardo F., Sansone A., Romanelli F., Paoli D., Gandini L., Lenzi A. The role of antioxidant therapy in the treatment of male infertility: An overview. Asian Journal of Andrology 2011; 13, 690–697.

[63] Park S., Park N.Y., Valacchi G., Lim Y. Calorie restriction with a high-fat diet effectively attenuated inflammatory response and oxidative stress-related markers in obese tissues of the high diet fed rats. Mediators of Inflammation 2012; doi: 10.1155/2012/984643.

[64] Tremellen K. Oxidative stress and male infertility – A clinical perspective. Human Reproduction Update 2008; 14; 243–258.

[65] Shang X.J., Li K., Ye Z.Q., Chen Y.G., Yu X., Huang Y.F. Analysis of lipid peroxidative levels in seminal plasma of infertile men by high performance liquid chromatography. Archives of Andrology 2004; 50; 411–416.

[66] Aitken R.J., Harkiss D., Buckingham D. Leukocytic infiltration into the human ejaculate and its association with semen quality, oxidative stress, and sperm function. Journal of Reproduction Fertility 1993; 98; 257–265.

[67] Loft S., Kold-Jensen T., Hjollund N.H. Oxidative DNA damage in human sperm influences time to pregnancy. Human Reproduction 2003; 18; 1265–1272.

[68] Agarwal A., Makker K., Sharma R. Clinical relevance of oxidative stress in male factor infertility: An update. American Journal of Reproductive Immunology 2008; 59; 2–11.

[69] Said T.M., Kattal N., Sharma R.K. Enhanced chemiluminescence assay vs colorimetric assay for measurement of the total antioxidant capacity of human seminal plasma. Journal of Andrology 2003; 24; 676–680.

[70] Ferramosca A., Pinto Provenzano S., Montagna D., Coppola L., Zara V. Oxidative stress negatively affects human sperm mitochondrial respiration. Urology 2013; 82(1); 78–83.

[71] O'Flaherty C.M., Beorlegui N.B., Beconi M.T. Reactive oxygen species requirements for bovine sperm capacitation and acrosome reaction. Theriogenology 1999; 52; 289–301.

[72] Gordon I. Capacitating bovine sperm. In Gordon I (ed.) Laboratory production of cattle embryos (2nd ed.). CABI Publishing, CAB International, Wallingford, 2003; 158–175.

[73] Aitken R.J., Clarkson J.S. Cellular basis of defective sperm function and its association with the genesis of reactive oxygen species by human spermatozoa. Journal of Reproduction and Fertility 1987; 81; 459–469.

[74] Aitken J., Fisher H. Reactive oxygen species generation and human spermatozoa: The balance of benefit and risk. Bioessays 1994; 16; 259–267.

[75] Aitken R.J., Marshall G.J. Human spermatozoa: The future of sex. Nature 2002; 415; 963.

[76] Griveau J.F., Le Lannou D. Reactive oxygen species and human spermatozoa: Physiology and pathology. International Journal of Andrology 1997; 20; 61–69.

[77] Ben Abdallah F., Dammak I., Attia H., Hentati B., Ammar-Keskes L. Lipid peroxidation and antioxidant enzyme activities in fertile men: Correlation with semen parameter. Journal of Clinical Laboratory Animal 2009; 23; 99–104.

[78] Tavilani H., Goodarzi M.T., Vaisi-raygani A., Salimi S., Hassan-Zadeh T. Activity of antioxidant enzymes in seminal plasma and their relationship with lipid peroxidation of spermatozoa. International Brazil Journal of Urology 2008; 34; 485–491.

[79] Ball B.A., Medina V., Gravance C.G., Baumber J. Effect of antioxidants on preservation of motility, viability and acrosomal integrity of equine spermatozoa during storage at 5°C. Theriogenology 2001; 56; 577–589.

[80] Ball B.A., Vo A.T., Baumber J. Generation of reactive oxygen species by equine spermatozoa. American Journal of Veterinary Research 2001; 62; 508–515.

[81] Cocchia N., Pasolini M.P., Mancini R., Petrazzuolo O., Cristofaro I., Rosapane I., Sica A., Tortora G., Lorizio R., Paraggio G., Mancini A. Effect of sod (superoxide dismutase) protein supplementation in semen extenders on motility, viability, acrosome status and ERK (extracellular signal-regulated kinase) protein phosphorylation of chilled stallion spermatozoa. Theriogenology 2011; 75(7); 1201–1210.

[82] Cocchia N., Ciani F., El-Rass R., Russo M., Borzacchiello G., Esposito V., Montagnaro S., Avallone L., Tortora G., Lorizio R. Cryopreservation of feline epididymal spermatozoa from dead and alive animals and its use in assisted reproduction. Zygote 2010; 18(1); 1–8.

[83] LeBlanc M.M., Causey R.C. Clinical and subclinical endometritis in the mare: Both threats to fertility. Reproduction in Domestic Animals 2009; 44(3); 10–22.

[84] Cocchia N., Corteggio A., Altamura G., Tafuri S., Rea S., Rosapane I., Sica A., Landolfi F., Ciani F. Superoxide dismutase (SOD) addition to transport media during storage of cat ovaries 4°C. Reproductive Biology, 2015; 15(1):56-64.

# 4

# Antiluteolytic Strategy for Bovine Embryo Transfer Programmes

Néstor Isaías Tovío Luna, Arturo Duica Amaya and
Henry Alberto Grajales Lombana

**Abstract**

This paper presents a comprehensive review of the problematic issue of embryonic mortality in cattle and develops possible strategies towards a hormonal antiluteolitic. A recent and extensive investigation using eCG is also described.

The paper evaluates the effect of the application of 400 IU of equine Chorionic Gonadotrophin (eCG) on day 5 or 8 of a synchronization protocol for embryo transfer upon follicular development (day 9), luteal development (day 17), progesterone concentration "$P_4$" (9 and 17) and percentage of pregnancy (day 52) in 70 Holstein heifers. The relationships between dominant follicle diameter (DFD) (day 9) and the luteal volume (VL) (day 17), as well as the concentration of P4 (day 17) are analysed without eCG treatments; the DFD (day 9), VL (day 17) and concentration of $P_4$ (day 17) versus percentage of pregnancy (day 52) are then analysed with the treatment. There was no effect ($P > 0.05$) of the day of eCG administration (5 or 8) on the number of dominant follicles, but $P < 0.05$ for diameter. The day of eCG administration (5 or 8) had no effect ($P > 0.05$) on the number of corpora lutea, VL, $P_4$ concentration (9 and 17) or pregnancy (day 52). There was no relationship ($P > 0.05$) between the DFD (day 9) and VL, but $P < 0.05$ between the VL and $P_4$ levels (day 17). In analysing the relationship between treatments (eCG day 5 or 8), the DFD (day 9), VL (day 17) and the concentration of $P_4$ (day 17) versus percentage of pregnancy (day 52), we observed that the only positive correlation ($P < 0.1$) existed between this variable and the concentration of $P_4$.

**Keywords:** eCG, Corpus luteum, Dominant Follicles, Progesterone, Embryo Transfer

## 1. Introduction

About 25-40% of embryonic losses are detected during the first days of pregnancy in female recipients of bovine embryos [1]. It is observed that most of these females return to heat on the expected date after 20-22 days, showing a whole and normal sexual cycle (oestrus cow repeaters) [2]; it is therefore suggested that embryo mortality (EM) might arise between days 7 and 17, the period from embryo transfer (ET) to the maternal recognition of pregnancy (MRP) [3]. As for pregnancy losses occurring between days 28 and 98 (at the occurrence of MRP), percentages ranging between 7% and 33% have been calculated [4].

It has been suggested that during pregnancy establishment there is a well defined "critical period" from day 15 to day 17 [3]; we can suppose that reproductive biology during this period would be multifactorial and complex, where the endometrium receives a non-suitable antiluteolytic signal, of course without blocking prostaglandin $F_{2\alpha}$ ($PGF_2\alpha$) endometrial production, triggering the lysis of the corpus luteum (CL) (maintaining pregnancy depends upon CL functionality) [1]. At that point, antiluteolytic signal is generated by the embryo into mononuclear trophoblast cells, which secrete interferon *tau* (IFN-τ), thereby blocking $PGF_2\alpha$ synthesis produced at endometrial level [5]. The latter process suggests that embryo loss could occur because of a weak or inadequate signal due to an asynchrony between a decreasing progesterone ($P_4$) and the degree of embryo development, so it does not inhibit the synthesis of uterine $PGF_2\alpha$ [6].

The critical nature of the period of recognition, apposition and adhesion of the embryo to uterine endometrium during implantation demands strict synchronization between the transferred embryo and the recipient, emphasizing the importance of both the uterine environment and the embryo signals generating MRP [7] [8]. These signals must be released at the time and concentration required to guarantee CL structure and function maintenance, generating continuous $P_4$ production for embryotrophic environment maintenance to support the normal development of the conceptus (the embryo including all the linked layers) [2].

In relation to the influence of $P_4$ on certain events related to pregnancy maintenance from early stages and the ability of $PGF_2\alpha$ to instigate luteolysis, a number of hormonal strategies to maintain pregnancy have been proposed and developed [9] [10]. These tend to be based on making the $P_4$ secretion capacity of the CL more effective: the secretion should be timely, thus ensuring a proper uterine environment for development of the embryo transplanted to the recipient bovine female. All of this is aimed at increasing the pregnancy rate in ET programmes [2].

According to some reports, the higher the plasma $P_4$ concentration, the better the uterine environment for developing conceptus [11]. It should be noted in this context that any variation of $P_4$ concentration is crucial to modulate expression and secretion of growth factors, cytokines and proteins that affect the uterine environment for endometrial receptivity and embryo viability processes [12].

Consequently, it has been proposed that by providing direct or indirect $P_4$ sources to females during the first days of pregnancy, thus improving the uterine environment to enable the conceptus to develop appropriately, the percentage of embryo loss will be decreased. This leads to better synthesis and more timely secretion of IFN-τ, as long as this secretion is influenced by the embryo development status [13].

## 2. Use of equine Chorionic Gonadotropin (eCG) in bovine embryo transfer programmes

The relationship between pregnancy rate and plasma $P_4$ concentration, according to the CL size in recipients of bovine embryos, has been much debated in the literature. Some researchers have verified a positive correlation between these variables, establishing that the greater the CL area, the greater the plasma $P_4$ concentration, and, subsequently, the higher the pregnancy rate [10] [14]. Other reports, however, have not been able to observe this relationship and effect [15].

Similarly, plasma $P_4$ concentration during dioestrus has been positively correlated to an embryo's ability to secrete IFN-τ, thus triggering increased pregnancy rates [16] [17]. This might suggest that increased $P_4$ concentration during the "critical period" improves the uterine environment for a developing embryo, generating an effective MRP process as it stimulates the secretion of IFN-τ and antiluteolytic agents at the right time by trophoblast cells [18].

One can thus see $P_4$ as a forerunner of the various components making up the embryotrophic environment; therefore, any change in its concentration is critical to modulate expression and secretion of growth factors, cytokines and proteins that affect the uterine environment for endometrial receptivity and embryo viability processes [19]. Accordingly, we may assume that by providing direct or indirect $P_4$ sources to females during the first days of pregnancy, percentage of embryo loss may be decreased due to having an improved uterine environment where the embryo might follow a proper development process (blastocyst stage) with synchronized synthesis and secretion of IFN-τ. This latter is undoubtedly influenced by the status of an embryo's development [13].

In order to increase pregnancy rates, hormone treatments have been used in females included in programmes of fixed-time artificial insemination (TAI) and fixed-time embryo transfer (FTET) using equine chorionic gonadotropin (eCG) [10], [20].

eCG, formerly known as pregnant-mare serum gonadotropin (PMSG) is a glycoprotein hormone with a molecular weight of 45 kDa. It has a three-day span life and is produced by endometrial calyces in pregnant mares from day 40 to day 130 [21]. The hormone is composed of two subunits, $\alpha$- and $\beta$. Subunit $\alpha$ is encoded by a gene common to any glycoprotein; the gene coding for subunit $\beta$ gives the hormone specificity [22].

This hormone binds to FSH and LH follicle recipients as well as LH recipients of CL, thereby creating conditions for follicle growth, ovulation and luteinization [20]. The prevalent action is given by FSH, leading to a formation of accessory corpora lutea, typical for a pregnant mare [23].

eCG application at the expected time of a new wave of follicle growth has been shown to lead to excellent ovulation efficiency (per dosage) and development of a larger-diameter dominant follicle, thus determining a greater number of corpora lutea or a larger corpus luteum [10]. Higher plasma $P_4$ concentrations and a higher rate of conception and pregnancy are seen in comparison to treatments without application of this hormone, both in *Bos taurus* and *Bos indicus* cattle and their crossbreed [24] [11]. However, other researchers have reported no difference between plasma $P_4$ concentration and the number of corpora lutea in pregnant females; in fact, we established higher pregnancy losses in females with double ovulation, suggesting that too much plasma $P_4$ could alter the hormonal uterine balance, damaging the embryotrophic environment for a developing embryo [25].

It has been verified that with eCG application on day 8 (as dominant follicle established), within a synchronization protocol of bovine embryos in recipient females (*Bos indicus/Bos taurus*), one-time larger corpora lutea are achieved in comparison to application of the same hormone on day 5 (as growth of a new follicle wave begins), but no differences have been determined between the treatments in the produced plasma $P_4$ concentration or pregnancy rates [26]. Related reports have confirmed that rate of use (transferred females/synchronized females*100) improves when eCG application occurs on day 8 within a fixed-time embryo transplant protocol with *Bos indicus* recipients [27].

For eCG application on day 8 of synchronization, double ovulation of only 2% has been reported in embryo recipients, but it is evident that application of this hormone can achieve one-time larger corpus lutea, thus increasing the pregnancy rate [13]. Similarly, Quezada and Ortiz [27] established that eCG application on day 8 improves the utilization rate; however, they were unable to establish that the hormone enhances the CL area.

Other hormone strategies have been used in several studies to increase plasma $P_4$: cows and buffaloes have been used for treatments with Gonadotropin-Releasing Hormone (GnRH), Luteinizing Hormone (LH), human Chorionic Gonadotropin (hCG), and $P_4$ slow-release devices [28].

hCG (produced in the trophoblastic syncytium of pregnant women) has been applied to synchronization treatments on day 6, resulting in higher pregnancy rates compared to groups without application of this hormone [29]. These results also suggest that hCG, which has LH action, induces ovulation and formation of accessory corpus luteum (co-dominance), which increases the plasma $P_4$ concentration and pregnancy rate in recipient females of bovine embryos [2].

In addition, eCG has an advantage over other gonadotropins used to support hormone cattle in its stimulation by carbohydrates, especially sialic acid, in relation to subunit alpha, which gives a higher lifespan (see Table 1). This feature, allied to the hormone's molecular weight, makes glomerular filtration harder, thus increasing its lifespan even more [30].

| Hormone | Molecular Weight ng/ml | Carbohydrates (%) | Sialic Acid (%) | Span Life |
|---|---|---|---|---|
| Luteinizing (LH) | 28000 - 34000 | 12 - 24 | 1 - 2 | 30 minutes |
| Stimulating Follicle (FSH) | 32000 - 37000 | 25 | 5 | 2 hours |
| Human Chorionic Gonadotropin (hCG) | 38000 | 32 | 8 -5 | 11 hours |
| Equine Chorionic Gonadotropin (eCG) | 68000 | 48 | 10.4 | 26 hours |

**Table 1.** Features of gonadotropic hormones. Adapted from Knobil and Neill, 2006.

### 2.1. Effect of eCG upon pregnancy rate among recipient heifers of bovine embryos

A study was proposed and developed in order to assess the effect of applying a treatment of equine Chorionic Gonadotropin (eCG) on day 5 or day 8 within a synchronization protocol for a fixed-time embryo transfer (FTET) upon development (number and mm diameter) of dominant follicles on day 9, luteal development (number and volume in $mm^3$) on day 17, plasma $P_4$ concentration (ng/ml) on days 9 and 17, and pregnancy rate (%) on day 52, using 70 Holstein heifers (eCG day 5, n = 42 and eCG day 8, n = 28) as embryo recipients in high tropical areas in Colombia.

To meet the research goal two treatments were proposed in control protocols for the oestrus cycle, where only the eCG application day was changed (day 5 or 8) (Figures 1 & 2).

Regardless of synchronization treatment (eCG day 5 and eCG day 8), we determined $P_4$ profiles for three samples (days 5, 9 and 17) for every heifer in the analysis (n=70). A relationship between volume of corpus luteum and plasma $P_4$ concentration on day 17 (sample 3) was established.

By a logistic function the treatment effects (eCG days 5 and 8) upon follicle diameter (dominant follicle – day 9), total luteal volume (day 17), and $P_4$ concentration (day 17) were determined upon pregnancy diagnosis (day 52).

#### *2.1.1. Number of dominant follicles (day 9)*

This analysis shows that every female used for both treatment 1 (eCG day 5) and treatment 2 (eCG day 8) had at least dominant follicle as a variable with no evident differences (P>0.05) (see Table 2).

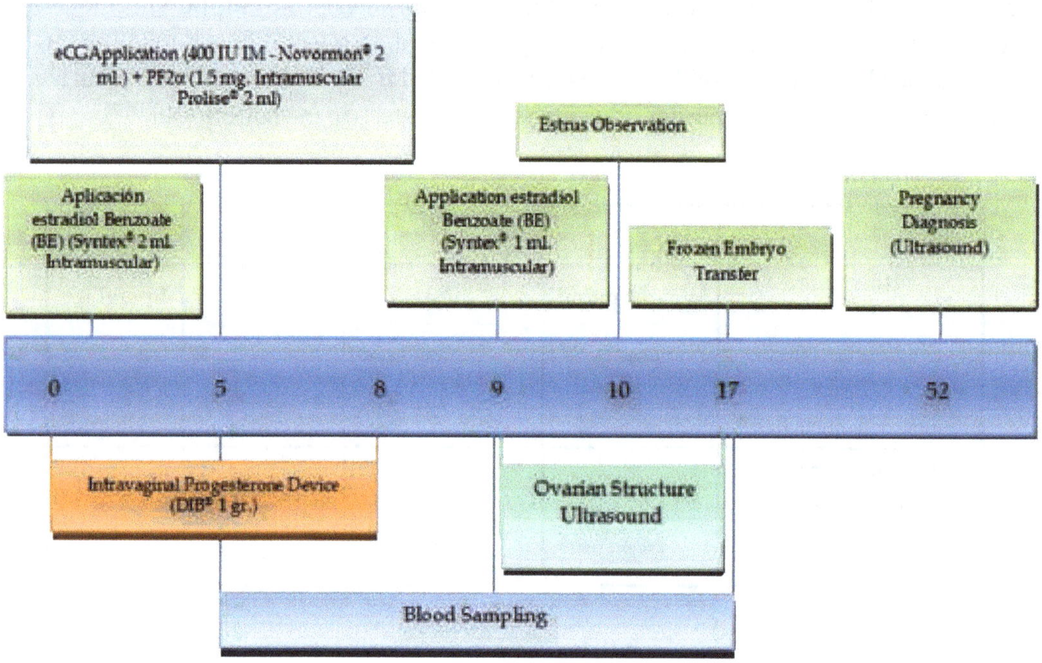


**Figure 1.** Treatment 1: Synchronization protocol of oestrus cycle using eCG application on day 5 (in relation today 1 protocol).

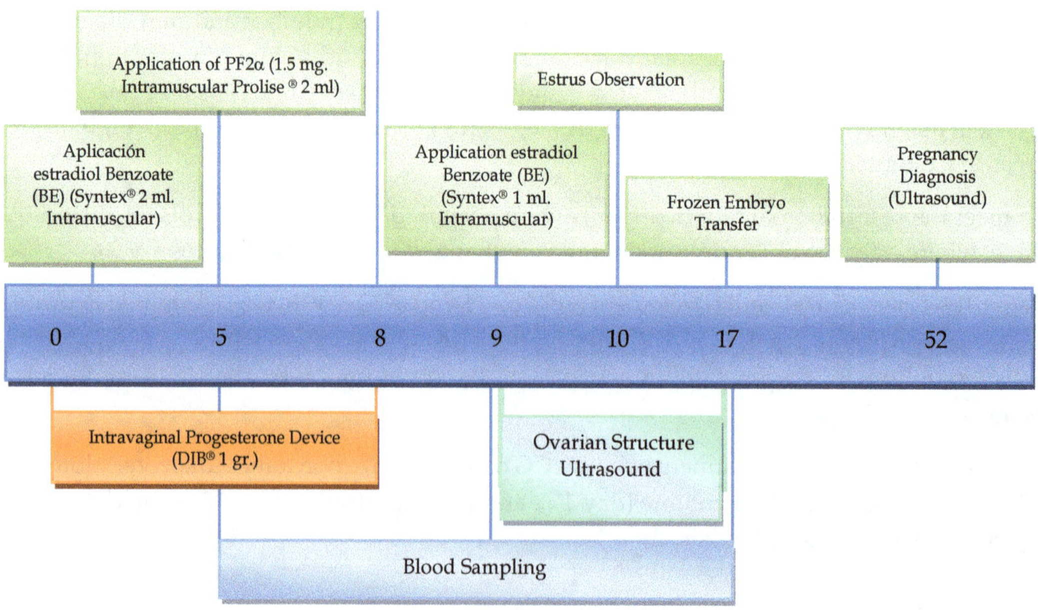


**Figure 2.** Treatment 2: Synchronization protocol of oestrus cycle using eCG application on day 8 (in relation to protocol day 1).

| Treatment | Dominant Follicle (Number) day 9 | | | Diameter (mm) Dominant Follicle day 9 | | |
|---|---|---|---|---|---|---|
| | Min. | Max. | Avrg.[1] | Min. | Max. | Avrg.[1] |
| eCG day 5 (n=42) | 1 | 2 | 1.1 ± 0.3 a | 10 | 19 | 11.7 ± 054 a |
| eCG day 8 (n=28) | 1 | 1 | 1 ± 0 a | 9.2 | 16 | 10.1 ± 0.6 b |
| Total Sample (n=70) | 1 | 2.0 | 1.1 ± 0.2 | 9.2 | 19 | 10.9 ± 0.41 |

**Table 2.** Dominant follicles on sampling day 9. [1]Results of follicle diameter are expressed as an average (mean) ± Standard error of the mean (SEM) while follicle values are expressed as an average ± Standard Deviation (SD).

This result differs from previous studies where addition of eCG on day 5 in a synchronization protocol for the oestrus cycle caused a reflection cascade at molecular level, triggering development of more than one dominant follicle [31]. Since these control oestrus cycle treatments, where a follicle wave growth using $P_4$-and-oestradiol implant is synchronized (as in this work), the emergence of a new follicle wave occurs after four to five days, an effect perhaps caused by blood hormone levels required to provoke a negative feedback. This affects the synthesis and secretion of gonadotropin-releasing hormone (LH) and alters the normal follicle development, which suggests a leading regression of growing follicles (FSH-dependent) and hinders progress of the phenomenon of dominant follicle ovulation (LH-dependent), generating a regression and starting a new follicle wave [32].

When eCG is applied on day 5, the follicle wave is at a very early stage of development; consequently, the eCG could lead to stimulation in recruitment and selection of more than one dominant follicle with increasing mRNA synthesis coded for gonadotropic hormone recipients (FSH and LH) at theca-and-granulosa cell level [10]. This effect in this study was only observed in four of 42 heifers (9.5%).

In relation to the above, Nasser et al. [26] applied 400 IU of eCG to two groups of Nellore/ Angus -crossbreed recipient heifers (eCG day 5 versus eCG day 8) of 22-30 months in age; this was supplemented with 2 kg/day concentrate, establishing differences (P<0.05) according to the number of dominant follicles on day 8, with a higher number of follicles applied on day 5 (start of a new wave of follicle growth), thus demonstrating the follicle-stimulating action of eCG. The hormone stimulates the mRNA synthesis encoded for FSH follicle recipients in developing follicles [33]; therefore, more than one follicle is chosen because there are no dominant follicles at that time (day 5 of application in relation to the start of the control protocol of the oestrus cycle) that could inhibit other developing follicles. For eCG applied on day 8 (follicle dominance established) only one dominant follicle stimulation (eCG linking FSH and LH follicle recipients) was observed [34]; statistical differences were observed in that work.

On the other hand, since there are no statistical differences of this variable in our analysis one might acknowledge the species factor, where there are differences regarding hormone sensitivity [31], which differentiates *Bos indicus* and relevant crossbreeds, which are more sensitive than *Bos taurus* [35]. Taking this into account, one might infer that concentrations of

400 IU of eCG will trigger a different effect on both species; however, such sensitivity was not noticeable in this study, where we worked with *Bos taurus* heifers. Therefore we might conclude it is possible to work with different dosages according to the above factors since dosages of 400 IU of eCG, as used in this research, may be less likely to stimulate the growth of a large number of follicles dosages used in other studies of this subject, which have used 1000 IU [36] and 800 IU [37], and have used both heifers and cows, which could dramatically influence results [38].

When eCG treatment is provided on day 8, follicle dominance may already be established [37] and may only generate stimulation of the dominant follicle (in some cases, the largest subordinate follicle) [31]. In this study, evidence of a dominant follicle was found only for the group of heifers on treatment 2 (eCG day 8), maximum one (1) and minimum one (1), so one might infer the stimulus to this single dominant follicle (see Table 2).

*2.1.2. Dominant follicle diameter, day 9*

All used heifers (treatment 1 – eCG day 5; treatment 2 – eCG day 8 had at least one dominant follicle (follicle ≥ 9 mm). Accordingly, differences were established ($P<0.05$) between both treatments, e.g., a higher follicular diameter for eCG day 5 (treatment 1) (see Table 2). Some researchers working with the same type reported higher values. Sousa et al. [24] applied 400 IU of eCG on day 8 to a group of Holstein cows (in relation to starting day of synchronization), and established a dominant follicle size of 14.7 ± 0.6 mm, compared to 13.1 ± 0.6 mm in cows without eCG. Using Holstein heifers and lactating cows, Sartori et al. [35] established an ovulatory follicle size of 14.9 ± 0.2 mm for heifers, and 16.8 ± 0.5 mm for cows. (Animals with this CL were not treated with any hormone; GnRH was given to others.)

Other studies have applied $PGF_2\alpha$ with an 11-day interval. Lynch et al. [39] used crossbred *Bos taurus* cows, synchronized with application of two dosages of PF2$\alpha$ (an 11-day interval), establishing pre-ovulatory follicles of diameter 14.1 ± 1.9 mm. Thus, based on the results of different studies one might suggest elements such as treatments or dosages used, development stages (heifers, cows), number of births, and so on, may somehow explain the different effects established [40].

Nutrition factors may somehow influence follicular dynamics of heifers [41]. One may suppose that the heifers used in this study were grazing without any additional supplement to guarantee total coverage of their physiological needs; therefore, there might be an imbalance that would generate an initial effect at the hypothalamus, and subsequently the anterior pituitary (adenohypophysis), which affects synthesis and secretion of gonadotropic hormones, and follicle growth and development could be affected [40].

Furthermore, it should be noted that follicle measurements were made on the morning of day 9 in this work (before application of oestradiol benzoate); then, each heifer was given 1 ml (5 mg) of oestradiol benzoate in order to stimulate synthesis and secretion of FSH and LH to facilitate both the final follicle development and ovulation [10]. Therefore, we can suppose that the final development stage of the pre-ovulatory follicle is not yet completed where action by gonadotropic hormones increases final diameter, and follicle diameter averages may be lower compared to the results of most studies cited, where measurements were performed at the time of maximum follicle development (day 9 in the afternoon) [35] [42].

In relation to the effect ($P<0.05$) with treatment 1 (eCG day 5 – starting day of synchronized cycle follicle wave) given by this study, eCG seems to trigger an outbreak of event cascade at molecular level, resulting in a further development of dominant follicle [31]. Here we must take into account of course that eCG stimulates the mRNA formation encoding FSH and LH recipients, whose stimulation increases as the follicle is at a very early stage of dominance. During this period eCG continues to operate with a three-day lifespan [43], which virtually guarantees its action during the time that the follicle is becoming dominant, and allows an increased density of FSH and LH recipients, which is associated to follicle growth [44]. On the other hand, compared with heifers of treatment group 2 (eCG day 8), whose application was made with follicle dominance practically established, the stimulating effect of eCG would be very short.

Table 3 shows the results of variables corpus luteum (number) and luteal volume ($mm^3$) on day 17, plasma $P_4$ concentration (ng/ml) on days 9 and 17, and percentage pregnancy (%) on day 52, with a comparison between treatments (eCG day 5 versus eCG day 8). Analysis and discussion of variables by luteal volume on day 17, $P_4$ concentration on day 17, and pregnancy rate on day 52 (see Table 3) are provided to analyse thoroughly the variable pregnancy rate for a greater understanding of studies related that deal with these three variables together.

| Treatment | Corpus Luteum (Number) Day 17 | | | Luteal Volume ($mm^3$) day 17 | | | Progesterone Concentration (ng/ml) | | | | | | Pregnancy (%) Day 52 |
|---|---|---|---|---|---|---|---|---|---|---|---|---|---|
| | | | | | | | Day 9 | | | Day 17 | | | |
| | Min. | Max. | Avg[1] | Min. | Max. | Avg[1] | Min. | Max. | Avg[1] | Min. | Max. | Avg[1] | |
| eCG day 5 (n=42) | 1 | 2 | 1.1 ± 0.3 a | 375 | 16443.6 | 5023.6 ± 512.4 a | 0 | 0.84 | 0.28 ± 0.03 b | 1.98 | 10.1 | 5.12 ± 0.31 a | 69 (29/42) a |
| eCG day 8 (n=28) | 1 | 1 | 1 ± 0 a | 1150.35 | 18057.3 | 5554.9 ± 758.6 a | 0 | 0.86 | 0.33 ± 0.05 b | 2 | 9.6 | 5.52 ± 0.30 a | 64 (18/28) a |
| Total Sample (n=70) | 1 | 2 | 1.1 ± 0.2 | 375.4 | 18057.3 | 5236.1 ± 429.7 | 0 | 0.9 | 0.3 ± 0.03 | 2 | 10 | 5.2 ± 0.22 | 67 (47/70) |

**Table 3.** Performance of luteal structures, progesterone concentration and pregnancy rate. [1]Results by luteal volume and progesterone concentration are expressed as average (mean) ± SEM while other values are expressed as mean ±DS.

### 2.1.3. *Corpus luteum (Amount)*

All heifers (70/70) of two experimental groups in this research (42 heifers of treatment 1 –eCG on day 5; 28 heifers of treatment 2 – eCG day 8) had at least one functional corpus luteum consolidated on day 17 (dioestrus stage) with application of control protocols of oestrus cycle proposed (see Table 3); therefore we can suppose that all heifers ovulated, taking into account of course that all of them had at least one dominant follicle on day 9 (see Table 2).

According to the average of this variable there was no difference ($P>0.05$) between treatments used (Table 3); there were parallels regarding average dominant follicles evidenced (Table 2) during the experiment.

A similar study by Nasser et al. [26] accounted for significant differences between both treatments used (eCG on day 5 or day 8), which provided 400 IU of such a hormone to Nellore/Angus-crossbreed recipients, synchronized for fixed-time embryo transfer, where 1.44 ± 0.18 corpora lutea were obtained (eCG day 5) compared to 1.03 ± 0.03 corpora lutea (eCG day 8), using more sensitive animals in relation to hormone dosages used (*Bos indicus* breed). However, established values in that analysis when eCG was applied on day 8 are similar to this report, maybe due to similar synchronization treatments used.

In a study by Baruselli et al. [37], which used a control treatment (no eCG), statistical differences were evidenced in recipients of Zebu-cross embryos, which were given 800 IU of eCG (day 5 in relation to start of synchronized cycle – growth of a new follicle wave). This study reports 2.58 ± 2.93 corpora lutea in animals with eCG, but 0.5 ± 0.5 corpora lutea in animals without eCG. This finding may demonstrate a super-ovulatory action of eCG following a dosage of 800 IU, given on starting-growth day of the follicle wave. Such a super-ovulatory effect has also been seen in other experiments conducted by Fuentes and De la Fuente [36], who worked with Holstein heifers applying 1000 IU of eCG on day 5 (in relation to treatment start). That study reveals that the hormone significantly increased the number of corpora lutea (between two and five structures for each ovary at the transfer time). Following the variable in several studies, these results could also be indicating different actions of eCG according to dosage used, breed type, and development status of the animal (cow or heifer), which could influence the results for number of follicles (see explanation above) [35].

#### 2.1.4. Luteal volume

For this variable there was no difference (P>0.05) between treatment groups (see Table 3). This highlights a synchrony due to evidence of luteal structures established on day 17, so it is evident that 100% of heifers in both treatments (treatment 1 – eCG day 5, 42/42; eCG day 8, 28/28) had at least one consolidated luteal structure. For a better understanding of the results, a discussion related to luteal volume on day 17, $P_4$ concentration on day 17 and pregnancy rate is carried out to analyse the variables by pregnancy rate.

#### 2.1.5. Progesterone concentrations

It should be clear that the first day of sampling (day 5) certainly could not have any effect of treatment using eCG for this variable, because at the time of sampling the hormone was not applied to treatment group 1 (eCG day 5); in treatment group 2 eCG was only applied on day 8. However, the behaviour of $P_4$ concentration on day 5 is shown in Figures 4 & 5) in order to analyse trends among groups of heifers. Figure 4 shows ranges between minimum and maximum values, which can be associated to data scattering caused by an irregularity of oestrus-cycle phases, where heifers of the experimental group were subjected to synchronization treatments. This group showed a significant percentage with corpora lutea starting treatments, which might support reports in the literature whereby approximately 40 or 50% of a group of reproductive fit females had luteal structures after carrying out a reproductive examination [44]. Therefore in this analysis we expected a significant percentage of heifers showing $P_4$ levels higher than 1ng/ml (Figure. 4). It should be noted that a slow release device of $P_4$, applied on day 0 of the control protocol for the oestrus cycle, expedited somehow a concentration (residual) of this hormone [45], evident during the first sampling (day 5). In relation to a $P_4$ concentration on day 9, there was no difference (P> 0.05) among treatments assessed (see Table 3).

It should be noted that on day 5, to start the synchronization protocol, prostaglandin F2$\alpha$ was applied, which triggered a functional and structure regression of any corpus luteum [46]. Therefore, performing an ovarian ultrasound examination during day 9 (sample 2), we did not find any structure consistent with corpora lutea, which was confirmed by observing plasma $P_4$ concentration of heifer groups afterwards. In the absence of luteal structures we could suppose that on day 9 blood $P_4$ (a synchronized cycle) levels should be very close to basal levels, ≤0.3 ng/ml [2].

These basal $P_4$ concentrations (Figure 3) concur with those reported by authors such as Kastelic et al. [47], who worked with a group of Holstein heifers, and related measures of corpus luteum with plasma $P_4$ concentration, resulting on day 9 in a maximum decrease in levels ≤ 0.3 ng/ml. Perry et al. [48], studying a group of crossbred cows with beef characteristics and a hormone therapy applied to synchronize the oestrus cycle (GnRH, $PGF_2\alpha$, GnRH) reported $P_4$ concentration values of 0.2 ng/ml, both in groups of pregnant females and in non-pregnant ones. Similar values were reported by Chagas et al. [49], working with Holstein heifer recipients of embryos, which were not subject to a control treatment of oestrus cycle (embryo transfer with observed heat), 0.21 ± 0.01 ng/ml.

These results by several authors seem consistent to the data of this study, since there are numerical trends which allow us to observe that on the day of maximum follicle development, plasma $P_4$ levels dropped to baseline. This is associated to application of prostaglandin F2$\alpha$ (day 5 of a synchronized cycle), which favours a dramatic reduction of blood flow to the ovary, triggering a cascade of luteolytic mechanisms [50]. Therefore, on day 9 we would expect to find a corpus albicans at ovarian level and therefore $P_4$ baseline [51]. In this study, $PGF_2\alpha$ had a luteolytic effect on both groups of treated females; there were thus no statistical differences in relation to $P_4$ concentration (day 9). As for $P_4$ concentration on day 17, there were no differences (P>0.05) between treatments assessed (see Table 3).

As could be expected at ovary level during third sampling, there is at least one functional and developed corpus luteum whose plasma $P_4$ levels had a tendency to be spread (Figure 4), which is consistent with the difference between sizes of luteal structures shown.

Figure 3 shows an estimated function by regression analysis, which was significant (P<0.05) for a relationship between CL volume and plasma $P_4$ concentration on day 17 (sample 3), regardless of treatments of eCG used (eCG day 5 and eCG day 8) on any heifer used during this work (n=70). Analysis shows a positive correlation between these two variables, indicating that an increased CL volume involves a $P_4$ concentration; therefore a greater $P_4$ involves a greater luteal volume which produced it. Probably, catkins is a possibility to adapt a better embryotrophic environment needed for embryos to be synchronously developed and send signals for maternal recognition, which could possibly trigger higher pregnancy rates [52].

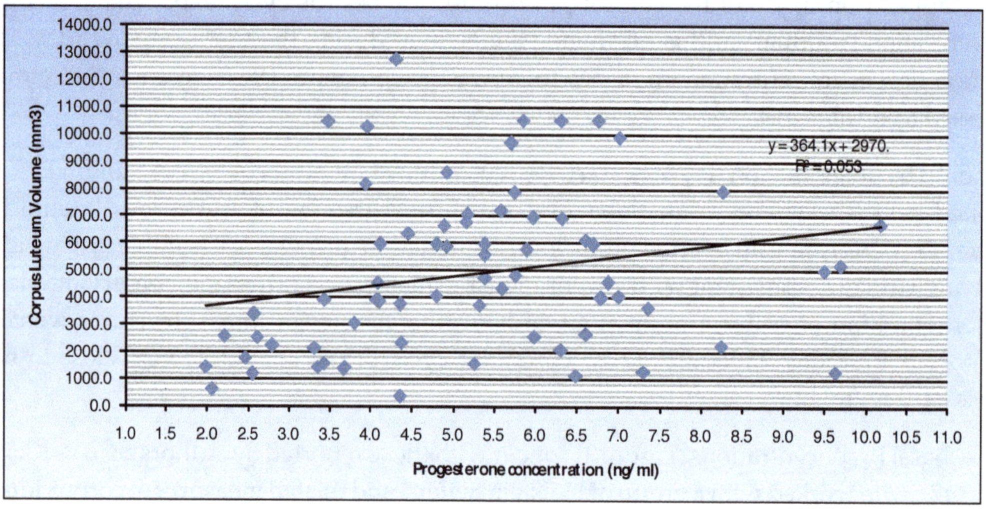


**Figure 3.** Estimated relationship of progesterone concentration (ng/ml) as a function of a luteal volume (day 17).

According to the above, Spain et al. [53] established a correlation (P<0.001) between plasma $P_4$ concentration and a luteal area of Holstein cows. The authors proposed that luteal area may be associated to plasma $P_4$ levels and this, in turn, to a pregnancy diagnosis. Sartori et al. [54] working with lactating cows, dry cows and Holstein heifers, gave them $PGF_2\alpha$ on day 7 of the oestrus cycle, also establishing a correlation between luteal volume and plasma $P_4$ concentration. Likewise, Rodriguez et al. [55] in an analysis conducted in the central and low Colombian tropical areas, using several species and crossbreeds, reported a positive correlation between both variables. This also coincides with a report by Duica [44], who worked with embryo recipients, Holstein heifers to which eCG was applied on day 5 (in relation to the synchronized cycle). Other studies have related the corpus luteum weight to the plasma $P_4$ concentration. In this regard, authors such as Mann, [17] using multiparous Holstein cows, established on day 5 (in relation to heat) a strong relationship between the corpus luteum weight and plasma $P_4$ concentration. However, this relationship was not present on day 8 (in relation to heat), unlike in our work.

Other studies have established a variation of this correlation, and authors such as Howell et al. [56] report a seasonal variation. Other authors have also shown a positive correlation between the total CL area and $P_4$ in dairy [57]. However, others have observed insufficient correlation coefficients between these two variables [58] [59].

According to the results presented in several works, authors such as Kastelic et al. [60] suggest that assessment by ultrasonography of corpora lutea becomes a viable alternative to establish $P_4$ concentration for an assessment of a luteal function of Holstein heifers.

In relation to variations reported in some analysis one might say that the amount of luteal tissue formed by small and large luteal cells producing $P_4$ is related to a concentration of the hormone in plasma; however, CLs are not always functional, since the probable cell alterations mentioned or modifications of some inner components may alter their secretion [44]. It should also be noted that correlation between plasma $P_4$ and luteal area is not constant throughout the oestrus cycle [61]; therefore, during luteal regression phase this index will lose relevance. This has not been reported here because there was indeed a correlation on sampling day 3 (day 17 in relation to the start of treatment synchronization – embryo transfer): a luteal volume of one or more functional CL(s) was detected in all heifers post-ovulating. Other studies have reported similarly on this topic [62] [44].

Figure 4 shows the performance curve by $P_4$ concentration established for three samples conducted with total heifers (n=70) (sample 1 – day 5; sample 2 – day 9; sample 3 – day 17).

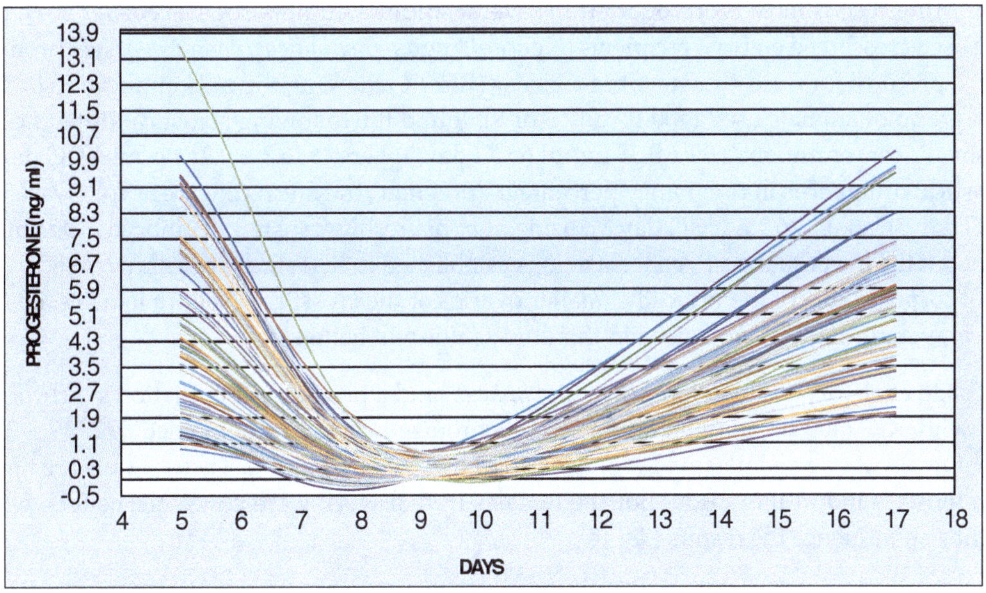


**Figure 4.** Progesterone performance during three samples taken with total heifers (n=70)

In Figure 4, we can infer that the $P_4$ level on day 5 is caused by functional corpora lutea before application of $PGF_2\alpha$, since 98.6% (69/70) of total heifers of this study had ≥1 ng/ml $P_4$ concentration during first sampling (day 5). We might also argue there is a residual effect caused by slow-release implants of $P_4$ on the first sampling day (day 5). Considering that prostaglandin F2$\alpha$ was applied on day 5, immediately after sample 1, the curve (sample 2 – day 9) shows decreasing $P_4$ levels due to a functional and structural luteolysis caused by a luteolytic factor by prostaglandin [46], allowing follicle development and dominance [29]. Figure 4 also shows a behaviour pattern of dispersion in the data range at the beginning and end (days 5 and 17), taking into account the above explanation in relation to possible corpora lutea established at the beginning of the control protocol of oestrus cycle (day zero) and synchronization of wave growth achieved on day 5 [45]. Additionally, controlled ovulation allowed a generation of corpora lutea on day 17 (sample 3), which differed in volume (5236.1 ± 429.7) and was reflected at the end of the curve according to several $P_4$ concentrations established (>1 ng/ml.).

### 2.1.6. Pregnancy rate

In relation to pregnancy percentage there are no differences (P>0.05) between treatments (see Table 3), which is consistent with behaviour established between both variables discussed (luteal volume and plasma $P_4$ concentration). Therefore, the hypothesis *"The day of application of equine Chorionic Gonadotropin (eCG) determines a luteal development, a progesterone concentration, and a pregnancy rate to recipient females of bovine embryos"* is not entirely supported statistically. One might note that the heifers undergoing treatment 1 (eCG day 5) showed 5% more pregnancy than heifers undergoing treatment 2 (eCG day 8), but we cannot legitimately adopt a conclusion.

Conflicting results have been reported in several studies. Authors such as Nasser et al. [26], who used crossbreed embryo recipients (Nellore/Angus – *Bos indicus/Bos taurus*), synchronized with a protocol for fixed-time embryo transfer (FTET), changing the eCG application day for each group of animals used (400 IU day 5 or 8), found the following statistical differences of plasma $P_4$ concentration: 2.69 ± 0.38 ng/ml (eCG day 5) versus 1.63 ± 0.21 ng/ml (eCG day 8). Statistical differences in pregnancy percentage (pregnant/transferred) were as follows: 63.4% (eCG day 5) versus 36.1% (eCG day 8), using *in vitro*, freshly transferred embryos. One might point out the lower plasma $P_4$ concentrations established in that study, possibly caused by the small corpora lutea of the typically smaller ovaries of the crossbred Nellore females, i.e., *Bos indicus*, versus the *Bos taurus* used in this study (Holstein heifers).

Machado et al. [62] used Nellore cows (*Bos indicus*) and a protocol for ovulation synchronization with eCG (400 IU) applied on day 9 (synchronized cycle), and obtained 6927.49 ± 05.86 $mm^3$ luteal volume and plasma $P_4$ concentration of 8.15 ± 0.64 ng/ml. These results are higher than those found in this study, but the females in that work were cows, not heifers, which might also influence the results [38].

A plasma $P_4$ concentration higher than that reported here has also been observed in other studies conducted by Marques et al. [63], who set out to analyse the effects of eCG applied at the time of implant removal with $P_4$ in Brangus cows, and reported statistical differences of 8.6 ± 0.4 ng/ml in cows with eCG compared to 6.4 ng/ml in cows without eCG, confirming the previous evidence by Baruselli et al. [37], who synchronized crossbred embryo recipients by applying 800 IU of eCG on day 5, in relation to a synchronized cycle (growth of a new follicle wave), establishing that any eCG application generates larger corpora lutea (>13 mm) on the day of embryo transplant (84% of animals) and a pregnancy rate of 42% (with eCG) versus 34% (without eCG). These results show luteal development may be appropriate when eCG is applied; $P_4$ synthesis could thus be increased, aiding embryonic development. The period of maternal recognition of pregnancy might benefit. This is evident in the pregnancy rates found in previous studies [26] [64].

There may also be discrepancies here with the results of other researchers. For example, Siqueira et al. [65] established no significant differences with crossbred cows (*Bos Taurus/Bos indicus*) when applying eCG on day 5 (in relation to start of protocol). In that study, $P_4$ concentration values reported on day 17 (in relation to a synchronized cycle) were 5.2 ± 5.0 ng/ml; the luteal area was 72.4 ± 12.0 $cm^2$ in pregnant cows and 71.4 ± 11.3 $cm^2$ in cows that were no pregnant. It can be observed that the obtained $P_4$ concentration values were very similar to those obtained in this work – contrary to what we might expect, since one might assume that the ovarian structures and $P_4$ concentration of crossbred cows (*Bos indicus/Bos taurus*) would be smaller than those established in our work, i.e., 5.12 ± 0.31 ng/ml, using pure *Bos taurus* females (Holstein heifers). Heifers' structures may be smaller than those in cow females [62].

Working with *Bos indicus* cows, but with no embryo transfer programme or hormone treatments, Aguirre et al. [66] reported 45% pregnancy, a rate similar to other studies, such as that by Fuentes and De la Fuente [36], who used Holstein heifers treated hormonally (1000 IU eCG on day 5 in relation to the treatment start), and reported pregnancy rates with frozen embryos in glycerol of 54%, ethylene glycol 48%, and fresh 52% (no statistical differences). Rodrigues et al. [67], working with recipient cows of Nellore embryos, reported pregnancy rates of 56% (including eCG) compared to 37.8% (not including eCG); these rates are higher than those reported by Pita et al. [68] working with Zebu crossbred heifers, who found rates of 44% with frozen embryos using eCG on day 5 of the protocol, and 30% using eCG on day 8 of the protocol. These figures are lower than those reported by Peixoto et al. [69] using recipient crossbred Zebu and Holstein heifers (*Bos indicus/Bos taurus*), where eCG was not applied in synchronization treatment – 63.7%, a similar percentage to that obtained here. Other approaches have verified a range of figures for corpora lutea related to pregnancy rate. Siqueira et al. [65] using a synchronization treatment for fixed-time embryo transfer (FTET) on crossbred recipients (*Bos taurus taurus/Bos taurus indicus*) with fresh embryos (eCG applied on day 5 in relation to the protocol start), established a pregnancy rate of 42.9% (in recipients with a single corpus luteum) versus 61.9% (recipients with multiple corpora lutea). They concluded that higher luteal tissue was accompanied by a higher $P_4$ synthesis, and accordingly a higher pregnancy rate, but this effect was not demonstrated in our study.

There are several related studies. Their results are mostly contradictory in relation to the argument that the higher the luteal volume or area, the higher the synthesized plasma $P_4$ concentration, and the higher pregnancy rates [70] [71]. Studies have used different protocols, and some have applied equine Chorionic Gonadotropin (eCG) as hormonal support. In this research, when eCG was provided on day 5 we were trying a follicle recruitment and selection [72] which allows the stimulation of more than one follicle, culminating in multiple ovulation and, in turn, generating greater luteal tissue [73]. This would synthesize a higher $P_4$ concentration [10] and lead to a better embryotrophic environment [19] where embryonic development would be appropriate, favouring the maternal recognition of pregnancy. On the other hand, treatment with eCG applied on day 8, when the follicle domain is established, seeking a greater stimulation of dominant follicles (in some cases the largest subordinate follicle) generates a greater luteal tissue, a greater plasma $P_4$ concentration, and a higher pregnancy rate [73]. Accordingly, one can say that treatment 1 (eCG day 5) and treatment 2 (eCG day 8) are beneficial for pregnancy rates, taking into account the results cited. This result could stem from increased plasma $P_4$ concentration caused by eCG [51], which may have stimulated embryo growth and optimized synchronization and secretion of IFN-τ; therefore, maternal recognition of pregnancy happened at appropriate times [74]. This may have been produced by a luteotrophic action caused by applying 400 IU of eCG [10].

Since there are no differences (P>0.05) between treatments (eCG day 5 vs. eCG day 8) in this research in terms of variables analysed in Table 3 (luteal volume day 17, $P_4$ concentration day 17, pregnancy rate day 52), one might speculate on probable factors which could play an important role during performance of treatments applied in the studies cited. These might include dietary factors among others, which undoubtedly affect physiological reproductive performance [40]. We should also take into account the species factor, by which there are differences in hormone sensitivity [75]. Thus, one might infer that concentrations of 400 IU of eCG will trigger different effects in *indicus*, *taurus* and their crossbreeds [38].

Figure 5 shows an overall average $P_4$ performance for all heifers used in the study with three samples (days 5, 9 and 17). This behaviour is evidenced by the reproductive status of heifers (pregnant or not pregnant), where we can observe significantly higher concentrations during the third sampling (day 17), compared to pregnant heifers – an average of 40.6% (1.585 ng/ml) more plasma $P_4$.

In relation to these concentrations, Siqueira et al. [65] used a synchronization treatment for fixed-time embryo transfer (FTET), which used eCG applied on day 5 (in relation to protocol start) in crossbred recipients (*Bos taurus taurus/Bos taurus indicus*). On day of transfer (day 17 related to a synchronized cycle) a $P_4$ concentration of 5.2 ± 5.0 ng/ml in pregnant heifers was established, compared to 3.8 ± 2.4 ng/ml for non-pregnant heifers; these results are similar to those found in our research.

Other works, in which eCG has not been used, as in the study of Chagas et al. [49] who worked with recipient Holstein cows and heifers which were transferred embryos at standing heat, established a $P_4$ concentration on day 0 (day of maximum follicle development) for pregnant females of 0.22 ± 0.01 ng/ml, and for non-pregnant females of 0.21 ± 0.02 ng/ml, values similar to our research. On transfer day (day 17 of this study) these authors established o2.92 ± 0.08 ng/ml for recipient pregnant females versus 2.88 ± 0.08 ng/ml for non-pregnant females. These values are lower than those found in our study, where eCG seems to favour a luteinizing process, influencing $P_4$ synthesis and release [76].

Another study, by Lopes et al. [14], who used Holstein cows synchronized to Ovsynch, established a $P_4$ concentration on day of artificial insemination of 0.19 ± 0.01 ng/ml in pregnant cows and 0.24 ± 0.02 ng/ml in non-pregnant ones, suggesting this hormone could be affecting fertility even at these low concentrations. Moreira et al. [77] suggests low pregnancy rates for cows with an inadequate corpus luteum regression after an injection of $PGF_2\alpha$. This is because $P_4$ concentrations may cause incomplete maturation of pre-ovulatory follicles due to low LH circulating levels (alteration in mode of release), which compromises the follicle ovulation with sensitization of follicle cells changing to luteal status, altering the oocyte release. There could also be a change in $P_4$ secretion, changing the uterine environment so that it may no longer be appropriate for embryonic development; thus the concentration of IFN-$\tau$ may not be suitable at the time of the "critical period" to generate an effective signal of maternal recognition of pregnancy due to the asynchrony given in its growth.

As discussed above, our analysis shows that prostaglandin applied on day 5 (in relation to the synchronized cycle) seems to have been effective in all heifers (eCG treatment 1, day 5, and

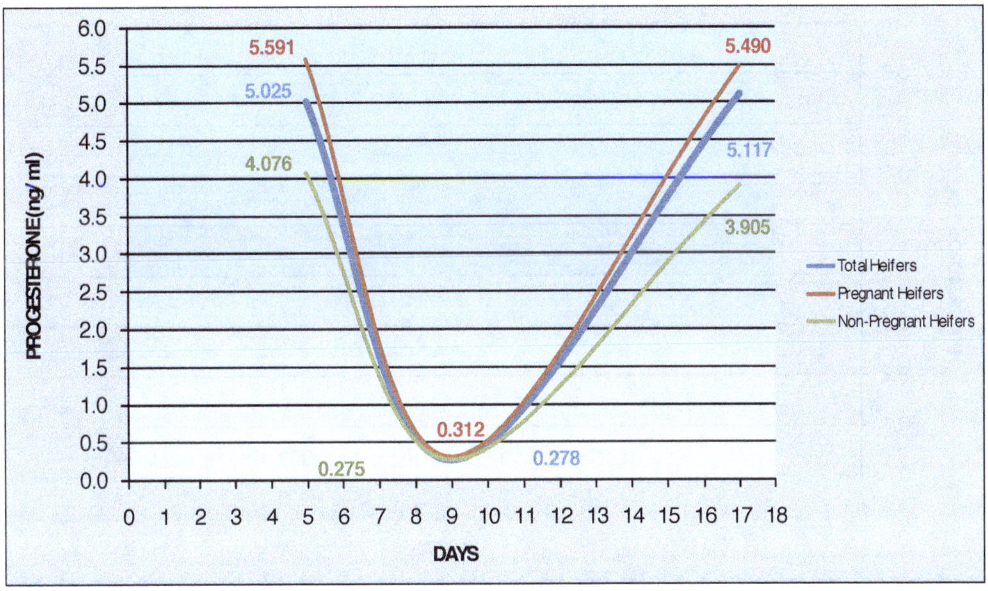


**Figure 5.** Progesterone levels in relation to reproductive status.

eCG treatment 2, day 8), since there was no evidence of luteal structures on the day of sample 2 (day 9 – maximum follicle development). Therefore, one might assume there was a pre-ovulatory LH peak, taking into account of course the measurable concentration of $P_4$ on that day (day 9); one might also assume that this came from a luteinizing process during a dominance period of the ovulatory follicle [2] or a residual status of the $P_4$ implant used [32], for example. In conclusion, $P_4$ may directly affect LH synthesis and release [78], which is evident from Figure 6.

Moreover, in some cases plasma $P_4$ concentration on day of embryo transfer (day 17) was higher (numerically) in successfully pregnant females compared to those not pregnant (Figure 5). In this context, Duica [44] has shown a potential impact upon recipient Holstein heifers treated with eCG on day 5 (in relation to treatment synchronization start), establishing differences ($P<0.05$) between pregnant and non-pregnant females, which might somewhere involve appropriate support in the uterine environment provided by $P_4$ to the embryos transferred, which are efficient in IFN-τ synthesis and secretion throughout their development [19], aiding maternal recognition of pregnancy [18].

Figure 6 shows $P_4$ concentration on day 9 of 33% (23/70) in successfully pregnant heifers. It is evident that 17% (4/23) of these heifers showed $P_4$ concentration lower than 0.1 ng/ml. In contrast, 83% (19/23) of heifers had a $P_4$ concentration higher than 0.1 ng/ml.

Of the 23 heifers that did not successfully become pregnant, 57% (13/23) belonged to treatment group 1 (eCG day 5) and 43% (10/23) to treatment group 2 (eCG day 8). Of those in group 1 (eCG day 5) on day 9, 15% (2/13) showed decreased $P_4$ concentration at values lower than 0.1 ng/ml, while 85% reported higher concentrations. Of those in group 2 (eCG day 8) on day 9,

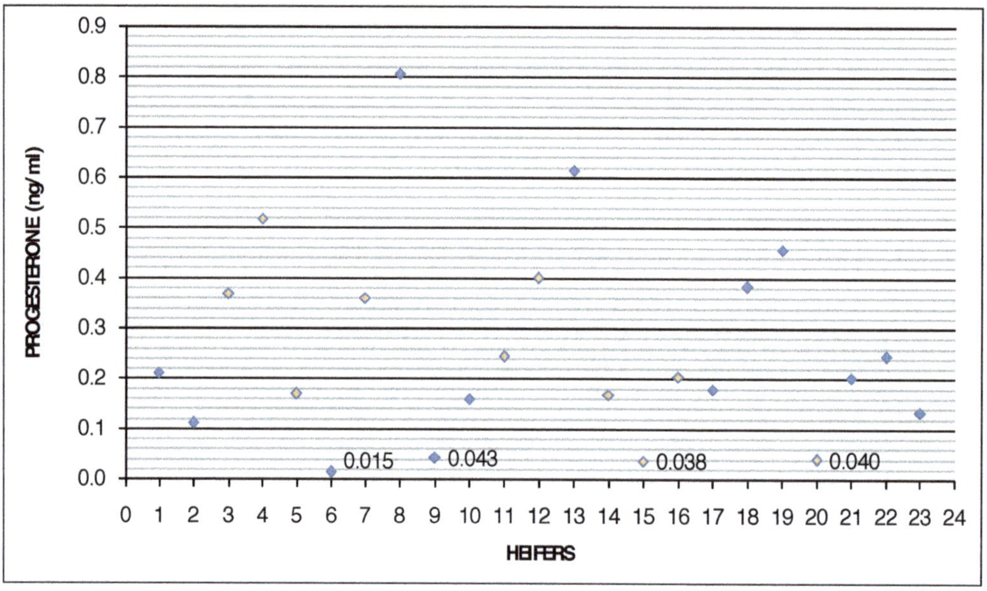


**Figure 6.** Progesterone concentration – non-pregnant heifers (sample 2 - day 9).

20% (2/10) showed decreased $P_4$ concentration at values lower than 0.1 ng/ml, while 80% reported higher concentrations.

Based on these results, we can suppose that a stronger decrease of $P_4$ on the day of maximum follicle development (sample 2 – day 9) to minimum levels should improve pregnancy rates. This is because the expected LH peak may occur without difficulty with subsequent, appropriate luteinization and ovulation [79]; cows that present supra-basal $P_4$ levels may not become fertilized. Additionally, this may affect ovulatory follicle luteinization, and thus the life structuring or programming of the corpus luteum and $P_4$ synthesis. Finally, it should be noted that the uterus might also be damaged – there is evidence of imbalance between the steroid hormones $P_4$ and oestradiol, for example [80].

Figure 7 shows logistic function according to the treatment effect (eCG day 5 and eCG day 8) of follicle diameter (dominant follicle – day 9), total luteal volume (day 17), and progesterone concentration levels (day 17) upon pregnancy diagnosis. Only plasma progesterone concentration on day 17 (third sample) was significant ($P<0.1$) in terms of pregnancy probability.

As we can observe (10.1 ng/ml) one might infer there is an increasing probability of pregnancy to the maximum $P_4$ concentration value. We should also note that this increased probability of pregnancy may increase to the maximum $P_4$ level for the total animals used in this research (treatment 1, eCG day 5; treatment 2, eCG day 8) in the range of values reported; however, we cannot always expect that an increased $P_4$ value increases the likelihood of pregnancy [25]. This can happen regardless of indications that blood $P_4$ levels and uterine environment during luteal phase favour pregnancy establishment and maintenance conditions [51].

In contrast to the results of this research, other works have not shown any significant effect of $P_4$ upon pregnancy. Siqueira et al. [65] used a synchronization treatment for a fixed-time

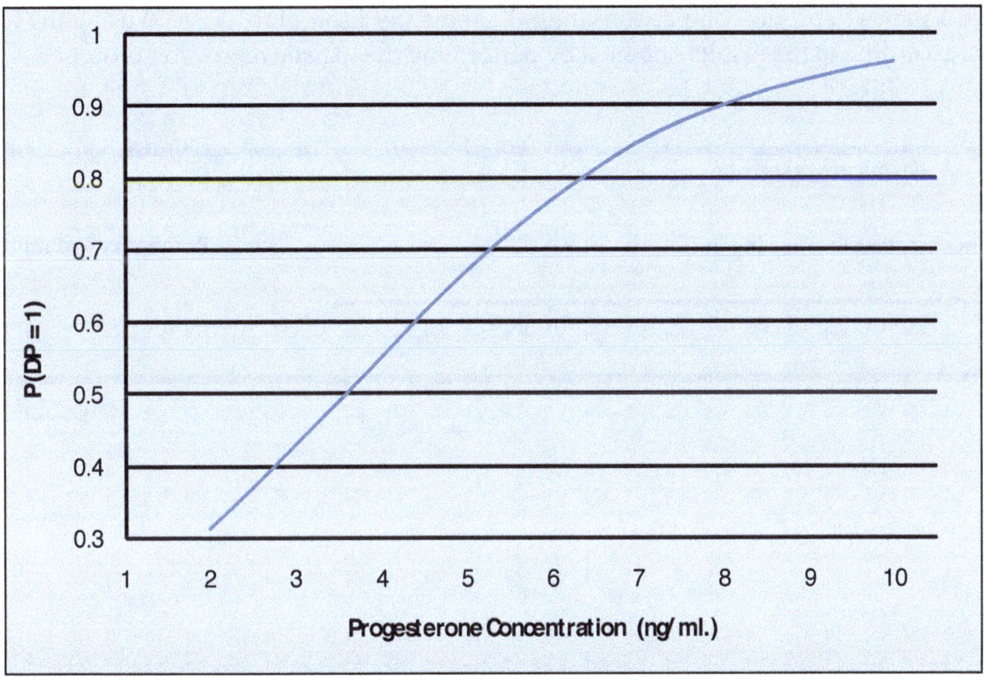


**Figure 7.** Logistic function for the range of values of progesterone concentration

embryo transfer (*in vivo* and *in vitro* embryos), applying eCG on day 5 (in relation to the protocol start) in crossbred recipients (*Bos taurus taurus/Bos taurus indicus*), applying a logistic regression model, and showed that the only variable (P=0.0002) significantly affecting pregnancy was the embryo type produced (*in vivo* and *in vitro*), not $P_4$ concentration, corpus luteum echo texture and area, animal category, embryo quality, or embryo development stage.

Rodriguez et al. [55] used several species and crossbreeds as recipients with transferred fresh and frozen embryos, then assessed the effect of other independent variables (CL diameter, $P_4$ concentration, embryo stage, embryo quality and species) upon pregnancy diagnosis. They did not establish any effect of any of these variables upon pregnancy diagnosis.

Other works have tried to relate pregnancy to other variables. For example, Peixoto et al. [69] used crossbred Holstein and Zebu heifers (*Bos indicus/Bos taurus*) as embryo recipients to determine which explanatory variables (transfer years: 1992-1999; season: autumn, winter and spring; embryo species; embryo stage; embryo quality; and synchrony between donors and recipients) might have a direct impact upon pregnancy. They established that the best logistic model to explain pregnancy included effects of year, transfer time, embryo stage, quality, and oestrus synchrony between donor and recipient.

Including other explanatory variables, Perry et al. [42] worked with synchronized crossbred heifers under a CO-Synch protocol for artificial insemination, and established that a pre-ovulatory follicle size (≥12.8 mm) predicted pregnancy at about 68.0 ± 4.9%, which decreased with follicle size.

Table 4 shows $P_4$ profile comparisons (ng/ml) on the third sampling (day 17) using the Odds ratio, according to the results obtained by performing the logistic regression proposed.

| **Plasma Progesterone Concentration Profiles (ng/ml)** | | **Pregnancy Probability** |
|---|---|---|
| Profile 1 | Profile 2 | |
| 6 | 4 | 2.72 |
| 5 | 2 | 4.48 |
| 4 | 2 | 2.72 |
| 8 | 4 | 7.4 |

**Table 4.** Contrasting progesterone profiles – pregnancy Odds ratio

Based on the results shown in the table, we might compare a heifer with a $P_4$ concentration of 6 ng/ml (profile 1) to a heifer with a $P_4$ concentration of 4 ng/ml (profile 2), and establish an Odds ratio of 2.72, indicating that it is 2.72 times more likely that the profile-1 cow should become pregnant than the profile-2 cow; therefore, pregnancy probability increases in line with $P_4$ concentration.

## 3. Conclusions

This study allows us to conclude that:

There was no effect of the day of application of eCG (day 5 or 8) on the number of dominant follicles; however, the eCG did affect the follicular diameter when applied on day 5, relating to the start of an oestrus synchronization protocol.

There was no effect of the day of application of eCG on the plasmatic progesterone levels on days 9 and 17 in protocols of oestrus synchronization in Holstein heifers. In the same way, the day of application of eCG does not affect the pregnancy rate evaluated on day 52 in Holstein heifers.

Further works should focus on antiluteolitic strategies that allow pregnancy rates in heifer and cow recipients involved in embryo transfer programmes to be improved.

## Author details

Néstor Isaías Tovío Luna*, Arturo Duica Amaya and Henry Alberto Grajales Lombana

*Address all correspondence to: nitoviol@unal.edu.co

Groups Researchers Biologia de la adaptacion de los animales al tropico, Facultad de Medicina Veterinaria y de Zootecnia, Universidad Nacional. UYWAY, Facultad de Ciencias Agrarias, programa de Zootecnia, Fundacion Universitaria Agraria de Colombia, Bogota, Columbia

## References

[1] Santos J, Thatcher W, Chebel R et al. The effect of embryonic death rates in cattle on the efficacy of estrus synchronization programs. Animal Reproduction Science. 2004; 83: pp. 513-535.

[2] Grajales H, Tovío N, Duica A. *Fundamentos de fisiología reproductiva en la hembra bovina*. 1 ed. Bogota, D.C: Editorial Universidad Nacional de Colombia; 2011

[3] Binelli M, Thatcher W, Mattos R, Baruselli P. Antiluteolytic Strategies to Improve Fertility in Cattle. Theriogenology. 2001; 56: pp. 1451-1463.

[4] Silke V, Diskin M, Kenny D et al. Extent, pattern and factors associated with late embryonic loss in dairy cows. Animal Reproduction Science. 2002; 71: pp. 1-12.

[5] Grajales H, Tovío N. Aspectos Básicos del ciclo estral de la vaca. Revista Genética Bovina. 2009; 15: pp. 32-36.

[6] Tovío N, Duica A, Grajales H. Mortalidad embrionaria en bovinos. Revista Genética bovina. 2010; 19: pp. 34-38.

[7] Tovío N, Duica A, Grajales H. Desarrollo embrionario y estrategias antiluteoliticas hormonales en programas de transplante de embriones bovinos. Revista MVZ Córdoba. 2008; 13 (1): pp. 1240-1251.

[8] Silva R, Rodriguez C, Marques M et al. Efeito do eCG e do GnRH na taxa de prenhez de vacas Nelore lactantes inseminadas em tempo fixo. Acta Scientiae Veterinariae. 2004; 32 (Suplemento): pp. 221.

[9] Duica A, Tovío N, Grajales H. Factores que afectan la eficiencia reproductiva de la hembra receptora en un programa de transplante de embriones bovinos. Journal de Medicina Veterinaria Universidad de la Salle. 2007 Jul; 14: pp. 107-124

[10] Baruselli P, Bó G, Reis E et al. Introducción de la IATF en el manejo reproductivo de rebaños de ganado de engorde en Brasil. Congreso Internacional de Reproducción Bovina Intervet. 2005; Bogotá, Colombia.

[11] Figueira M, Pegorer R, Ereno R et al. Neither plasma progesterone concentrations nor exogenous eCG affects rates of ovulation or pregnancy in fixed-time artificial insemination (FTAI) protocols for puberal Nellore heifers. Theriogenology. 2011; 75: (1): pp. 17-23.

[12] Peña M, Góngora A, Estrada J. Factores de crecimiento en el desarrollo folicular, embrionario temprano e implantación. Implicaciones en la producción de embriones bovinos. Journal MVZ Córdoba. 2007; 12 (1): pp. 942-954.

[13] Tovío N. Efectos de la aplicación de eCG (Día 5 u 8) sobre del cuerpo lúteo, nivel de progesterona y tasa de preñez en hembras receptoras de embriones bovinos. Tesis de Maestria. Facultad de Medicina Veterinaria y de Zootecnia, Universidad Nacional de Colombia; 2011.

[14] Lopes A, Butler S, Gilbert R et al. Relationship of pre-ovulatory follicle size, estradiol concentrations and season to pregnancy outcome in dairy cows. Animal Reproduction Science. 2007; 99: pp. 34-43.

[15] Moreira F, Badinga L, Burnley C et al. Bovine somatotropin increases embryonic development in super ovulated cows and improves post-transfer pregnancy rates when given to lactating recipient cows. Theriogenology. 2004; 57: pp. 1371-87.

[16] Kerbler T, Buhr M, Jordan L et al. Relationship between maternal plasma progesterone concentration and interferon-tau synthesis by the conceptus in cattle. Theriogenology.1997; 47: pp. 703-714.

[17] Mann G. Corpus luteum size and plasma progesterone concentration in cows. Animal Reproduction Science. 2009; 115: pp. 296-299.

[18] Vasconcelos J, Sartori R, Oliveira H et al. Reduction is size of the ovulatory follicle reduces subsequent luteal size and pregnancy rate. Theriogenology. 2001; 56: pp. 307-314.

[19] Gonella A, Grajales H, Hernández A. Ambiente receptivo uterino: control materno, control embrionario, muerte embrionaria. Journal MVZ Córdoba. 2010; 15 (1): pp. 1976-1984.

[20] Filho M, Ayres H, Ferreira R et al. Equine chorionic gonadotropin and gonadotropin-releasing hormone enhance fertility in a norgestomet-based, timed artificial insemination protocol in suckled Nellore (*Bos indicus*) cows. Theriogenology. 2010; 73: pp. 651-658.

[21] Bousfield G, Butnev V. Identification of twelve O-glycosylation sites in equine chorionic gonadtropin beta and equine luteinizing hormone by solid-phase Edman degradation. Biology Reproduction. 2001; 64: pp. 136-147.

[22] Forcada F, Ait Amer-Meziane J, Abecia M et al. Repeated super ovulation using a simplified FSH/eCG treatment for in vivo embryo production in sheep. Theriogenology. 2011; 75 (4): pp. 769-776.

[23] Everton L and Baruselli P. Sincronización de receptoras cruce por cebú en condiciones tropicales. IV Seminario de Reproducción de Grandes Animales, CGR, Biotecnología Reproductiva, Bogotá, Colombia, 2003.

[24] Souza A, Viechnieski S, Lima F et al. Effects of equine chorionic gonadotropin and type of ovulatory stimulus in a timed-AI protocol on reproductive responses in dairy cows. Theriogenology. 2009; 72: pp. 10-21.

[25] Melanie J, Starbuck A, Dailey E et al. Factors affecting retention of early pregnancy in dairy cattle. Animal Reproduction Science. 2004; 84: pp. 27-39.

[26] Nasser L, Reis E, Oliveira M et al. The use of hormonal treatments to improve reproductive performance of anestrous beef cattle in tropical climates. Animal Reproduction Science. 2004; 82: pp. 479-486.

[27] Quesada J and Ortiz J. Sincronización de receptoras de embriones tratadas con CIDR, benzoato de estradiol, D Cloprostenol asociado o no a eCG. VII Simposio internacional de reproducción animal – IRAC; Córdoba, Argentina. 2007.

[28] Campanile G, Di Palo R, Neglia G. et al. Corpus luteum and embryonic mortality in buffaloes treated with a GnRH agonist, hCG and progesterone. Theriogenology. 2007; 67: pp. 1393-1398.

[29] Baruselli P, Marques O, Nasser L et al. Effect of eCG on pregnancy rates of lactating zebu beef cows treated with CIDR–B devices for timed artificial insemination. Theriogenology. 2003; 59: p. 214.

[30] Berisha, B. and Schams, D. Ovarian function in ruminants. Domestic Animal Endocrinology. 2005; 29: pp. 305-317.

[31] Knobil E and Neill J. *Physiology of reproduction*. Third ed. Elsevier. United States of America. 2006.

[32] Bó G, Colazo M, Martínez M et al. Sincronización de la emergencia de la onda folicular y la ovulación en animales tratados con progestágenos y diferentes esteres de estradiol. 2o Simposio Internacional de Reprodução Animal Aplicada; Córdoba, Argentina. 2006.

[33] Kuran M, Hutchinson J, Broadbent P. The response of bovine granulosa cells to different gonadotrophins in culture. Animal Reproduction Science. 1991; 45: pp. 1-12.

[34] Cameron A, Batt P. PMSG may directly stimulate ovulation in female goats. Animal Reproduction Science. 1991; 25: pp. 233-239.

[35] Sartori R, Haughian J, Shaver R et al. Comparison of Ovarian Function and Circulating Steroids in Estrous Cycles of Holstein Heifers and Lactating Cows. Dairy Science. 2004; 8: pp. 905-920.

[36] Fuentes S, De la Fuente J. Tasas de gestación de novillas receptoras sincronizadas con Gonadotropina Coriónica Equina u Hormona Folículo Estimulante. Acta Scientiae Veterinariae. 2007; 35 (3): pp. 767-772.

[37] Baruselli P, Marques M, Hothnann E et al. Increased pregnancy rates in embryo recipients treated with CIDR-B devices. Theriogenology. 2011; 55, p. 157.

[38] Nogueira M, Melo D, Carvalho L et al. Do progesterone concentrations decrease pregnancy rates in embryo recipients synchronized with PGF2 and eCG? Theriogenology. 2003; 61 (7): pp. 1283-1290.

[39] Lynch C, Kenny D, Childs S et al. The relationship between periovulatory endocrine and follicular activity on corpus luteum size, function, and subsequent embryo survival. Theriogenology. 2010; 73: pp. 190-198.

[40] Rekwot P. Effects of feeding maize stover and cottonseed cake on onset of puberty in Bunaji (*Bos indicus*) heifers. Tropical Animal Health and Production. 2004; 36: pp. 637-644.

[41] Roche J. The effect of nutritional management of the dairy cow on reproductive efficiency. Animal Reproduction Science. 2004; 96: pp. 282-296.

[42] Perry G, Smith M, Roberts A et al. Relationship between size of the ovulatory follicle and pregnancy success in beef. Journal Animal Science. 2005; 85: pp. 684-689.

[43] Bó G, Alonso A, Caicedo J et al. Actualización sobre fisiología de la reproducción de la vaca. Especialización en reproducción bovina. IRAC, CGR, Universidad de Córdoba, Argentina; 2004.

[44] Duica a. Efecto del diámetro del folículo ovulatorio, tamaño del cuerpo lúteo y perfiles de progesterona sobre la tasa de preñez en la hembra receptora de embriones bovinos. Tesis de Maestria. Facultad de Medicina Veterinaria y de Zootecnia, Universidad Nacional de Colombia; 2011.

[45] Bó G. Sincronización de celos para programas de Inseminación Artificial y Transferencia de embriones Bovinos. Instituto de Reproducción Animal de Córdoba Argentina; 2003.

[46] Barnea E, Choi Y and Leavis P. Embryo maternal signaling prior to implantation. In: Textbook of Obstetrics Gynecology, 1 ed. Boston; pp.64. 2005.

[47] Kastelic J, Pierson R, Ginther O. Ultrasonic Morphology of a corpora lutea and central luteal cavities during the estrous cycle and early pregnancy in heifers. Theriogenology.1990; 34 (3): pp. 487-498.

[48] Perry G, Smith M, Lucy M et al. Proceedings of the national academy of sciences of the United States of America Current (PNAS). 2005; 102 (14), pp. 5268-5273.

[49] Chagas J, Lopes L, Robalo J. Plasma progesterone profiles and factors affecting embryo-fetal mortality following embryo transfer in dairy cattle. Theriogenology. 2002; 58: pp. 51-59.

[50] Sakase M, Kawate N, Nakagawa C, Fukushima M, Noda M, Takeda K, Ueno S, Inaba T, Kida, K and Tamada H. Preventive effects of CIDR-based protocols on premature ovulation before timed-AI in Ovsynch in cycling beef cows. The Veterinary Journal. In press; 2006.

[51] Shams D, Berisha B. Regulations of corpus luteum function in cattle – an overview. Reproduction Domestic Animals. 2004; 39: pp. 241-251.

[52] Gonella A. Posible relación de los niveles séricos ováricos (17 Beta estradiol y Progesterona), sus respectivos receptores endometriales (ER-1 alfa y PGR) y los cambios histológicos del endometrio durante el ciclo estral en hembras cíclicas de tres razas bovinas. Tesis de Maestria. Facultad de Medicina Veterinaria y de Zootecnia, Universidad Nacional de Colombia; 2011.

[53] Silva R, Rodriguez C, Marques M et al. Efeito do eCG e do GnRH na taxa de prenhez de vacas Nelore lactantes inseminadas em tempo fixo. Acta Scientiae Veterinariae. 2004; 32: pp. 221.

[54] Sartori G, Rosa M, Wiltbank M. Ovarian Structures and Circulating Steroids in Heifers and Lactating Cows in Summer and Lactating and Dry Cows in Winter. Journal Dairy Science. 2002; 85: pp. 2813-2822.

[55] Rodríguez J, Giraldo J, Castañeda S et al. Análisis multifactorial de las tasas de preñez en programas de transferencia de embriones en Colombia. Revista MVZ Córdoba. 2007; 12 (2): p. 978.

[56] Howell J, Fuquay J, Smith A. Corpus luteum growth and function in lactating Holstein cows during spring and summer. Journal Dairy Science. 1994; 77, pp. 735-739.

[57] Sprecher D, Nebel R, Whitmn S. The predictive value, sensitivity and specificity of palpation per rectum and transrectal ultrasonography for the determination of bovine luteal status. Theriogenology. 1998; 31: pp. 1165-1172.

[58] Badinga L, Thatcher W, Wilcox C et al. Effect of season on follicular dynamics and plasma concentrations of estradiol-17 beta, progesterone and luteinizing hormone in lactating Holstein cows. Theriogenology.1994; 42: pp. 1263-1274.

[59] Viana J, Torres C, Fernandes C et al. Avaliaçao ultra-sonográfica do corpo lúteo em novilhas mestiças utilizadas como receptoras de embriao. Archivos de Reproducción Animal. 1998; 5: pp. 42-47.

[60] Kastelic P, Bergfelt D, Ginther O. Relationship between ultrasonic assessment of the corpus luteum and plasma progesterone concentration in heifers. Theriogenology. 1990; 33 (6): pp. 1269-1278.

[61] Tom J, Pierson R, Adams G. Quantitative echotexture analysis of bovine ovarian follicles. Theriogenology. 1998; 50: pp. 339-346.

[62] Battocchio M, Gabai G, Mollo A et al. Agreement between ultrasonographic classification of the CL and the plasma progesterone concentration in dairy cows. Theriogenology. 1999; 51: pp. 1059-1069.

[63] Marques M, Reis E, Filho E et al. Efeitos da adminiatracao de eCG e de benzoato de estradiol para sincronizacao da ovulacao em vacas Bos taurus taurus X Bos taurus indicus no periodo pós parto. Simposio Internacional de Reproducción Animal; Huerta Grande; 2003.

[64] Bó G. and Cutaia L. Implementación de programas de inseminación artificial en rodeos de cría. Argentina. VI Simposio Internacional de Reproducción Animal. Instituto de Reproducción Animal; Córdoba Argentina. 2005; pp. 326-332.

[65] Siqueira L., Torres C, Souza E et al. Pregnancy rates and corpus luteum-related factors affecting pregnancy establishment in bovine recipients synchronized for fixed-time embryo transfer. Theriogenology. 2009; 72: pp. 949-958.

[66] Aguirre G, Pardo C, Góngora A. Inicio del celo, tasa de gestación y relación del tiempo de inseminación con los niveles de progesterona en vacas brahmán. Revista MVZ Córdoba. 2006; 11 (1): pp. 766-772.

[67] Rodrigues C, Ayres H, Reis E et al. Aumento de taxa de prenhez em vacas Nelore inseminadas em tempo fixo com o uso de eCG em diferentes periodos pós-parto; Acta Scientae Veterinariae. 2004; 32: p. 220.

[68] Pita F, Matute R, Tribulo R et al. Efecto de la aplicación de la Gonadotropina Coriónica Equina (eCG) y PGF2 alfa sobre la tasa de aprovechamiento y tasa de preñez en un protocolo de transferencia de embriones a tiempo fijo. VIII Simposio internacional de reproducción animal – IRAC; Córdoba, Argentina; 2009.

[69] Peixoto M, Bergmann J, Suyama E et al. Logistic regression analysis of pregnancy rate following transfer of *Bos indicus* embryos into *Bos indicus/Bos taurus* heifers. Theriogenology. 2007; 67: pp. 287-292.

[70] Moura M, Marques M, Frare J et al. Sincronizacao da ovulacao com Crestar ® e CIDR ® para inovulacao de embrioes bovinos em tempo fixo. VII Simposio internacional de reproducción animal; Cordoba, Argentina; 2001.

[71] Marques M et al. Follicular dynamics and pregnancy rates in Bos Taurus xBos indicus embryo transfer recipients treated to increase plasma progesterone concentrations; 2012. 9: p. 11-119.

[72] Barret D, Bartlewski P, Duggaathi R et al. Suppression of follicle wave emergence in cycle ewes by supraphysiologic concentrations of estradiol 17 beta and induction with a physiologic dose of exogenous ovine follicle stimulating hormone. Biology Reproduction. 2006; 75: pp. 633-641.

[73] Bó G. and Caccia M. *Ultrasonografía reproductiva en el ganado bovino*. Argentina. Instituto de Reproducción Animal de Córdoba (IRAC); 2003.

[74] Mann G, Lamming G. The influence of progesterone during early pregnancy in cattle. Reproduction Domestic Animals. 1999; 34: pp. 269-274.

[75] Sartori R, Barros A. Reproductive cycles in *Bos indicus* cattle. Animal Reproduction Science. 2011; 124 (3): pp. 244-250.

[76] Niswender G, Juengel J, Silva P et al. Mechanisms controlling the function and life span of the corpus luteum. Physiological Reviews. 2000; 222 (80): pp. 1-29.

[77] Moreira F, Risco C, Pires M et al. Use of bovine somatotropin in lactating dairy cows receiving timed artificial insemination. Journal Dairy Science. 2000; 83: pp. 1237-1247.

[78] Olivera M. Gestación. In: Galina C. Reproduccion de los animals domesticos. 1 ed. Mexico: Limusa. 2006; pp. 165-187.

[79] Lucy M, Savio J, Badinga L et al. Factors that affect ovarian follicular dynamics in cattle. Journal Animal Science. 1992; 70: pp. 3615-3626.

[80] Drawash A. The importance of milk progesterone concentrations during early pregnancy in the cow. Journal of Animal Breeding. 1998; 2: pp. 41-43.

5

# A Novel Discipline in Embryology—Animal Embryo Breeding

Bin Wu, Linsen Zan, Fusheng Quan and Hai Wang

### Abstract

The modern animal biotechnologies, such as animal cloning, transgenesis, sex determination, stem cells, designing new livestock, must be performed on animal gametes including sperm and oocytes, and embryos based on embryology theory. Currently, some key biotechnologies in embryology have become the most powerful tool for animal scientists and breeders to improve genetic construction of animal herds. Here, authors put forward a new concept of **Animal Embryo Breeding** Science to describe this discipline formation, development, and application in animal genetic improvement and breeding. The relationship of embryo breeding with other disciplines has been profiled. Thus, animal scientists and breeders can easily understand and apply embryo breeding theory and related key techniques to accelerate animal improvement speed, to modify genetic construction of animal population, and to design and create new animal individual or breed.

**Keywords:** Discipline, embryo breeding, biotechnology, livestock

## 1. Introduction

Animal breeding sciences concern the management and care of farm animals by humans for profit. Not only does it refer to the practice of selectively breeding and raising livestock to promote desirable traits in animals for utility, sport, pleasure, or research [1], but also it refers to the efficient exploitation of a species in agriculture advantageous to humans. The genetic improvement of livestock depends on defining breeding objectives and accurately identifying the right animals to be used for future breeding. Traditional breeding programs involve 1) the design of animal breeding goals including improvement traits, such as milk, wool, growth, carcass and fertility, females vs. males, progeny test and nucleus vs. commercial animal population; 2) application techniques, such as artificial insemination and embryo transfer, are used as methods not only to guarantee that females breed regularly but also to help improve herd genetics; 3) based on quantitative genetics theory, estimation of breeding value by phenotype, pedigree, BLUP (best linear unbiased prediction) method, and genetic markers; 4) selection and culling of individuals based on genetic evaluation, balancing rate of change, and inbreeding; and 5) determining mating system. This is a long-term process for livestock genetic improvement.

As modern biotechnology develops, some new techniques can be applied to animal breeding programs 1) to accelerate genetic progression by shortening generation interval and increasing female reproduction; 2) to add new genetic trait to animal body by transgenic technology or to remove bad traits from animal body by gene knockout method [2]; and 3) to create new animal individual or breed by modern biotechnologies including nuclear transfer, cloning, and genetic modification. These new technologies will make it easier to manipulate animal genomes, but food products from genetically engineered animals face a long road to market. Examples of biotechnology applications of particular interest to the department include cell culture, genomics, molecular-marker-assisted breeding, cloning, bioprocessing, and diagnostic testing, as well as gene technology (genetic modification). Genetic modification deliberates change of an organism's genetic material by moving, introducing, or eliminating specific genes, such as taking a single gene from an animal cell and inserting it into another animal cell to give the second cell a desired characteristic. The terms "gene technology," "genetic engineering" and "genetic manipulation," "genetic enhancement," "gene splicing," "transgenics," or the use of "recombinant DNA" are used to describe genetic modification processes. Genes can be found in and moved between different plants, animals or microorganisms such as viruses or bacteria, for example, transferring worm fat-1 gene to pig to produce more omega-3 fat acid in pork meat [3]. Genes can also be changed within a specific plant or animal individual. For instance, "knocking out" an undesirable characteristic gene such as susceptibility to a particular disease can be beneficial to the plant or animal life.

In mammals, the realization of these goals must depend upon *in vitro* manipulation of animal oocytes and embryos. Thus, embryology has become a core of these biotechnologies (Figure 1). Currently, embryo biotechnology, which most people call **embryo bioengineering,** has gradually become the most powerful tool for animal scientists and breeders to improve genetic construction of their animal herds or populations. Embryo transfer in cattle has recently gained considerable popularity with seedstock dairy and beef producers. Many kinds of species have been cloned and some transgenic animals have been produced. Thus, embryology has become a core of modern biotechnologies in animal genetic modification and breeding. Combining the new advances in modern biotechnology with future application, authors put forward the new concept of **Animal Embryo Breeding Science** to describe embryology development and application in animal genetic improvement and breeding.

## 2. Concept of animal embryo breeding

Breeding is the reproductive process, which is producing of elite offspring in animals or plants. Animal breeding programs involve the selection or culling of parents (such as bull and cow)

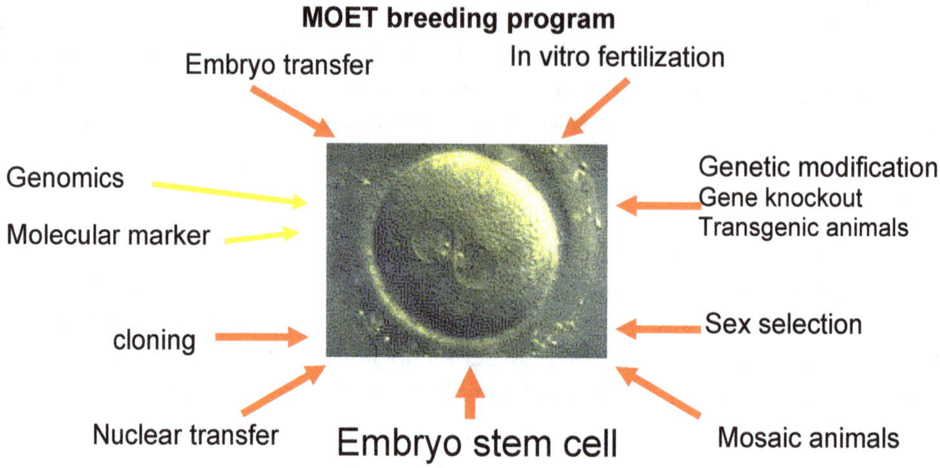


**Figure 1.** Embryology has become a core of modern biotechnologies in animal genetic modification and breeding. Any new developed biotechniques such as nuclear transplantation, cloning, and transgenesis, finally must be performed on animal oocytes or embryos. MOET represents multiple ovulation and embryo transfer.

and then determination of mating system. They must be female and male sex combination. However, **Animal Embryo Breeding** is an asexual reproduction of specific oocytes or embryos artificially by current developed biotechnology. The Science of Animal Embryo Breeding is to study how to use the embryo manipulation technologies to improve, create, and clone new animal individual or breed. Current developed techniques include nuclear transfer, cytoplasmic transfer or replacement, in vitro fertilization (IVF), sperm cytoplasmic injection (ICSI), parthenogenesis and androgenesis, embryo cloning, sex selection, transgenesis, gene knock out, stem cells and somatic cell cloning, etc. Although embryo breeding is a branch of traditional animal breeding discipline, the science of animal breeding is concerned with the application of the principles of population genetics and qualitative genetics to the improvement of domestic animals. However, Animal Embryo Breeding is concerned with application of the developed embryo biotechnologies to new animal individual creation, genetic cloning and preservation of animal breeds. The research main body of this discipline focuses on sperm, oocyte and embryo. After the desired animal type (genetic improved goal) has been designed, by means of a serial micromanipulation on oocyte or embryo, such as nuclear transfer, foreign DNA microinjection to egg pronucleus and stem cell technique, a modified improved embryo may be produced in vitro and then transferred into animal uterine cavity so that a new animal individual could be created. In the last couple of decades, many kinds of animals including transgenic pigs, cattle, sheep, and goat, have been produced [4].

## 3. The relationship of animal embryo breeding science with other disciplines

As a new developing subject, Animal Embryo Breeding Science mainly depends upon modern biotechnology development, especially molecular biology, genetics, and reproductive biology with embryology. However, it also has a close association with other subjects such as reproductive biology and embryology, animal genetics and breeding (Figure 2).

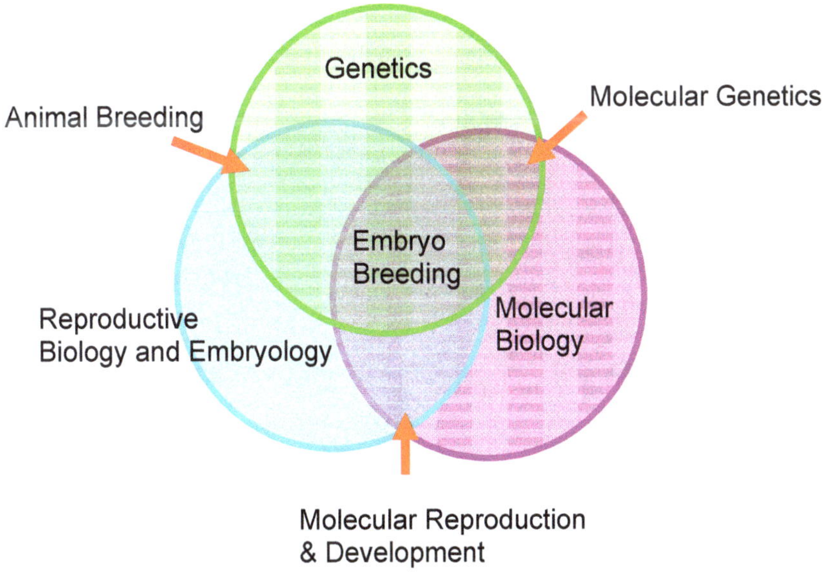


**Figure 2.** The designed relationship of Animal Embryo Breeding with other disciplines. The Embryo breeding is a core subject which combines molecular biology/genetics with animal genetics and breeding as well as reproductive biology and embryology.

The goal of animal breeding program can be realized by the current embryo breeding technology. Using molecular biological technique, a specific gene type for the desired animal may be designed. The new developed biotechnologies to attempt to modify animal genetic traits must be conducted on animal oocyte and embryo. The embryo in vitro production and animal individual birth must depend upon animal reproductive technology. Embryology may supply a good condition to produce many high-quality embryos. Thus, the Embryo Breeding is a core subject which combines molecular biology/genetics with animal genetics and breeding as well as reproductive biology and embryology.

## 4. Major research scope and content of animal embryo breeding

Animal Embryo Breeding Science is based on the current developed embryo biotechnology. The core of current embryo biotechnology is oocyte in vitro fertilization (IVF). As human IVF technique rapidly develops in infertility treatment, not only animal IVF has offered a very valuable tool to study mammalian fertilization and early embryo development, but also its commercial applications have being increased. Based on IVF research, some new developed embryo technologies consisting of nuclear transfer, transgenesis, cloning, and stem cells, etc., can be used to create new animal individual or population, and accelerate genetic progression of animal population during the period from early oocyte stage (oogenesis) to preimplantation embryo stage (Figure 3).

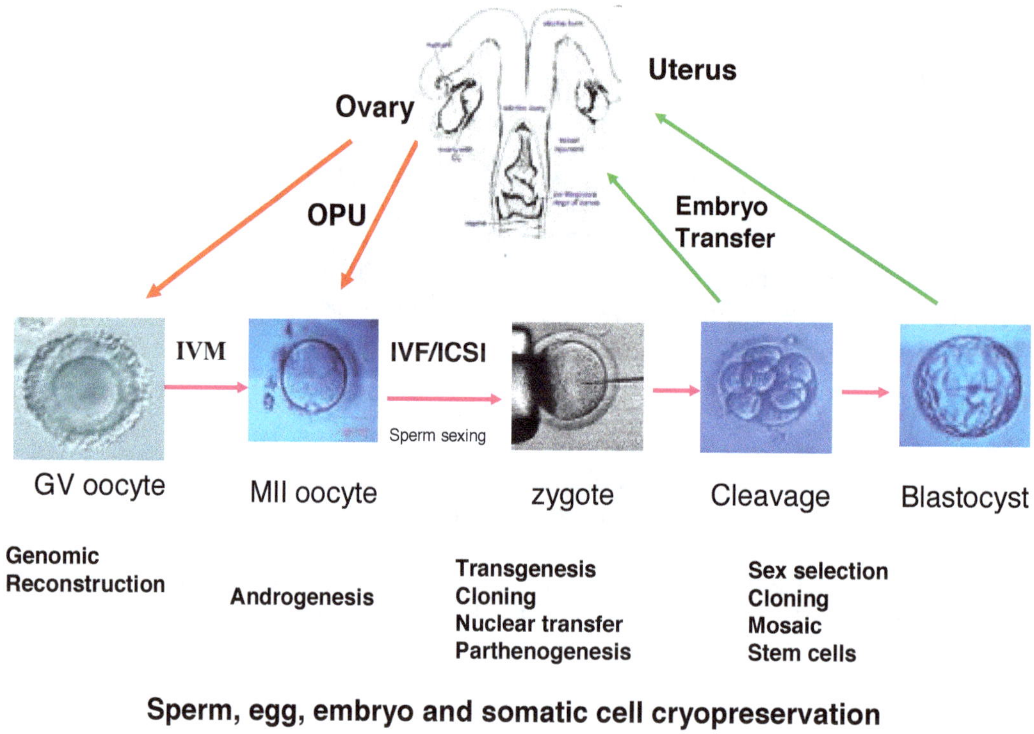


**Figure 3.** Schematic representation of main embryo biotechnologies which can impact on the genetic improvement programs on animal embryo breeding.

Based on this schematic picture, we may focus on several fields for Animal Embryo Breeding research. In the early stage of oogenesis and oocyte maturation, some key techniques such as genomic reconstruction, nuclear transfer, androgenesis and parthenogenesis, cytoplasm replacement, etc., may be used to change animal genetic construction [5]. At the fertilization stage, the sexing sperm may be used to produce specific-sex (female or male) animal population to achieve better economic results [6]. Using intracytoplasmic sperm injection (ICSI) technique may make an elite performance bull with a very few sperm produce a lot of offspring. At the pronuclear stage, the foreign DNA may be injected to zygote to produce transgenic animals. In the preimplantation cleavage and blastocyst stage, preimplantation genetic diagnosis (PGD) or preimplantation genetic screening (PGS), embryo cloning, mosaic animal and embryo stem cell techniques may be used to produce various different types of animals. Also, at any stage, sperm, egg and embryo, as well as somatic cells may be cryopreserved for future use [7]. Thus, we may profile the outline of Animal Embryo Breeding study as shown in Table 1 (Table 1).

| | |
|---|---|
| **Early Gamete Manipulation** | |
| | *Artificial Insemination* |
| | Semen collection and its storage |
| | Sperm sexing |
| | Ovulation control |
| | Superovulation |
| | Ultrasound-guided oocyte retrieval (TVOR) or nonsurgical ovum pick up (OPU) |
| | *Oocyte and egg cryopreservation* |
| **Embryo Transfer** | |
| | Multiple ovulation (superovulation) |
| | Multiple ovulation with embryo transfer (MOET) |
| | Embryo splitting |
| | Embryo sexing |
| | Embryo transfer technique |
| ***In vitro embryo production (IVP) technology*** | |
| | *In vitro* maturation (IVM) of oocytes |
| | *In vitro* fertilization (IVF) of oocytes |
| | Intracytoplasm sperm injection (ICSI) |
| | Culture of *in vitro* fertilized embryos |
| | Preimplantation embryo diagnosis |
| **Embryo Cloning** | |
| | Embryo blastomere cloning |
| | Somatic cell nuclear Transfer (Dolly) |
| | Embryonic stem cell nuclear transfer |
| | Induced pluripotent stem cells (iPS) nuclear transfer |
| **Transgenic animals** | |
| | **Transfer gene construct** |
| | Inserting genes |
| | Knockout genes |
| | **Strategies for gene transfer** |
| | a) Directly inject a gene into egg pronucleus |
| | b) Sperm-mediated gene transfer |
| | c) Stem-cell-mediated gene transfer (transfection) |
| | d) Retrovirus and viruses vector for gene transfer |

| | |
|---|---|
| | e) Transfer of animal cells/embryo |
| | f) Targeted gene transfer |
| | g) Liposomes or spheroplasts as vector |
| | h) Other techniques such as electroporation, use of complexes, of DNA with polycations or lipids; a particle gun, DNA with polycations or lipids, etc. |
| | **Production of various transgenic animals** |
| | a) Cow or cattle |
| | b) Sheep and goat |
| | c) Fish |
| | d) Pig |
| | e) Other animals |
| | **Animal bioreactor and molecular farming** |
| | **Transgenic breeding strategies** |
| | **Transgenic effect and cost** |
| **Genomic reconstruction** | |
| | Germinal vesicle (GV) transfer |
| | Androgenesis |
| | Parthenogenesis |
| | Three-parent baby |
| | Ova-plasma transfer |
| **Preimplantation embryo diagnosis/screening (PGD/PGS)** | |
| | Fluorescent *in situ* hybridization (FISH) |
| | Polymerase chain reaction (PCR) |
| | Microarray |
| | Comparative Genomic Hybridization (CGH) |
| | Gene chips |
| **Mosaic animal creation** | |
| | Heteromorphosis |
| **Rare animal individual or breed preservation** | |
| | Sperm cryopreservation |
| | Egg cryopreservation |
| | Somatic cell cryopreservation |

**Table 1.** Outline of Animal Embryo Breeding discipline

## 5. Research category of animal embryo breeding

As a new discipline, animal scientists and breeders can apply Animal Embryo Breeding Science theory to animal population to improve genetic traits, to add new benefit traits to animal body and to remove some harmful traits from animal body. Major research categories involve the following several aspects:

1. The objective of embryo breeding study is to create new animal individual or improve animal population. Based on the objective of the animal breeding program – what kind of animal traits you need in the breeding program – you may adopt an appropriate method of embryo biotechnique. For instance, if you want to add new genetic trait into animal body, you may use transgenic method to insert this gene into embryo. If you need to produce a complete same animal, clone method may be used as embryo cloning or nuclear transfer technique to clone this animal somatic cell.
2. The technique selection of embryo breeding: based on your breeding objective, a specific technique should be selected; for instance, in transgenic program, what gene and which method should be used to produce transgenic animals. In the animal cloning program to increase animal population homogeneity, various cloning methods should be evaluated for the best cloning technique, such as embryo cloning, stem cell, or somatic cell cloning.
3. Inserting embryo breeding into animal breeding program. In practice, embryo breeding is a trick to produce a specific animal. By the means of transgenic tactics, a given target gene vector may be constructed and transformed to chromosome in cell. Then, a given aim-gene embryo may be formed by nucleus transfer technique. By means of the genetic screening and diagnosis on cell levels, an expected embryo with a specific genotype embryo may be determined on embryonic level. Then, this expected embryo with a specific modified gene may be transferred into animal uterus to produce a specific animal. After individual level diagnosis, the ideal animal may be placed in animal population to expend its reproduction as traditional breeding program.

## 6. Application of Embryo Breeding in animal improvement program

1. Genomic reconstruction by somatic cloning and parthenogenesis to produce specific animal population

When a bull or cow with elite production performance in beet cattle population is discovered, the breeding aim will be to accelerate this cow or bull reproduction to propagate a new breed of cattle. By normal breeding mating, this cow may lose half its inherent genes in its offspring. However, by the means of cloning techniques, many individuals of the same genotype can be theoretically produced. Thus, the accuracy of evaluation may be greatly increased. In spite of low cloning efficiency, many scientists are still interested in animal cloning techniques, which will eventually be used to clone very valuable animals, such as breeding stock, transgenic animals, and endangered species.

By the means of cell nucleus transfer technology, a new animal can be produced using androgenesis method [7]. Androgenesis is a male parthenogenesis in which only paternal chromosomes are kept in the embryo with the removal of the egg nucleus at the fertilization [8]. This is a reproductive pattern from two male parents. After an oocyte nucleus has been removed, a male diploid cell is transferred into this egg in which the oocyte cytoplasm will induce this diploid cell going through meiosis to become a haploid MII oocyte. After inducement, a male sperm is injected into this oocyte to produce a paternal embryo. Finally, this modified embryo will be transferred into receipt cow to produce a new individual bull with two male parents.

2. Create new genetic variation in population by genomic modification during embryogenesis

The current animal breeding strategies are mainly based on the principle of selective breeding including the morphology of animal body, the application of quantitative genetics theory, the estimation of breeding value by phenotype, pedigree, BLUP (best linear unbiased prediction) method, and genetic markers. These methods mainly add genetic improvement by increasing the frequency of advantageous alleles of many loci, but actually very few of gene loci are identified. These techniques do not change gene movement from different species or genera due to reproductive barrier, while the new developed transgenic technique can remove the breeding barriers between different species or genera.

The most efficient method of transgenesis in mammals is the genetic manipulation of the pronuclear stage embryo [9]. By injecting foreign DNA into one of the two pronuclei of the zygote, the birth offspring may contain a functional foreign gene in the genome. In the last 20 years, many kinds of transgenic species have been produced for agriculture and medicine application [10]. For example, the transgenic technology in beef cattle industry may improve animals for faster growth, higher quality beef products, or disease resistance [11-13].

The transgenesis first starts with identification of the genes of interest. Current molecular biotechnology may help us to search for some interesting markers used as reference points for mapping relevant genes. These molecular markers can also be used for identification of the animals carrying the transgenes. Most of the quantitative genetic loci (QTL) are polygenic in nature but the manipulation of transgenesis is a single gene trait [14,15]. The technology holds promises in the future in moving polygenic QTL across the breeding barriers of animals. However, it is expected that molecular markers will serve as a potential tool to geneticists and breeders to evaluate the existing germplasm, and to manipulate it to create animals of desired traits [16].

3. Shorten generation interval by embryo in vitro production

As the oocyte in vitro maturation (IVM) and in vitro fertilization (IVF) techniques rapidly develop, the ultrasound-guided oocyte retrieval (TVOR) or nonsurgical ovum pick up (OPU) technique can retrieve many oocytes repeatedly from a cow or a heifer. As many as 1000 oocytes have been collected from one female cattle in a year [17-19]. Thus, the embryo in vitro production (IVP) technology has been able to promote a cow to produce more than one hundred offspring in a year and greatly accelerate herd genetic improvement speed [20]. In order to improve ordinary cattle herd, slaughterhouse ovaries also may be used as in vitro embryo production. A lot of oocytes could be obtained from slaughter house cow ovaries. After maturation, these oocytes may be inseminated with elite bull semen for in vitro fertilization [21]. Although the detail genetic backgrounds of these slaughterhouse animals are not known, these embryos have a very high genetic merit from elite bulls. Using these embryos, an ordinary cow herd could obtain at least 50% genetic improvement.

The multiple ovulation and embryo transfer (MOET) was used initially to produce more embryos from genetic elite cows in shorter time periods. Currently, the MOET breeding schemes have widely established in many countries and their use accounts for about 80% of cattle embryos transferred commercially [22]. Currently, the application of transvaginal ultrasonically guided OPU technique may significantly improve MOET scheme efficiency because about 1000 oocytes may be collected and 300 embryos may be produced *in vitro* from a cow in a year at frequent intervals using IVF technology [19]. Also, oocytes may be collected from prepubertal heifers and cattle generation interval may be shorted for 2-3 years. The combination of MOET program with OPU/IVF technique is providing a more efficient way to produce more embryos from an individual donor donor than superovulation stimulation program [23]. Thus, OPU/IVF technique greatly increases MOET breeding scheme efficiency in milk and beef industry.

**4.** Increased economy from animal population by sex selection

Animal sex selection may increase animal economical value for humans. Embryo breeding theory may provide several ways for animal sex selection, including sperm sex selection and preimplantation embryo sex selection. Sperm sex selection is to try to separate semen into X- or Y-bearing chromosome sperm by flow cytometry [24, 25]. Current sorted sperm has been successfully used in IVF for in vitro embryo production and artificial insemination in cattle [6, 26].

Another sexing pathway is to determine the sex of an embryo prior to transfer. Preimplantation genetic diagnosis (PGD) technique has become an efficient method for sex selection. Y-specific chromosome probe for polymerase chain reaction (PCR) and Fluorescent *In Situ* Hybridization (FISH) are two common methods in animal sex determination. On the ordinary farm, cattle embryos may be sexed by complete cell biopsy and PCR technique. Our clinic farm practice [7] showed that a few of trophoectoderm cells could be microbiopsied from blastocyst embryos by transzonal incision using a microsurgical blade. The mini-tube PCR was carried out for 30 minutes and the gel electrophoresis was run for 20 minutes. The sexing result could be obtained in 2 hours. These results clearly demonstrate that the microsurgical technique and subsequent PCR sex analysis allow the rapid commercial exchange of genetic resources on the basis of fresh or frozen sex-desired embryos in embryo transfer programs.

Fluorescent *in situ* hybridization (FISH) technique has also been used as embryo chromosome set (karyotype) diagnosis. A blastomere is removed from an embryo by micromanipulation, and then used to examine the embryo X/Y chromosomes by FISH. Recently, new developed technologies in PGD allow examining of all chromosomes and identifying certain genes or genetic mutations, such as the competitive genomic hybridization (CGH) and microarray analysis. More recently, novel developed Next Generation Sequencing (NGS) for preimplantation genetic screen (PGS) is now being offered clinically to provide comprehensive, accurate screening of all 24 chromosomes for selections of euploid embryos. PGS results generated are comparable to those achieved with the CGH technology, with improved accuracy, sensitivity, and resolution for more accurate detection of euploid embryos, aneuploidies, chromosome imbalances (translocations), and embryo mosaicism. NGS is a superior technology because it looks at close to 1.1 million data points on the genome compared to around 3,000 with CGH.

**5.** Preservation breeding

Many animal breeders are interested in preserving bloodlines of animals, either of a rare breed, or of rare pedigrees within a breed. Therefore, Rahbek [27] put forward a preservation breeding concept to describe the purpose of preservation breeding, which is to protect genetic diversity within a species, and to preserve valuable genetic traits that may not be popular or in fashion in the present, but may be of great value in the future. In the animal embryo breeding program, two kinds of cells including reproductive cells and somatic cells may be cryopreserved in liquid nitrogen for future use. Reproductive cell cryopreservation is an important branch of embryo breeding science because it involves the preservation of gametes (sperm and oocytes), embryos, and reproductive tissues (ovarian and testicular tissues) for future use in the assisted reproductive technology. Practically, animal embryo breeding program may provide a sperm and embryo bank with the objective of avoiding genetic dilution and irreplaceable gene losses of the valuable "naturalized breeds" germplasm. It is much lower in cost than normal animal breeding, preserving rare native animal breed plan. At present, many countries have set up gene banks to store frozen embryos and semen of various animal species including native cattle, pig, and some endangered animals.

The development of embryo freezing technologies has revolutionized cattle breeding. Since then, advancements in cryobiology, cell biology, and domestic animal embryology have enabled the development of embryo preservation methodologies for our other domestic animal species, including sheep and goats. Currently, use of preserved embryos has become a routine breeding alternative for all domestic animal species. This freezing and storage methodology may provide for maternal germplasm, global genetic transport, increased selection pressure of herd genetics, and genetic resource rescue.

In the conventional breeding program, an outstanding bull may maintain normal mating for 5 years. However, if this bull semen is cryopreserved, it will extend the bull's breeding time. In embryo breeding program, when some elite bulls leave very few sperm, we may use intracytoplasmic sperm injection (ICSI) technique to inject a single sperm to an oocyte so that genetic merit embryos are obtained [28]. Also, sperm cell genome cloning technique may be used to produce many copies of a specific sperm [8]. The application of this technique to beef and dairy cattle industry has greatly increased merit bull spread in animal herd [29].

Like normal reproduction, somatic cell nuclear transfer (SCNT) starts with an egg or oocyte, but here the nucleus of the egg needs to be removed. Then the nucleus from a somatic (skin) cell is transferred into the enucleated egg which would be analogous to the sperm entering the oocyte. As this develops into a blastocyst, cells from the inner cell mass can be isolated and purified to serve as a source for pluripotent stem cells. In animal embryo breeding, somatic cell is also an important genetic resource. Therefore, the somatic cells, such as skin, hair, and other cells from rare and endangered animals may be collected and cryopreserved so that they can be used in the future.

## 7. Conclusions

Currently, the following biotechnologies in embryology have been applied or will be applied in animal genetic improvement [9]: 1) Genomic reconstruction by somatic cloning and parthenogenesis can produce specific animal population; 2) new genetic variation in population can be created by genomic modification during embryogenesis, such as transgenic breeding strategies; 3) animal generation interval may be shortened by embryo in *in vitro* production; 4) economy efficiency from animal population may be significantly increased by embryo sex selection; and 5) a rare breed, or of rare pedigrees within a breed, may be efficiently preserved at low cost in liquid nitrogen. Thus, the development of modern biotechnology has brought into being the concept and theory of **Animal Embryo Breeding Science.** Understanding and applying its theory and technology will be helpful to animal scientists and students as well as animal breeders to accelerate animal improvement speed, to modify genetic construction of animal population, and to create new animal breeds.

## Author details

Bin Wu[1,2], Linsen Zan[3], Fusheng Quan[4] and Hai Wang[1,2]

1 Arizona Center for Reproductive Endocrinology and Infertility, Tucson, Arizona, USA

2 Yunnan Jiuzhou Hospital, Kunming, Yunnan, China

3 College of Animal Science and Technology, National Beef Cattle Improvement Center, China

4 College of Veterinary Medicine, Northwest A&F University, Yangling, Shaanxi, China

## References

[1] Jarman, MR, Clark G, Grigson C, Uerpmann HP, Ryder ML, 1976: Early animal husbandry. *The Royal Soc.* 275 (936): 85-97.

[2] Wolfer DP, Crusio WE, Lipp HP, 2002: Knockout mice: simple solutions to the problems of genetic background and flanking genes. *Trends Neurosci* 25(7):336-40.

[3] Lai L, Kang JX, Li B, Wang J, Witt WT, Yong HY, Hao Y, Wax DM, Murphy CN, Rieke A, Sanuel M, Linville ML, Korte SW, Evans RW, Starzl TE, Prather RS, Dai Y, 2006: Generation of cloned transgenic pigs rich in omega-3 fatty acids. *Natur Biotechnol* 24: 435-436.

[4] Wheeler MB, Rutledge JJ, Fischer-Brown A, Van Etten T, Malusky S, Beebe DJ, 2006: Application of sex semen technology to in vitro embryo production in cattle. *Theriogenology* 65:219-227.

[5] Lillico SG, Proudfoot C, Carlson DF, Slverakova D, Neil C, Nlain C, King TJ, Richie WA, Tan, W, Mileham A, Mclaren DG, Fahrenkrug SC, Whitelaw BA, 2013: Live pigs produced from genome edited zygotes. *Sci Rep* 3:2847.

[6] Seidel GE Jr, 2007: Overview of sexing sperm. *Theriogenology* 68:443-446.

[7] Wu B, Zan L, 2012: Enhance beef cattle improvement by embryo biotechnologies. *Reprod Dom Anim* 47:865-871.

[8] Wu B, Gelety TJ, Shi JZ, 2012: Advances in fertility options of azoospermic men. In: Bin Wu (eds.), *Advances in Embryo Transfer*. Croatia: InTech Press 2012: p. 115-132.

[9] Wilmut I, Hooper ML, Simons JP, 1991: Genetic manipulation of mammals and its application in reproductive biology. *J Reprod Fert 92* 245-279.

[10] Niemann H, Kues WA, 2003: Application of transgenesis in livestock for agriculture and biomedicine. *Anim Reprod Sci*. 79:291-317.

[11] Greger M, 2010: Transgenesis in animal agriculture: Addressing animal health and welfare concerns. *J Agric Environ Ethics*. DOI 10.1007/s10806-010-9261-7

[12] Wheeler MB, 2003: Production of transgenic livestock: Promise fulfilled. *J Anim Sci*. 81(Suppl. 3):32–37.

[13] Wheeler MB, 2007: Agricultural applications for transgenic livestock. *Trends Biotechnol* 25(5):204-210.

[14] Anderson SJ, Noyes HA, Agaba M, Kemp SJ and Archibald AL, 2007: A transgenic approach to QTL analysis in a trypanotolerant mouse model. In: International Symposium on Animal Genomics for Animal Health, 23-25 October 2007, OIE HQ, World Organisation for Animal Health, 12 Rue de Prony, Paris France (unpublished).

[15] Cao Z, Ding WD, 2013: Homologous rearranged DNA can change phenotype and genotype of the host by transgenic method and a QTL related to weight was obtained from it. *Adv J Food Sci Technol*. 5(3): 295-302

[16] Beuzen ND, Stear MJ, Chang KC, 2000: Molecular markers and their use in animal breeding. *Vet J*. 160(1):42-52.

[17] Taneja M, Yang X, 1998: Promises and problems of in vitro production of embryos by TVOR-IVF scheme in cows and heifers. *Embryo Transf Newslett.16* 10-12.

[18] Machado SA, Reichenbach HD, Weppert M, Wolf E, Gonçalves PB, 2006: The variability of ovum pick-up response and in vitro embryo production from monozygotic twin cows. *Theriogenology*. 65(3):573-583.

[19] Presicce GA, Xu J, Gong GC, Moreno JF, Chaubal S, Xue F, Bella A, Senatore EM, Yang XZ, Tian XC, Du FL, 2011: Oocyte source and hormonal stimulation for *In vitro* fertilization using sexed spermatozoa in cattle. *Vet Med Int*. Published online 2010 September 5. Vet Med Int. 2011; 2011: 145626.

[20] Martinez HR, 2012: Assisted reproductive techniques for cattle breeding in developing countries: A critical appraisal of their value and limitations. *Reprod Dom Anim* (47), SI, 21-26.

[21] Wu B, Ignotz G, Currie WB, Yang X, 1997: Dynamics of maturation-promoting factor and its constituent proteins during in vitro maturation of bovine oocytes. *Bio Reprod* 56:253-259.

[22] Thibier M, 2005: The zootechnical applications of biotechnology in animal reproduction: current methods and perspectives. *Reprod Nutr Dev*. 45:235-42.

[23] Betteridge KJ, 2006: Farm animal embryo technologies: Achievements and perspectives. *Theriogenology*. 65:905-913.

[24] Blondin P, Beaulieu M, Fournier V, Morin N, Crawford L, Madan P, King WA, 2009: Analysis of bovine sexed sperm for IVF from sorting to the embryo. *Theriogenology*. 71: 30-38.

[25] Underwood SL, Bathgate R, Ebsworth M, Maxwell WMC, Evans G, 2010: Pregnancy loss in heifers after artificial insemination with frozen-thawed, sex-sorted, re-frozen-thawed dairy bull sperm. *Anim Reprod Sci* 118(1):7-12

[26] Pontes JHF, Silva KCF, Basso AC, Rigo AG, Ferreira CR, Santos GMG, Sanches BV, Porcionato JPF, Vieira PHS, Faifer FS, Sterza FAM, Schenk JL, Seneda MM, 2010: Large-scale *in vitro* embryo production and pregnancy rates from *Bos taurus, Bos indicus,* and *indicus-taurus* dairy cows using sexed sperm. *Theriogenology*. 74:1349-1355.

[27] Rahbek C, 1993: Captive breeding-a useful tool in the preservation of biodiversity. *Biodivers Conserv*. 2, 426-437.

[28] Hara H, Abdalla H, Morita H, Kuwayama M, Hirabayashi M, Hochi S, 2011: Procedure for bovine ICSI, not sperm freeze-drying, impairs the function of the microtubule-organizing center. *J Reprod Dev*. 57(3):428-432.

[29] Abu NMAR, 2010: Intracytoplasmic sperm injection-revolution in human and animal assisted reproduction: A review. Biotechnology 9(2): 392-410.

# 6

# Influence of ROS on Ovarian Functions

Francesca Ciani, Natascia Cocchia,
Danila d'Angelo and Simona Tafuri

**Abstract**

High level of ROS (Reactive Oxygen Species), due to an increased production of oxidant species and/or a decreased efficacy of antioxidant system, can lead to oxidative stress (OS) an emerging health risk factor involved in the aging and in many diseases, either in humans or in animals. ROS are a double-edged sword – they serve as key signal molecules in physiological processes, but also have a role in pathological processes involving the female reproductive tract.

ROS affect multiple physiological processes in reproduction and fertility, from oocyte maturation to fertilization, embryo development and pregnancy. Several studies indicate that follicular atresia in mammalian species due to the accumulation of toxic metabolites often results from oxidative stress. It has been suggested that ROS under moderate concentrations play a role in signal transduction processes involved in growth and protection from apoptosis. Conversely, increase of ROS levels is primarily responsible for the alteration of macromolecules, such as lipids, proteins and nucleic acids, that lead to significant damage of cell structures and thereby cause oxidative stress. To prevent damage due to ROS, cells possess a number of non-enzymatic and enzymatic antioxidants. Non-enzymatic antioxidants include vitamin C, glutathione and vitamin E. Enzymatic antioxidants consist of superoxide dismutases (MnSOD and Cu/ZnSOD) that convert superoxide into hydrogen peroxide; glutathione peroxidase (GPX) and catalase (CAT) which neutralize hydrogen peroxide. Intracellular homeostasis is ensured by the complex interaction between pro-oxidants and antioxidants.

This chapter describes gathering evidence that oxidative stress is involved in ovarian physio-pathology caused by diverse stimuli. There is strong evidence that ROS are involved in initiation of apoptosis in antral follicles caused by several chemical and physical agents, in the fluid follicular environment, influencing the folliculogenesis and the steroidogenesis. Although less attention has been focused on the roles of ROS in primordial and primary follicle death, several studies have shown protective effects of antioxidants and/or evidence of oxidative damage, suggesting that ROS may play a role in these smaller follicles as well. Oxidative damage to lipids in the oocyte has been implicated as a cause of persistently poor oocyte quality. Developing germ cells in the fetal ovary have also been shown to be sensitive to toxicants and ionizing radiation, which induce oxidative stress. Recent studies have begun to elucidate the mechanisms by which ROS mediate ovarian toxicity. It has been investigated the role of antioxidant enzymes, such as catalase, glutathione peroxidase and the SOD isoforms in maintaining low levels of oxidative stress.

The literature provides some evidence of oxidative stress influencing the entire reproductive cycle. OS plays a role in multiple physiological processes from oocyte maturation to fertilization and embryo development. An increasing number of published studies have pointed towards increased importance of the role of OS in female reproduction. Of course, there is much to learn about this topic, whereby it cannot be underestimated.

**Keywords:** Assisted reproductive technologies (ART), reactive oxygen species, ovary functions

## 1. Introduction

High level of ROS (Reactive Oxygen Species), due to an increased production of oxidant species and/or a decreased efficacy of antioxidant system, can lead to oxidative stress (OS) an emerging health risk factor involved in the aging and in many diseases, either in humans or in animals. ROS are a double-edged sword – they serve as key signal molecules in physiological processes, but also have a role in pathological processes involving the female reproductive tract.

ROS affect multiple physiological processes in reproduction and fertility, from oocyte maturation to fertilization, embryo development and pregnancy. Several studies indicate that follicular atresia in mammalian species due to the accumulation of toxic metabolites often results from oxidative stress. It has been suggested that ROS under moderate concentrations play a role in signal transduction processes involved in growth and protection from apoptosis. Conversely, increase of ROS levels is primarily responsible for the alteration of macromolecules, such as lipids, proteins and nucleic acids, that lead to significant damage of cell structures and thereby cause oxidative stress. To prevent damage due to ROS, cells possess a number of non-enzymatic and enzymatic antioxidants. Non-enzymatic antioxidant include vitamin C, glutathione and vitamin E. Enzymatic antioxidants consist of superoxide dismutases (MnSOD and Cu/ZnSOD) that convert superoxide into hydrogen peroxide; glutathione peroxidase (GPX) and catalase (CAT) which neutralize hydrogen peroxide. Intracellular homeostasis is ensured by the complex interaction between pro-oxidants and antioxidants.

This chapter describes gathering evidence that oxidative stress is involved in ovarian physiopathology caused by diverse stimuli. There is strong evidence that ROS are involved in initiation of apoptosis in antral follicles caused by several chemical and physical agents, in the fluid follicular environment, influencing the folliculogenesis and the steroidogenesis. Although less attention has been focused on the roles of ROS in primordial and primary follicle death, several studies have shown protective effects of antioxidants and/or evidence of oxidative damage, suggesting that ROS may play a role in these smaller follicles as well. Oxidative damage to lipids in the oocyte has been implicated as a cause of persistently poor oocyte quality. Developing germ cells in the fetal ovary have also been shown to be sensitive to toxicants and ionizing radiation, which induce oxidative stress. Recent studies have begun to elucidate the mechanisms by which ROS mediate ovarian toxicity. It has been investigated the role of antioxidant enzymes, such as catalase, glutathione peroxidase and the SOD isoforms in maintaining low levels of oxidative stress.

The literature provides some evidence of oxidative stress influencing the entire reproductive cycle. OS plays a role in multiple physiological processes from oocyte maturation to fertilization and embryo development. An increasing number of published studies have pointed towards increased importance of the role of OS in female reproduction. Of course, there is much to learn about this topic, whereby it cannot be underestimated.

## 2. Follicular development and ovary functions

The study of folliculogenesis and factors involved in its function is important in order to develop techniques able to increase the effectiveness of therapies or biotechniques included in assisted reproductive technologies (ART).

The follicle and oocyte development in mammals starts in fetal life. Briefly the primordial germinal cells undergo to mitosis until the ovogonias formed become primary oocytes. The meiotic development starts and at the birth the progression stops to the diplotene phase of the first meiotic division [1]. It will continue at the puberty. During the period of meiosis interruption the chromosomes become relaxed and nuclear structure so formed is named germinal vescicle (GV). At the puberty the GV disappears, the chromatin is recondensed, the pairs of homologous chromosomes are separated and half of them are expelled forming the first polar body. At this point the meiosis is interrupted again (metaphase II - MII). In this moment the oocyte is mature and fertile [2-4]. Luteinizing hormone (LH) is responsible of resumption of meiosis [5, 6]. The oocytes included in primordial follicles form a finite stock which leave this stage just when they are stimulated [7]. However, it was found that young adult rats have mitotic activity in germinative cells in order to maintain the follicular pool. The mechanisms involved in growing are not yet known [8].

During folliculogenesis the ovarian steroids, estradiol (E2) and progesterone (P), and the peptide hormone, inhibin, are synthesized in the granulosa cells and theca cells. These hormones feed back to regulate the synthesis and secretion of GnRH, LH, and FSH. The majority of ovarian follicles do not ovulate, but undergo an apoptotic process of degeneration called atresia at the small antral follicle stage [9].

Growth of the antral follicles, in most cases, can be divided into two phases. In the first phase, characterized by slow growth stage, early growth of follicles can be attributed to an increase in the number of granulose cells and therefore an increase in the surface of the granulose layer [10]; this stage is critical for the development of oocyte capacity, in which it reaches the final size and competence [11, 12]. In the second phase, characterized by fast growth, in follicles larger than 2-5 mm, follicular growth appears to result from antrum development rather than an increase of the number of granulosa cells. This exponential increase in the antrum surface extends up to a possible ovulation of this follicle [13]. Modest are the information about the endocrine dependence or influence on the growth of small antral follicles. Several were the experiments performed to determine which hormone(s) is involved in this process. In cows, the immunization of GnRH, hence inactivation of the hormone, demonstrated that the first stage of the antral follicular growth can occur in an environment characterized by basal levels of follicle stimulation hormone (FSH) and without luteinizing hormone (LH) pulses [14-16]. It has not been demonstrated how the growth of small antral follicles is possible under basal levels of FSH. In mice the follicular wall is not responsive to FSH up to follicles develop from pre-antral stage to small antral follicles [17]. In any case, the second phase is absolutely under FSH control and adequate pulse of LH [18]. Stimulation of preovulatory follicle development in rodents via injection of equine chorionic gonadotropin (eCG, also called pregnant mare's serum gonadotropin), which has FSH and LH receptor-binding activity, followed 46–48 h later by an ovulatory dose of human chorionic gonadotropin (hCG), which has only LH receptor-binding activity, is commonly used in experiments assessing the effects of gonadotropin hormones on ovarian gene expression and other endpoints and for generating preovulatory follicles or ovulated oocytes for other studies [19].

In mammalian species, the main function of the corpus luteum (CL) is the synthesis of progesterone which is required for the establishment of a uterine environment suitable for the development of peri-implantation conceptus (embryo and associated extra-embryonic membranes) and the successful progression and maintenance of pregnancy [20]. Progesterone acts on the endometrium to regulate the synthesis of growth factors, cytokines, transport and adhesion proteins, protease inhibitors, hormones and enzymes which are primary regulators of conceptus implantation, survival and development [21]. Thus, compromised CL progesterone production Although the mechanisms of CL rescue from cell death and maintenance of progesterone production are very complex and vary among mammalian species [22], there is substantial evidence that reactive oxygen species (ROS) are key factors in determining the CL lifespan [23] and that antioxidants play significant roles in CL physiology during the oestrous/menstrual cycle [24-27]. Luteal ROS production and propagation depends upon several regulating factors, including luteal antioxidants, steroid hormones and cytokines, and their crosstalk. However, it is unknown which of these factors have the greatest contribution to CL function. In addition, the sequence of events leading to the functional and structural luteal regression at the end of the oestrous/menstrual cycle is still not clear. The scarce in-vivo reports studying the CL of rats [29], women [28] and sheep [28, 29] have shown the importance of antioxidant enzymes in the control of CL function during the peri-implantation period. As a luteal phase defect can impact fertility by preventing implantation and early conceptus development in livestock and humans, this review attempts to address the importance of ROS-scavenging antioxidant enzymes in the control of mammalian CL function and integrity [30].

## 3. Reactive Oxygen Species (ROS): Chemical and Oxidative Stress (OS)

Free radicals are believed to play an important role in regulating the metabolic activity and functioning of some organs. There is a complex interaction of the pro-oxidants (free radicals) and antioxidants, resulting in the maintenance of the intracellular homeostasis. Whenever there is an imbalance between the pro-oxidants and antioxidants, favorable to free radicals, a state of oxidative stress (OS) is initiated. It is an emerging health risk factor involved in the aging and in many diseases, either in humans or in animals. Under normal conditions, paired electrons create stable bonds in biomolecules. A free radical is defined as any species capable of independent existence that contains one or more unpaired electrons in the outer orbit, independently upon the expressed electric charge. Depending on the distribution of the charge (electron cloud) and/or of its redox potential, free radicals have a more or less marked reactivity, linked to the spontaneous tendency to exist as entities having all the electrons arranged in pairs. This state corresponds to the chemical stability. The radicals are not equally reactive, in general the increase of charge and volume ratio of free radicals is directly proportional to their reactivity, therefore, they will tend to reach their own stability stripping electrons to any chemical species with which they are in contact and oxidize them [31].

Free radicals are classified on the basis the nature of the atom to which it belongs the orbital with the unpaired electron. There are, therefore, free radicals centered on oxygen, carbon, nitrogen, or chlorine, and so on. The present chapter, however, will reference mainly to free radicals centered on the oxygen, known more simply as oxygen free radicals. The latter, in fact, besides being one of quantitatively the most important elements of living matter, as well as the primary source of life itself, through a variety of mechanisms – not last the same cellular respiration – induces continuously the formation of chemical species with reactivity characteristics.

The oxygen free radicals are included into more large family of reactive oxygen species (ROS). This term indicates a class of reactive chemical species derived from oxygen, not necessarily radical, all united by more or less marked tendency to oxidize various organic substrates (carbohydrates, lipids, amino acids, proteins, nucleotides, etc.). Classic examples of radical origin of ROS are singlet oxygen and hydroxyl radical. The ozone and hydrogen peroxide, however, are not radical reactive oxygen species.

In living organisms, ROS are generated during normal cellular metabolic activity; some exogenous agents, however, can increase production, even with direct mechanism. It is possible to identify at least five sources of primary metabolic free radicals, in relation to the cellular site mainly interested in the production of ROS: the plasma membrane, mitochondria, peroxisomes, the smooth endoplasmic reticulum (microsomes) and the cytosol. In each of these locations ROS are produced either spontaneously or as a result of reactions catalyzed by enzymes or by transition metals (eg. iron or copper) [31].

The free radicals can be generated by different mechanisms and, once formed, generally give rise to a series of chain reactions, in the course of which the radicalic site can be transferred or inactivated [31, 32].

Free radicals are mainly generated by homolytic cleavage or interaction with the transition metals. The term homolytic cleavage refers to the division of the covalent bond of a molecule as effect of the administration energy (thermal or radiant), with generation of two new chemical species, each one with an unpaired electron, distinctive element of free radicals. A classic example of homolytic cleavage is the radiolysis or photolysis of water that generates an atom of hydrogen and a hydroxyl radical. This chemical reaction is different from the ionization observed, for example, after dissolved in water molecules having at least one covalent bond polarized (eg. HCl). In this case, the water molecules, because of their polarity and without any administration of energy, are able to crack one of the polarized covalent bonds of the molecule solute generating two chemical species loaded of opposite sign, a cation and an anion ($H^+$ and $Cl^-$, respectively, in the example considered). The ionization, unlike the homolytic cleavage, the doublet electronic binding of the original molecule is not separated but remains in one of the new ionic species (anion) [33].

In the interaction with the transition metals, the electron generated by oxidation of a metal transition in ionic form (eg. from $Fe^{2+}$ to $Fe^{3+}$ or $Cu^+$ to $Cu^{2+}$) breaks a covalent bond to a target molecule generating a radical free and an anion. Alternatively, the electron required for reducing a transition metal in ionic form (eg. from $Fe^{3+}$ to $Fe^{2+}$ or $Cu^{2+}$ to $Cu^+$) is extracted from the covalent binding of a target molecule, which is decomposed into a free radical and a cation. Through this mechanism, for example, iron ($Fe^{2+}$/$Fe3^+$) or copper ($Cu^+$/$Cu^{2+}$) act as catalysts in a sequence of redox reactions generating alkoxy radicals (RO*) and peroxyl (R-O-O*) from peroxides (R-O-O-R). In the simplest case - described for the first time by Fenton - one ferrous ion ($Fe^{2+}$), oxidizes to ferric ion ($Fe^{2+}$), transfers its electron to a molecule of hydrogen peroxide ($H_2O_2$) and it breaks one of covalent bonds, generating a free radical (the hydroxyl radical, HO*) and an anion (hydroxyl ion). In turn, the ferric ion ($Fe^{3+}$) is reduced - regenerating as any catalyst – to ferrous ion ($Fe^{2+}$), ripping an electron from a second molecule of hydrogen peroxide, which is split into a free radical (radical perhydroxyl (HOO*), and a cation (a hydrogen ion, $H^+$). Similarly, the hydroperoxides are split, for catalytic action of the iron, in the radical alkoxyl (RO*) and peroxyl (ROO*). In the absence of catalysts, the split of peroxides - which gives rise to a single species radical, the alkoxy - can take place only with energy consumption. A method of great biological relevance that gives rise to the formation of free radicals, includes the decomposition of nitrocompounds. In fact, alkyl radicals originate following the removal of molecular nitrogen ($N_2$) [31].

Once a radical reaction is triggered, it tends to propagate chain. There are four basic mechanisms of propagation of radical reactions: transfer, addition, fragmentation and rearrangement. The most common among these is the transfer. In this mode, the free radical - generated by one of previous reactions - attacks a molecule subtracting to it one of its atoms (generally a hydrogen atom). The result is the formation of a new reactive species and, in practice, radical site has been transferred. With this mechanism, for example, the hydroxyl radical (HO*), attacking an organic molecule (R-H), rips to this one atom of hydrogen and generates, with a molecule of water ($H_2O$), an alkyl radical (R*). With this mechanism, the radical site is transferred from the hydroxyl radical to the alkyl one.

Finally, a radical reaction chain may stop (term) by two mechanisms: combination or disproportion. In particular, in the combination, which is the homolytic cleavage of the reverse reaction, two radicals react with each other giving rise to a molecule not more reactive. The first radical acts as the oxidant, while the second acts as a generic antioxidant. This mechanism is exploited to block a radical reaction, and in general, any radical process chain can be interrupted by the intervention of agents called, generically, antioxidants.

In living organisms ROS are generated during normal cellular metabolic activity; some exogenous agents, however, may increase production, even with direct mechanism (figure 1).

As mentioned above, it is possible to identify at least 5 of primary metabolic free radical sources, in relation to cellular site: the plasma membrane, the mitochondria, peroxisomes, smooth endoplasmic reticulum (microsomes) and the cytosol (figure 2).

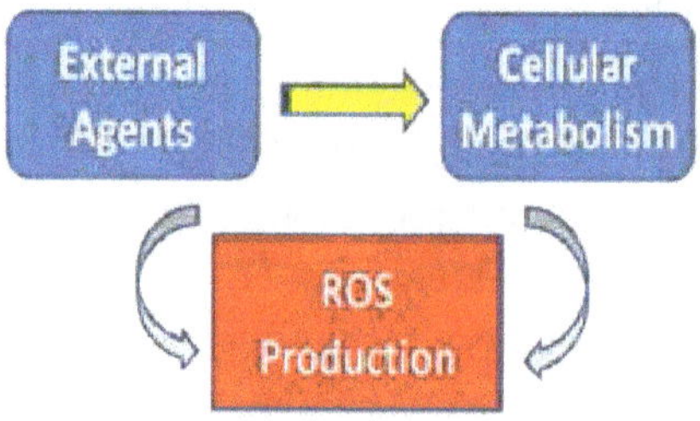


**Figure 1.** General mechanism of ROS production.

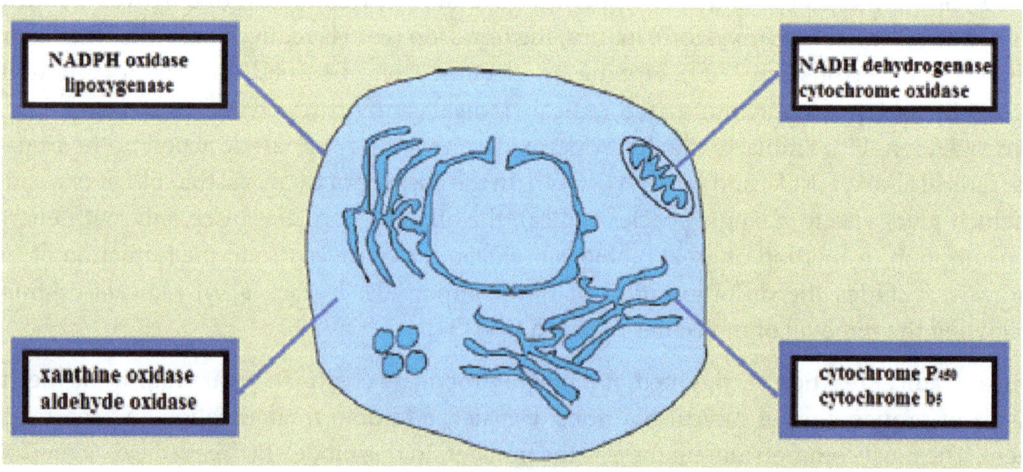


**Figure 2.** Primary source of ROS cell production

The plasma membrane is one of the most important sources of ROS, particularly (but not exclusively) in polymorphonuclear leukocytes (PMNs). In fact, in the plasma membrane of PMNs are located several enzymes, such as the NADPH oxidase and lipoxygenase, whose activation is accompanied by the production, respectively, of superoxide anion and metabolic intermediates with chemical characteristics of peroxides. The NADPH oxidase is an enzyme that catalyzes the formation of superoxide anion by NADPH ($H^+$) and molecular oxygen, after specific stimulation of PMNs, due, for example, to endotoxins, bacteria, or antibodies).

The reaction is made possible by the increased availability of NADPH ($H^+$), for the increased oxidation of glucose through the shunt of hexoses, and of molecular oxygen, under the so-called "respiratory burst". The system of lipoxygenase, localized also at the level of the plasma membrane, includes three enzymes, the 5-, 12-, and 15- lipoxygenase, which catalyze the formation, from arachidonic acid, of 5-, 12-, and 15-HPETE (hydroperoxyeicosatetraenoic acid), respectively. These substances are chemically hydroperoxides acids, theybelong to a group of ROS named ROM (reactive oxygen metabolites, ie metabolites or derived reactive oxygen). The production of ROS at the level of PMNs plasma membrane for activation NADPH oxidase and/or lipoxygenase, takes place, typically, in the course of reactive processes (eg. infections, immunoreactions pathogenic, inflammation) [31].

The mitochondria are the primary metabolic source of ROS because the enzyme complexes of respiratory chain are localized on their crests and are involved in oxidative phosphorylation. Ideally, the transfer of electrons from reduced NAD to cytochrome C and from the latter to oxygen should end with the production of $H_2O$, once synthesized ATP, (reduction tetravalent of molecular oxygen). However, already in normal conditions, this process is not perfect so, for not easily controllable reasons, a certain amount of electrons (1-2%) escapes the system transport of various coenzymes (eg. ubiquinone, flavoproteins, cytochromes, etc.) and reacts directly with molecular oxygen, generating, thus, superoxide anion and/or hydrogen peroxide (reduction uni- and bivalent molecular oxygen). In fact, this process, during a intense exercise in skeletal muscle, this electronic shunt can reach 15% of the oxygen used by mitochondria due to the intense stimulation of cellular metabolism. The phenomenon of the reduction in one or bivalent molecular oxygen takes place, in the mitochondria, without the intervention of enzymes, as opposed to what is observed in other cell locations. In other words, from a purely chemical point of view, the production of free radicals during oxidative phosphorylation is not just a mode of enzymatic production of reactive species. In fact, as it has just been mentioned, the generation of free radicals in living organisms is closely related to vital phenomena and, therefore, constitutes a "physiological" phenomenon that takes place continuously in the course of redox reactions through both enzymatic and non-enzymatic mechanisms. It should be stressed that, in addition to mitochondria, there are other sources of non-enzymatic free radicals in cells. For example, peroxynitrite spontaneously generates hydroxyl and nitroxide radicals. However, the most important non-enzymatic reactions from a biological standpoint for the production of free radicals are those catalyzed by transition metals. In these reactions, which generally require iron or copper in the reduced state (respectively $Fe^{2+}$ and $Cu^+$), hydrogen peroxide is split into hydroxyl radical and hydroxyl ion for incorporation of the electron ripped to transition metal, which is released in the oxidized form ($Fe^{3+}$ and $Cu^{2+}$, respectively), according to the mechanism discussed above of the interaction with transition metals. Hydroperoxides undergo a similar reaction, which generate the alkoxy radical. The enzymes that regenerate the transition metals in the reduced state constitute a complex indicated with MCO (metal-catalyzed oxidation systems). They include xanthine oxidase, NADPH and NADH oxidase, nicotinic acid hydroxylase, the cytochrome P450 system, the NADH reductase (with coenzyme quinone), the succinic-reductase (with coenzyme quinone) and an amount of iron-sulfur proteins non-heme. The quinones and reduced flavin prosthetic groups generated by these enzymes in their turn reduce the transition metals, resulting in the direct reduction of molecular oxygen to hydroxyl radical and/or peroxide hydrogen (through the mediation or not of superoxide anion).

In addition to the plasma membrane and mitochondria, peroxisomes also represent an important source of ROS. In these cell organelles, in fact, a particular process of fatty acid oxidation takes place, which is different from the conventional way (beta-oxidation). In the first stage of this sequence of reactions, a flavoprotein extracts a pair of hydrogen atoms from one molecule of activated fatty acid (acyl-CoA) by transferring it directly to molecular oxygen, with the formation of hydrogen peroxide (subsequently inactivated by catalase).

In the endoplasmic reticulum (microsomes) production of reactive species passes through the cytochrome P450. The latter plays a major role in detoxification processes. The cytochrome P450 acts as immediate donor of electrons in many reactions of hydroxylation, particularly those that take place within the hepatocytes and that are aimed to inactivation of hormones (eg. steroid) and not physiological compounds (xenobiotics, such as toxic and hydrophobic drugs which are thereby made more soluble and less toxic). The P450 is a heme iron protein localized not only in the endoplasmic reticulum of the liver but also in the mitochondria of the adrenal cortex that, in a process very complex and not yet fully clarified, acts as connection between NADPH ($H^+$) (electron donor) and the substrate that should be hydroxyled. In this complex reaction, a substrate able to be hydroxylated (SH) reacts with NADPH ($H^+$) and molecular oxygen ($O_2$) to form the corresponding hydroxylated derivative (S-OH), plus NADP $^+$ and water. A production of free radicals in the cell also occurs in the course of many other biochemical reactions, such as during oxidation of hypoxanthine to xanthine and xanthine to uric acid, which mark the final phase of the catabolism of purine nucleotides. Both of these reactions are catalyzed by xanthine dehydrogenase, a molybdenum enzyme. Under special conditions, such as during the so-called ischemia-reperfusion, xanthine dehydrogenase is converted to xanthine oxidase (probably for proteolytic cleavage calcium-dependent). The latter, using as a final electron acceptor the oxygen, generates hydrogen peroxide and superoxide anion, starting, respectively, from hypoxanthine and xanthine.

Other reactions that generate free radicals are described in the synthesis of catecholamines.

From the above, it is clear that ROS represent intermediate obligated cellular metabolism. And since their production is closely linked to the vital phenomena, they have been called "irreplaceable companions" of our existence.

It appears evident that in each cell site, the production of reactive species has its own specific function. In fact, it has been recognized that ROS play an important role "in the service of life" because they are not only involved in cell metabolism but also in the "reactive processes" such as infection and inflammation. Actually, the superoxide anion and other ROS are generated on the outer surface of the plasma membrane of activated leukocytes. These reactive species attack extraneous components such as bacteria, weakening the wall and making them more readily accessible to phagocytosis and, ultimately, to their destruction. These "immunological" activities are expressed not only in respect of extraneous components but also against "self" components, such as tissues or transplanted organs (rejection reaction). This strategy is also used in the course of healing of organs or tissues subject to trauma. In fact, the leukocytes migrate to the injured, are activated and begin bombing damaged cells with free radicals, that accelerate their destruction, remove lysis products, and promote the recovery (regeneration). The production of free radicals by the cells may sometimes undergo a considerable increase depending on external stimuli. In fact, physical, chemical and biological agents, alone or in combination, may also induce the generation of ROS or increase the "physiological" production through a specific metabolic stimulation. Ionizing and UV radiation are reported to be physical agents. Both these sources of energy can induce the phenomenon of homolytic cleavage of water, also called radiolysis or photolysis, depending on the type of radiation involved.

In this reaction, the water molecule absorbs energy and uses it to break one of its two covalent bonds with the hydrogen: the products will be two free radicals, the hydroxyl radical and the hydrogen atom. Considering that a living organism is made up primarily of water and he spends most of his life under the influence of radiation (UV or ionizing they are) it is clear how this phenomenon affects substantially the production of free radicals.

As chemical agent, capable of stimulating the production of free radicals, ozone (ROS) is to be quoted. It directly generates peroxyl radicals by interaction with phenolic compounds. The two cases considered so far (radiation and ozone) are examples of direct production of reactive species. Other chemical agents, however, such as polycyclic aromatic hydrocarbons, or certain drugs, induce increased production of free radicals through an indirect mechanism, activating the cytochrome P450 microsomal level. Biological agents that typically lead to increased production of ROS for metabolic activation are bacteria, as part of the physiological process of defense against infection, and certain antibodies, as part of some reactions immune-pathogen. In these cases, as mentioned with regard to the plasma membrane, the PMNs are directly implicate. They, in fact, possess NADPH oxidase and a series of enzymes directly involved in the production and, in part, inactivation of reactive chemical species, such as superoxide dismutase (SOD), myeloperoxidase (MPx), catalase (CAT) and glutathione peroxidase (GPx).

SOD catalyzes the conversion of superoxide anion into hydrogen peroxide which, in turn, can be inactivated to water by CAT or GPx. However, the availability of chlorides - even at physiological concentrations - makes the hydrogen peroxide a substrate for MPx. The end result is the production of a highly oxidising agent, the hypochlorous acid (HClO). The HClO can attack numerous organic substrates and, in particular, amino acids and proteins, to produce chloramines, a potential source of alkoxyl and peroxyl radicals. Finally, an increase in free radical production may be observed in "physiological " situations, such as after an intense muscular effort or in the course of many diseases. In the latter case, often, it is not clear how far the ROS are the cause or the effect of a certain pathology [31].

## 4. The antioxidant defense system

ROS are chemical species potentially detrimental. For this reason, living organisms have developed over millennia of evolution a complex antioxidant defense system, consisting of a set of enzymes, vitamins, trace elements and other vitamin-like substances. These antioxidants may be classified according to different criteria: on the basis of the origin, in endogenous and exogenous, on the basis of the chemical nature, in the enzymatic and non-enzymatic, and on the basis of the solubility in fat-soluble and water-soluble. On the basis, however, of the mechanism of action prevalent, physiological antioxidants can be easily assembled into four main groups: preventive antioxidants, scavenger, shelter agents and adaptation agents [34].

Preventive antioxidants are agents that, through various mechanisms, such as the chelation of transition metals, prevent the formation of reactive species.

The scavengers act through different mechanisms. They may be of hydrophilic nature (albumin, urate, ascorbate, urate) or lipophilic (carotenoids, vitamin E, ubiquinol). According to some researchers, the scavenger should be distinguished from antioxidants proper. In fact, while the scavenger (eg. A-tocopherol) are agents that reduce the concentration of free radicals removing them from the medium in which they are located, antioxidants (eg. Diphenylamine) are agents that inhibit the auto-oxidation process, e.g. the fat rancidity. This phenomenon, well known in food science, is called auto-oxidation since it occurs through a sequence of autocatalytic radical reactions in the presence of oxygen. Alternatively, you can use the term peroxidation, as the same process generates intermediates with characteristics of peroxides (R-O-OR).

Through this process some dietary fat rancid and cellular membranes of living organisms are oxidized.

Shelter agents include only enzymes involved after the damage from reactive species has been established. Their action - often sequential - provides first the identification of the molecular segment oxidized, then the separation of the fragment unusable and, finally, the synthesis and the insertion of a new segment in substitution of the damaged one. The category of shelter antioxidants includes hydrolases (glycosidases, lipases, proteases), and the transferase and polymerases, all essential for the repair of free radical damage of important molecules or cellular structures (eg. DNA, membranes, etc.).

Finally, the agents of adaptation include all substances or techniques or procedures through which it is possible to strengthen the physiological antioxidant system of an organism. For example, a proper physical exercise or the adoption of a proper and balanced diet are measures by itself able to check the oxidative metabolism by reducing the production of reactive species, and induction of enzymes with antioxidant activity.

The antioxidant defense system is regularly distributed in the body, both at the extracellular and intracellular levels.

In plasma, the set of substances potentially able to give equivalent reducing (hydrogen atoms or single electrons) so as to meet "the greed of electrons" that makes free radical constitutes unstable is the so-called barrier antioxidant. In the plasma, all protein and, in particular, albumin, bilirubin, uric acid, cholesterol, and various exogenous antioxidants introduced with food or in the form of dietary supplements (ascorbate, tocopherol, polyphenols etc.) are part of it. The thiol groups (-SH), commonly found in the cysteine side chain, play a role of particular importance in the context of this barrier. In addition, thiol groups, are the most chemically reactive sites on proteins, such as albumin, and have strong reducing properties [35, 36].

Inside the cells, the antioxidant system of cell defense has its precise compartmentalization (figure 3). The antioxidant system includes some enzymes (glutathione, superoxide dismutase, catalase) and a series of substances taken from outside (vitamins and substances similar to antioxidant activity, such as polyphenols, trace elements etc.). Some of these agents are fat-soluble (eg. tocopherols) and, entering the team of biomembranes, constitute the first line of defense against the attack of free radicals. Others, however, are water soluble (eg. ascorbate) and intervene especially in the context of soluble matrix of the cytoplasm and cellular organelles.

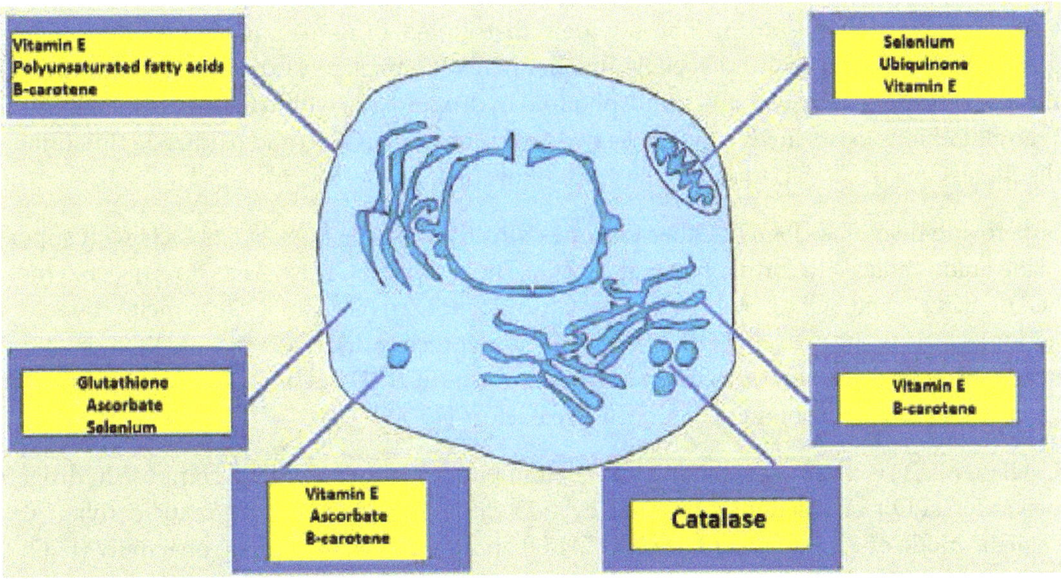


**Figure 3.** Compartmentalization of antioxidant system

Glutathione (GSH) is a tripeptide (L-g-glutamyl-L-cysteinyl-glycine, with multiple biological functions and that has been found in all mammalian cells [37-39]. Its biological activity is primarily related to the active thiol group of the cysteine residue [40]. The reduced and oxidized forms of glutathione (GSH and GSSG) act in concert with other redox-active compounds (e.g., NAD(P)H) to regulate and maintain cellular redox status. It is an abundant low-molecular-mass thiol antioxidant, which either interacts directly with reactive oxygen and nitrogen species (ROS and RNS, respectively) or serves as a cofactor for many antioxidant and associated enzymes such as peroxidases and transferases [41]. The chemical structure of GSH determines its potential functions and its broad distribution among all living organisms reflects its important biological role Probably most importantly, GSH is responsible for protection against ROS and RNS, and detoxification of endogenous and exogenous toxins of an electrophilic nature. Depletion of GSH results in DNA damage and increased $H_2O_2$ concentrations; as such, GSH is an essential antioxidant. During the reduction of $H_2O_2$ to $H_2O$ and $O_2$, GSH is oxidized to GSSG by glutathione peroxidase (GPx). Glutathione reductase participates in the reverse reaction, and utilizes the transfer of a donor proton from NADPH to GSSG, thus, recycling GSH [42]. Vitamin E ($\alpha$-tocopherol) protects GPx4-deficient cells from cell death. In addition, glutathione is (1) a storage form of cysteine in the cells and for interorgan transfer; (2) a storage form and transporter of nitric oxide (as GSNO); (3) involved in the metabolism of estrogens, leukotrienes, and prostaglandins, reduction of ribonucleotides to deoxyribonucleotides, and maturation of iron–sulfur clusters of proteins; (4) involved in the regulation of certain transcription factors from the environment to cellular transcription machinery; (5) involved in the detoxification of many endogenous compounds and xenobiotics (the mercapturate pathway); and (6) copper and iron transfer. Glutathione also can be used even for the detoxification of ions of transition metals such as chromium [43, 44].

Five isoforms of glutathione peroxidase exist in the body: GPx1, GPx2, GPx3, GPx4, and GPx5. GPx1 is the cytosolic isoform that is widely distributed in tissues, while GPx2 encodes a gastrointestinal form with no specific function; GPx3 is present in plasma and epididymal fluid. GPx 4 specifically detoxifies phospholipid hydroperoxide within biological membranes. Free glutathione exists in vivo mostly as two forms, reduced (GSH) and oxidized (glutathione disulfide; GSSG). GPx5 is found in the epididymis [39].

Superoxide dismutase (SOD): Other enzymes directly detoxify ROS. SOD reacts with superoxide anion radicals to form oxygen and $H_2O_2$. The enzyme SOD exists as three isoenzymes: SOD 1, SOD 2, and SOD 3. SOD 1 contains Cu and zinc (Zn) (Cu, Zn-SOD) as metal co-factors and is located in the cytosol. SOD 2 (Mn-SOD) is a mitochondrial isoform containing manganese (Mn), and SOD 3 encodes the extracellular form (ECSOD). SOD 3 is structurally similar to Cu, Zn-SOD, as it contains Cu and Zn as cofactors [45, 46].

Catalase (CAT) is a heme-containing homotetrameric protein. CAT can decompose hydrogen peroxide ($H_2O_2$) in reactions catalyzed by two different modes of enzymatic activity: the catalatic mode of activity ($2H_2O_2 \rightarrow O_2 + 2H_2O$) and the peroxidatic mode of activity ($H_2O_2 + AH_2 \rightarrow A + 2H_2O$). Although several substrates such as methanol and ethanol can be oxidized by the peroxidation reaction, the physiological significance of this catalase function is not understood. Decomposition of $H_2O_2$ by the catalatic activity of catalase follows the fashion of a first-order reaction, and its rate is dependent on the concentration of $H_2O_2$. In fact, catalase belongs to the group of enzymes that catalyze reactions at a rate near kinetic perfection; the reaction rate is only limited by the rate at which the enzyme collides with the substrate. Catalase is ubiquitously present in all prokaryotes and eukaryotes. With the exception of erythrocytes, it is predominantly located in peroxisomes of all types of mammalian cells where $H_2O_2$ is generated by various oxidases. However, a certain amount of catalase has also been found in mitochondria of rat heart. Since $H_2O_2$ serves as a substrate for Fenton reaction to generate the highly reactive hydroxyl radical, catalase is believed to play a role in cellular antioxidant defense mechanisms by limiting the accumulation of $H_2O_2$ [47-49].

The non-enzymatic antioxidants consist of dietary supplements and synthetic antioxidants such as vitamin C, GSH, taurine, hypotaurine, vitamin E, Zn, selenium (Se), betacarotene, and carotene [41]. Vitamin C (ascorbic acid) is a known redox catalyst that can reduce and neutralize ROS. Its reduced form is maintained through reactions with GSH and can be catalyzed by protein disulfide isomerase and glutaredoxins. Glutathione is a peptide found in most forms of aerobic life as it is made in the cytosol from cysteine, glutamate, and glycine [42]; it is also the major nonenzymatic antioxidant found in oocytes and embryos. Its antioxidant properties stem from the thiol group of its cysteine component, which is a reducing agent that allows it to be reversibly oxidized and reduced to its stable form [42]. Levels of GSH are regulated by its formation de-novo, which is catalyzed by the enzymes gamma-GCS and glutathione synthetase [4, 11]. Glutathione participates in reactions, including the formation of glutathione disulfide, which is transformed back to GSH by glutathione reductase at the expense of NADPH [17].

Cysteine and cysteamine (CSH) increase the GSH content of the oocyte. Cysteamine also acts as a scavenger and is an antioxidant essential for the maintenance ofhigh GSH levels. Furthermore, CSH can be converted to another antioxidant, hypotaurine [43, 44].

The concentrations of many amino acids, including taurine, fluctuate considerably during folliculogenesis. Taurine and hypotaurine are scavengers that help maintain redox homeostasis in gametes. Both neutralize lipid peroxidation products, and hypotaurine further neutralizes hydroxyl radicals [44].

Like GSH, the Thioredoxin (Trx) system regulates gene functions and coordinates various enzyme activities. It detoxifies $H_2O_2$ and converts it to its reduced state via Trx reductase [45]. Normally, Trx is bound to apoptosis-regulating signal kinase (ASK) 1, rendering it inactive. However, when the thiol group of Trx is oxidized by the SO anion, ASK1 detaches from Trx and becomes active leading to enhanced apoptosis. ASK1 can also be activated by exposure to $H_2O_2$ or hypoxiareoxygenation, and inhibited by vitamins C and E. The Trx system also plays a role in female reproduction and fetal development by being involved in cell growth, differentiation, and death. Incorrect protein folding and formation of disulfide bonds can occur through $H^+$ ion release from the thiol group of cysteine, leading to disordered protein function, aggregation, and apoptosis [2].

Vitamin E ($\alpha$-tocopherol) is a lipid soluble vitamin with antioxidant activity. It consists of eight tocopherols and tocotrienols. It plays a major role in antioxidant activities because it reacts with lipid radicals produced during lipid peroxidation [42]. This reaction produces oxidized $\alpha$-tocopheroxyl radicals that can be transformed back to the active reduced form by reacting with other antioxidants like ascorbate, retinol, or ubiquinol.

The hormone melatonin is an antioxidant that, unlike vitamins C and E and GSH, is produced by the human body. In contrast to other antioxidants, however, melatonin cannot undergo redox cycling; once it is oxidized, melatonin is unable to return to its reduced state because it forms stable end-products after the reaction occurs (see below for functions).

## 5. Commonly used markers of ROS-induced modification of cellular components

It seems that despite their high chemical reactivity most generated ROS do not lead to serious negative physiological consequences for organisms. That is mainly due to the action of highly efficient systems of ROS neutralization operating in concert with reparation and elimination of ROS-modified molecules always exists, that may be called the basal steady-state (stationary) level [37, 50]. Reactive oxygen species can modify most types of biomolecules including proteins, lipids, carbohydrates, nucleic acids, metabolic intermediates, etc. It is widely accepted that the use of only one type of modification to assess oxidative damage during oxidative stress is not sufficient. That is due to the different sensitivity, dynamics, and nature of ROS-promoted modifications. Instead, in order to evaluate the intensity of ROS-involving processes, several approaches for the evaluation of particular oxidatively modified molecules have been selected. They reflect the level of products of interaction between ROS and cellular components of different natures. "Classically", several essential markers are used. They are: (*i*) for lipids – the formation of malonic dialdehyde (MDA), isopsoralens, and lipid peroxides; (*ii*) for proteins – protein carbonyl groups; and (*iii*) for DNA – 8-oxoguanine. Malonic dialdehyde is commonly measured via its reaction with thiobarbituric acid (TBA). However, this reaction is not specific and many other compounds react with TBA under the assay conditions. The array of products formed is collectively called thiobarbituric acid reactive substances (TBARS) to reflect this low specificity. Certain amino acids, carbohydrates, aldehydes and other compounds interfere with the reaction measurement and, therefore, this method should be used with precaution and discussed taking into account the highlighted issues [50]. In the last decade, an HPLC technique was applied to evaluate MDA levels and this method, along with immunochemical identification [51] can now be recommended as more reliable than the TBARS assay. There are also many other approaches to evaluate the intensity of ROS induced lipid peroxidation and the measurement of lipid peroxides [51], 4-hydroxynonenal [52] are just some of them. Selection of methods depends on many things, particularly tools available [33]. Probably the most popular method for detection of ROS-modified proteins is the one based on the formation of additional carbonyl groups with their visualization due to their interaction with 2, 4-dinitrophenylhydrazine [53]. The hydrazones formed are measured spectrophotometrically. Specific antibodies that interact with carbonyl groups on proteins [54] have also been developed. In some cases, there is also the possibility to evaluate the amount of dityrosines and other products of free radical induced oxidation of proteins. Oxidation of nucleic acids also forms an array of products, but in this case there are some favorites that are relatively easy to quantify. These are mainly oxidatively modified guanine derivatives, of which 8-hydroxyguanine (8-OHG) is the most commonly used, but 8-oxo-7, 8- dihydro-2′-deoxyguanosine (8-oxodG) and 8-oxo-7, 8-dihydroguanine (8-oxoGua) can also be measured. Certainly, there are many more different markers of ROS-induced modification of cellular constituents, but those listed here are the most widely used and applied approaches.

## 6. Influence of ROS on reproductive functions

ROS affect multiple physiological processes in reproduction and fertility, from oocyte maturation to fertilization, embryo development and pregnancy. Several studies indicate that follicular atresia in mammalian species due to the accumulation of toxic metabolites often results from oxidative stress. It has been suggested that ROS under moderate concentrations play a role in signal transduction processes involved in growth and protection from apoptosis. Conversely, increase of ROS levels is primarily responsible for the alteration of macromolecules, such as lipids, proteins and nucleic acids, that lead to significant damage of cell structures and thereby cause oxidative stress. To prevent damage due to ROS, cells possess a number of nonenzymatic and enzymatic antioxidants. Nonenzymatic antioxidant include Vitamin C, glutathione, cysteamine, vitamin E. Enzymatic antioxidants consist of superoxide dismutases (MnSOD and Cu/ZnSOD, which are in the mitochondria and cytosol, respectively), that convert superoxide into hydrogen peroxide; glutathione peroxidase (GPX) and catalase (CAT) which neutralize hydrogen peroxide. Intracellular homeostasis is ensured by the complex interactions between pro-oxidants and antioxidants.

This chapter describes gathering evidence that oxidative stress is involved in ovarian physiopathology caused by diverse stimuli. There is strong evidence that ROS are involved in initiation of apoptosis in antral follicles caused by several chemical and physical agents, in the fluid follicular environment, influencing the folliculogenesis and the steroidogenesis. Although less attention has been focused on the roles of ROS in primordial and primary follicle death, several studies have shown protective effects of antioxidants and/or evidence of oxidative damage, suggesting that ROS may play a role in these smaller follicles as well. Oxidative damage to lipids in the oocyte has been implicated as a cause of persistently poor oocyte quality. Developing germ cells in the fetal ovary have also been shown to be sensitive to toxicants and ionizing radiation, which induce oxidative stress. Recent studies have begun to elucidate the mechanisms by which ROS mediate ovarian toxicity. It has been investigated the role of antioxidant enzymes, such as catalase, glutathione peroxidase and the SOD isoforms in maintaining low levels of oxidative stress.

The literature provides some evidence of oxidative stress influencing the entire reproductive cycle. OS plays a role in multiple physiological processes from oocyte maturation to fertilization and embryo development. An increasing number of published studies have pointed towards increased importance of the role of OS in female reproduction. Of course, there is much to learn about this topic, whereby it cannot be underestimated.

## 7. Role of ROS in folliculogenesis, ovulation, and corpus luteum function

The ROS should not always be coupled with negative effects [56]. Accumulating data have recently shown that reactive oxygen species can regulate cell function by controlling production or the activation of substances that have biological activities.

Numerous genes related to inflammation are induced in preovulatory follicles by the LH surge. The analogy of ovulation with an acute inflammation may suggest a role for ROS along this process. Because ROS are massively generated during the inflammatory process hypothesized that ROS could be involved in the signaling cascade leading to ovulation. The findings were that $H_2O_2$ mimicked the effect of LH, bringing about an extensive mucification/expansion of the follicle-enclosed cumulus–oocyte complexes; impaired progesterone production was observed in isolated follicles incubated with LH in the presence of antioxidant agents; furthermore, LH-stimulated up-regulation of genes, the expression of which is crucial for ovulation, was substantially attenuated upon ROS ablation. Together, these results provide evidence that ovarian production of ROS is an essential for preovulatory signaling events, most probably transiently triggered by LH [56].

The increase in steroid production in the growing follicle causes an increase in P450, resulting in ROS formation. Reactive oxygen species produced by the pre-ovulatory follicle are considered important inducers for ovulation. Oxygen deprivation stimulates follicular angiogenesis, which is important for adequate growth and development of the ovarian follicle. Follicular ROS promotes apoptosis, whereas GSH and follicular stimulating hormone (FSH) counterbalance this action in the growing follicle. Estrogen increases in response to FSH, triggering the generation of catalase in the dominant follicle, and thus avoiding apoptosis [26].

In ovaries, the corpus luteum is formed after ovulation and produces progesterone, which is necessary for the establishment and maintenance of pregnancy. When pregnancy occurs, the rescue of the corpus luteum and subsequent progesterone production are important for the maintenance of pregnancy. In contrast, when pregnancy does not occur after ovulation, the decline of progesterone production is important for the follicle development of the next reproductive cycle. The chance of conception occurring as soon as possible and as often as possible depends on how rapidly progesterone production declines. Therefore, the strategy for reproduction in the ovary is the rapid rescue of the corpus luteum when pregnancy occurs, and the rapid termination of the corpus luteum function when pregnancy does not occur after ovulation. Corpus luteum regression is defined as that the corpus luteum declines in function, decreases in volume, and thereafter disappears from the ovary. Corpus luteum regression consists of two stages of regression, functional luteolysis and structural luteolysis. Structural luteolysis is defined as structural involution of the corpus luteum, and is clearly distinguished from functional luteolysis which is characterized by depletion of progesterone production without structural changes such as loss of luteal cells and blood vessels. Rapid decline in progesterone production is important for follicle growth in the next reproductive cycle. It is therefore of interest to study the mechanism of functional luteolysis. ROS and SOD are involved in functional luteolysis. ROS are produced in the corpus luteum [26]. There are several potential sources of ROS in the corpus luteum. Macrophages and neutrophils, that are clear sources of reactive oxygen species, are well documented as residing in the corpus luteum [57-61] The increase in ROS in the corpus luteum is involved in functional luteolysis. The decrease in Cu, Zn-SOD expression could be one of the causes for the increase in reactive oxygen species in the regressing corpus luteum. It seems there is another possible mechanism able to increase ROS. PGF2$\alpha$ has been well recognized as a luteolysin since it increases in the corpus luteum during the regression phase [62] and inhibits the production of progesterone by luteal cells. A number of reports have shown so far that the inhibitory effect of PGF2$\alpha$ on progesterone production by the corpus luteum is, in part, mediated through the increase of ROS [63, 64]. ROS can activate phospholipase A2 activity and cyclooxygenase-2 expression in the corpus luteum which are key enzymes for PGF2$\alpha$ synthesis. Thus, there seems to be a close interrelation between PGF2$\alpha$ and ROS [65, 66].

Steroidogenic cells are also potential sources of reactive oxygen species because reactive oxygen species are generated as byproducts of normal metabolism. Intracellular sources of ROS include mitochondrial electron transport, endoplasmic reticulum, nuclear membrane electron transport systems and plasma membranes [67]. There is a significant co-relationship between Cu, Zn-SOD activities and serum progesterone concentrations. In contrast, lipid peroxide levels increase in the corpus luteum during the regression phase in the both rat models and show an opposite change from serum progesterone concentrations [68, 69]. Reactive oxygen species generated normally during steroidogenesis restrict the capacity of the corpus luteum to produce progesterone [70]. In pregnancy, the decrease in Cu, Zn-SOD expression causes the inhibition of progesterone production via the increase in ROS. Therefore, the increase in ability to scavenge ROS may be associated with the maintenance of luteal cell integrity and prolonged life span of the corpus luteum [71]. In other animals, such bovines, SOD and CAT have been reported to be correlated with progesterone production by the corpus luteum [72] It is plausible that the luteotropic substances, usually synthesized by placenta during pregnancy, stimulate the expression of molecules that protect luteal cells from ROS. Finally, the increase in Cu, Zn-SOD by placental luteotropins is an important mechanism to rescue the corpus luteum and maintain progesterone production [73].

Aerobic metabolism utilizing oxygen is essential for energy requirements of the gametes, and the free radicals play a significant role in physiological processes within the ovary. Many studies have demonstrated involvement of ROS in the follicular-fluid environment, folliculogenesis, and steroidogenesis [74]. The immunohistochemical distribution of the copper-zinc superoxide dismutase (Cu, Zn-SOD) in the human ovary was given by [74]. They found, for the first time, that the gestational corpus luteum, theca and granulosa lutein cells showed intensive and moderate staining activity, respectively, to Cu, Zn-SOD. Furthermore, they suggested that, as SOD catalyses the dismutation reaction of superoxide anion radicals, the theca interna cells play an important role in the protection of the developing oocyte from oxygen radicals by acting as a blood-follicular barrier during follicle maturation, [76] underlined the presence of manganese superoxide dismutase (Mn-SOD) and Cu, Zn-SOD in human ovaries and fallopian tubes, with different localizations and actions. The superoxide radical-SOD system might play an important role in ovulation and in the luteal function of the human ovary in the human ovary and fallopian tube, and to examine the role of superoxide radicals and SODs in the human ovulatory process. These enzymes can be considered as markers of cytoplasmic maturation [77].

Culture of small and large (preovulatory) antral rat follicles without gonadotropin support leads to apoptotic death within 24 h, while FSH suppresses apoptosis [78].To investigate if oxidative stress plays a role in granulosa cell apoptosis during follicular atresia in the immature rat ovary, healthy antral follicles obtained from rats were in the absence or presence of FSH, SOD, ascorbic acid (a free radical scavenger), N-acetyl-L-cysteine (a free radical scavenger and stimulator of endogenous glutathione peroxidase activity), or CAT. The results showed that each antioxidant was able to protect against apoptosis in rat large antral follicles cultured without gonadotropin support [79].

Markers of peroxidation were measured in follicular fluids and sera of women attending an in vitro fertilization (IVF), to assess the pro or anti oxidative status and the effects of the administration of antioxidants. The substances in follicular fluid were all significantly lower than those in serum, both in the presence or absence of antioxidants. In conclusion, the intensity of peroxidation in the Graafian follicle is much lower than that in serum. This gradient is the result of the lower rate of initiation of peroxidation in the follicular fluid due to, probably, the presence of efficient antioxidant defense systems in the direct milieu of the oocyte before ovulation [80].

The role of ROS and antioxidant enzymes was provided using immunohistochemical localization, mRNA expression, and thiobarbituric acid methods that suggested a complex role in ovulation and luteal function in the human ovary [80]. Oxidative stress has been shown to affect the midluteal corpus luteum and steroidogenic capacity both in vitro and in vivo. In a very interesting study, using corpora lutea collected from pregnant and nonpregnant patients, it was observed that during normal situations, Zn-SOD expression parallels the levels of progesterone, with a rise from early luteal to midluteal phase and decrease during regression of the corpus luteum. The mRNA expression, however, of Cu, Zn-SOD in the corpus luteum during pregnancy was much higher than those of midcycle corpora lutea. This factor enhanced SOD expression during pregnancy, possibly caused by increased human chorionic gonadotropin (HCG) levels, and may be the cause of apoptosis of the corpora lutea. Similarly, the antioxidant enzymes glutathione peroxidase and MnSOD are considered the markers for cytoplasmic maturation, as these are expressed only in metaphase II oocytes [6]. Decreased developmental potential of oocytes from poorly vascularized follicles has also been attributed to low intrafollicular oxygenation [8]. Studies demonstrate intensified lipid peroxidation in the preovulatory Graafian follicle and that glutathione peroxidase may help in maintaining low levels of hydroperoxides inside follicle, suggesting an important role of oxidative stress in ovarian function. Oxidative stress and inflammatory process have roles in the pathophysiology of polycystic ovarian disease and drugs such as Rosiglitazone maybe effective by decreasing the levels of oxidative stress [81].

Two groups have developed Cu, Zn-SOD null mice, and both groups reported that the female mice were subfertile; however, the mechanistic basis for the reduced fertility of female Cu, Zn-SOD null mice remains unclear. [82] reported that ovaries of adult female Cu, Zn-SOD null mice had reduced numbers of preovulatory follicles and corpora lutea. They concluded that these mice were subfertile because of a defect in late follicular development or ovulation. In contrast, [83] reported that Mn-ZnSOD null female mice had normal ovarian histology and ovulated similar numbers of ova during a natural estrous cycle but displayed increased postimplantation embryonic lethality. Perhaps the different genetic backgrounds of these two Cu, Zn-SOD knockout models accounts for these different findings. A study by [84] on copper chaperone for superoxide dismutase null mice, which have decreased ability to incorporate copper into Mn-ZnSOD, found a similar phenotype as [85], with abnormal development of antral follicles and no corpora lutea. Taken together, the evidence seems to support a role for Cu-ZnSOD in antral follicle development. Cu, Zn-SOD knockout is lethal prior to puberty. However, transplantation of ovaries from Mn-SOD knockout juvenile mice to the ovarian bursa of wild-type mice, in which the ipsilateral ovaries had been removed and the contralateral oviducts had been cut, resulted in all stages of follicular development, ovulation, and fertility, suggesting that this enzyme is not critical for ovarian function.

Superoxide, hydrogen peroxide and lipid peroxides are generated in luteal tissue during natural and prostaglandin-induced regression in the rat, and this response is associated with reversible depletion of ascorbic acid. ROS immediately uncouple the luteinizing hormone receptor from adenylate cyclase and inhibit steroidogenesis by interrupting transmitochondrial cholesterol transport. The cellular origin of oxygen radicals in regressing corpora lutea is predominantly from resident and infiltrated leukocytes, especially neutrophils. ROS are also produced within the follicle at ovulation and, as the corpus luteum, leukocytes are the major source of these products. Antioxidants block the resumption of meiosis, whereas the generation of reactive oxygen induces oocyte maturation in the follicle. Although oxygen radicals may serve important physiologic roles within the ovary, the cyclic production of these damaging agents over years may lead to an increased cumulative risk of ovarian pathology that would probably be exacerbated under conditions of reduced antioxidant status [87].

Melatonin appears to have some kinds of functions at different stages of follicle development, oocyte maturation, and luteal stage. Melatonin concentration in the growing follicle may be an important factor in avoiding atresia, because melatonin in the follicular fluid reduces apoptosis of critical cells. Melatonin also has protective actions during oocyte maturation reducing intrafollicular oxidative damage. An association between melatonin concentrations in follicular fluid and oocyte quality has been reported In the ovarian follicle, melatonin impacts the function of numerous cells, especially granulosa cells and the ovum (oocyte). The actions of melatonin in these cells are mediated via membrane receptors and also possibly via binding sites in the nucleus and in the cytosol. In addition to its receptor-mediated actions, melatonin also functions as a direct free radical scavenger to reduce oxidative stress at the level of the ovary; this beneficial action is carried out without an interaction with a receptor. Additional antioxidant functions of melatonin are achieved when the indole stimulates enzymes which metabolize free radicals to less toxic products. The antioxidative enzymes include superoxide dismutase (SOD), glutathione peroxidase (GPx) and catalase (CAT) in thecal cells, granulosa cells and in the follicular fluid. Via these actions, melatonin reduces free radical damage, which would be especially bad for the ovum, and maintains these elements in an optimally functional state. The origin of melatonin in the follicular fluid is the blood and from its local synthesis in granulosa cells [87-89].

## 8. Assisted Reproductive Techniques (ART) and ROS

Assisted reproductive techniques (ART) are advanced technological procedures, which are the treatments of choice in many cases of female and male infertility or assisted fertilization, included the use of medical techniques, such as drug therapy, artificial insemination, or in vitro fertilization, to enhance fertility. Expanded ART include any directed action taken by humans to enhance reproduction in animals, both through 1) Assisted reproduction with a technical component (mostly mammals), 2) assisted reproduction using various forms of population management. The two are not mutually exclusive.

ART include:

1. Artificial Insemination
2. Embryo transfer
3. In vitro fertilization
4. Semen/embryo sexing
5. Intra cytoplasm sperm injection (ICSI)
6. Gamete/embryo micromanipulation
7. Somatic cell nuclear transfer (SCNT)
8. Genome resource banking.

They function, in humans, as an alternative to overcome causative factors of infertility, such as endometriosis, tubal factor infertility, male factor infertility. They can be used in the veterinary field also [90]. ART, in fact, were recently accepted into the programs for the safeguard of endangered species from extinction [90-93]. In a feasible program it is necessary proceed in the following five steps: 1) Technique development in a domestic animal counterpart, if available; 2) characterization of species-specific reproductive biology in a targeted non-domestic animal; 3) assessment of technique feasibility for producing offspring; 4) demonstration of adequate efficiency for applied usage; 5) application of new tool for population management [90] Figs 4, 5, and 6 show cumulus oocyte complexes (COCs) from mare explanted ovaries: these tools are employed in ART to have genetic improvement in horses,

Oxidative stress is involved in ovarian physio-pathology caused by diverse stimuli caused by several chemical and physical agents: ROS are involved in initiation of apoptosis in antral follicles in the fluid follicular environment, influencing the folliculogenesis and the steroidogenesis. ROS may play a role in these smaller follicles as well. Oxidative damage to lipids in the oocyte has been implicated as a cause of persistently poor oocyte quality. Developing germ cells in the fetal ovary have also been shown to be sensitive to toxicants and ionizing radiation, which induce oxidative stress. Recent studies have begun to elucidate the mechanisms by which ROS mediate ovarian toxicity. It has been investigated the role of antioxidant enzymes, such as catalase, glutathione peroxidase and the SOD isoforms in maintaining low levels of oxidative stress [46]. It was demonstrated for the first time by [94] that high oxygen concentration compromises nuclear maturation rates and worsens the oxidative stress during in vitro maturation (IVM) of canine oocytes.

Incubated oocytes showed severely high quantities of superoxide dismutase (SOD), glutathione reductase (GSR), glutathione peroxidase (GPX1) and catalase (CAT) mRNA and this effect results in a protective mechanism against oxidative stress [95].

[45] studied the effect of ovary transport media supplementation with SOD on ovarian cell viability and apoptosis and in vitro embryo production (IVEP). They proposed, as mechanism of action, the intervention of SOD in inactivating the atmospheric $O_2$, potential deleterious precursor of free radicals.

With IVF, sperm-oocyte interaction occurs in culture media, leading to fertilization [32]. Reactive oxygen species may develop as a consequence of increased oocyte number per dish, spermatozoa, and cumulus cell mass. Cumulus cells demonstrate higher antioxidant activity at the beginning of culture than denuded oocytes do [96]. In ICSI, a single sperm is injected into an oocyte's cytoplasm [142]. It bypasses natural selection, thus allowing for the injection of damaged spermatozoon into the oocyte. Alternatively, the IVF process prevents fertilization by DNA-damaged spermatozoa [97].

Recently, OS has been identified as an important factor in ART success. Oocyte metabolism and a lack of antioxidants combined with the follicular and oviductal fluid of the embryo causes an increase in ROS levels [384]. Follicular fluid is the net result of both the transfer of plasma constituents to follicles and the secretory activity of granulose and theca cells [385]. The oocyte develops within the FF environment and this intimately affects the quality of oocytes and their interaction with sperm, thus affecting implantation and embryonic development [98]. Oxidative stress contributes to oocyte quality, and its degree can be assessed by biomarkers of lipid peroxidation [99]. The effects of OS may be may be further altered by environmental factors. A hyperoxic environment augments SO radical levels by promoting enzyme activity. Particularly in IVF, increased incubation time heightens exposure to O2 concentration [100]. As in biological systems, metallic cations act as exogenous sources of OS by stimulating ROS formation in ART culture media, and metal chelators such as EDTA and transferrin can ameliorate the production of ROS [43]. Furthermore, visible light can cause ROS formation, thereby damaging DNA [101]. Fertilization success in ART is determined by the quality of spermatozoa involved [32]. Although ROS contribute to normal sperm functions such as oocyte fusion, capacitation, and acrosome reaction, OS produced by spermatozoa may provoke oxidative damage to the oocyte, decreasing the likelihood for fertilization [81].

The in vitro environment exposes gametes and embryos to an excess of ROS with the absence of enzymatic antioxidant protection normally present during in vivo fertilization and pregnancy. Free radicals are thought to act as determinants in reproductive outcomes

due to their effects on oocytes, sperm, and embryos [95]. Oxidative stress disturbs human oocyte intracellular $Ca^{2+}$ homeostasis as well as oocyte maturation and fertilization. During ovulation, ROS are produced within the follicles, however, the excessive production of ROS may increase the risk for poor oocyte quality since oxidative stimulation promotes oocyte maturation and wall rupture within the follicle [390]. A physiologic amount of ROS in follicular fluid is indicative of a healthy developing oocyte [102]. In vitro fertilization can disturb the oxidant-antioxidant balance, rendering the culture media less protected against oxidation. The adverse effects of sustained OS and resulting loss of oocyte antioxidant content were shown to be improved by adding lipophilic and hydrosoluble antioxidants to the culture media to lessen OS [103]. Oral vitamin and mineral supplementation have been shown to increase serum concentrations of GSH and vitamins C and E; these antioxidants have been suggested to play a significant role in IVF outcomes [104].

Much research on IVEP has focused on the damaging effects of an oxidative environment and the inherent creation of reactive oxygen species that may impair embryo development. There are evidences that endoplasmic reticulum (RE) is significantly less reducing, consequently, excessive supplementation of reducing agents in media to offset oxidative damage has resulted in controversial outcomes as slight redox imbalances are detrimental for embryo development [73]. Conversely, an excess of ROS produced without sufficient antioxidant protection may lead to disequilibrium of the redox balance versus oxidative stress characterized by damaging DNA, RNA, protein and lipids [74]. Studies have been performed under high and low oxygen tension conditions and have resulted in controversial findings. Studies using antioxidants on swine model, indicated that the effect of the combination of GSH, β-ME and cysteine on embryo development. Treatment groups had a greater number of developing embryos than the control and the favorable result depended on the high $O_2$ culture conditions were used [105].

In contrast, guaiazulene (a component of various chamomile species with antioxidant properties) had no positive effect on embryo development under low oxygen tension (5 % O2) [106]. Furthermore, [94] found that low oxygen gas composition improves nuclear maturation rates and alleviates the oxidative stress for canine oocytes during in vitro maturation.

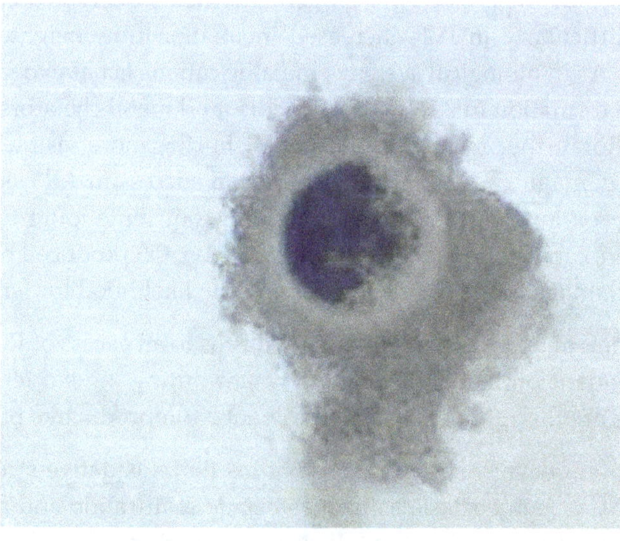

**Figure 4.** Cumulus Oocyte Complexes (COCs) of Pre Antral Follicle from explanted mare ovaries. Ooplama bipolarisation with a dark and a clear portion (ptical microscope, 100x)

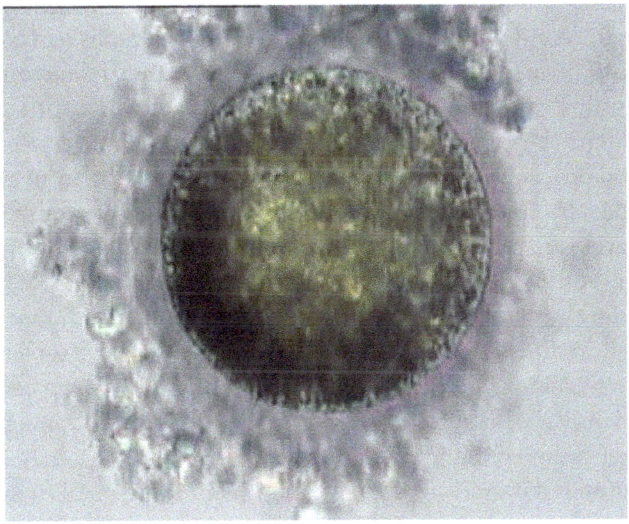

**Figure 5.** Cumulus Oocyte Complexes (COCs) of Pre Antral Follicle from explanted mare ovaries. COC stained with 5-carboxyfluorescein diacetate (cFDA) and trypan blue (with unviable cumulus cells and viable oocyte) (optical microscope 200x).

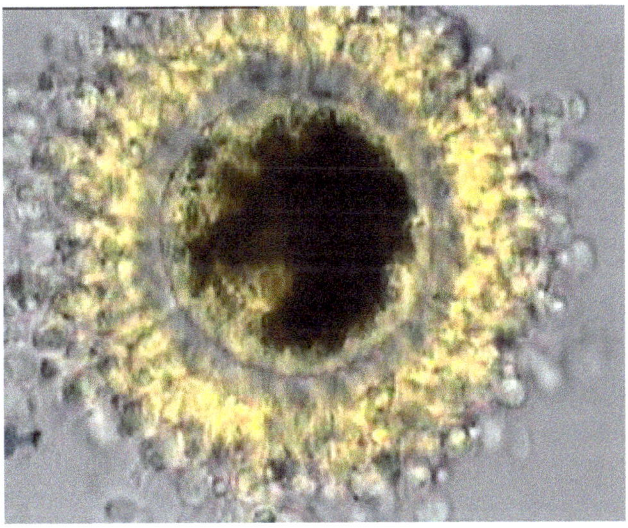

**Figure 6.** Cumulus Oocyte Complexes (COCs) of Pre Antral Follicle from explanted mare ovaries. Viable COC stained with 5-carboxyfluorescein diacetate (cFDA) and trypan blue (optical microscope 200x)

## 9. Conclusions

Oxidative stress has been extensively studied for about four decades. Substantial progress has been achieved to date – from descriptive characterization of this process to delineation of molecular mechanisms underlining adaptive responses and targeted manipulations of expected responses. In recent years, the importance of ROS synthesis in ovarian functions has been established also. Several data have recently shown that reactive oxygen species can regulate cell function by controlling production or the activation of substances that have biological activities. It has been suggested that ROS under moderate concentrations play a role in signal transduction processes involved in growth and protection from apoptosis. Conversely, increase of ROS levels is primarily responsible for the alteration of macromolecules, such as lipids, proteins and nucleic acids, that lead to significant damage of cell structures and thereby cause oxidative stress. Oxidative damage to lipids in the oocyte has been implicated as a cause of persistently poor oocyte quality after early life exposure to several toxicants. Developing germ cells in the fetal ovary have also been shown to be sensitive to toxicants and ionizing radiation, which induce oxidative stress. Recent studies have begun to elucidate the mechanisms by which ROS mediate ovarian toxicity. To prevent damage due to ROS, cells possess a number of nonenzymatic and enzymatic antioxidants. that include Vitamin C, glutathione, cysteamine, vitamin E, superoxide dismutases (SOD1, SOD2, and SOD3), glutathione peroxidase, and catalase. Intracellular homeostasis is ensured by the complex interactions between pro-oxidants and antioxidants. The bulk of evidence in support of therapeutic effects of antioxidants to date, has been observed through experimental studies on animals and humans ART, whose aim is depth knowledge of human reproductive functions, conservation of species in danger of extinction, and acceleration of life cycles using reproduction for purposes of genetic and productive.

In the future, the hope is to clarify the efficacy of antioxidants as potential therapies for infertility and in ART the use of specific antioxidants to improve multiple physiological processes from oocyte maturation to fertilization, embryo development and pregnancy.

## Author details

Francesca Ciani*, Natascia Cocchia, Danila d'Angelo and Simona Tafuri

*Address all correspondence to: ciani@unina.it

Department of Veterinary Medicine and Animal Productions – University of Naples Federico II, Naples, Italy

## References

[1] Baker TG, Franchi LL. The fine structure of chromosome in bovine primordial oocytes. J Reprod Fertil 1976, 14:511-513.

[2] Dekel N, Aberdan E, Goren S, Feldman B, Shalgi R. Mechanism of action of Ngr-induced oocyte maturation. J Reprod Fertil. 1989; 37 (suppl): 319-327.

[3] Fissore RA, He Cl, Woude GFV. Potential role of mitogen-actived protein kinase meiosis resumption in bovine oocytes. Biol Reprod 1996; 55:1261-1270.

[4] Homa ST. Calcium and meiotic maturation of the mammalian oocyte. Mol Reprod Dev 1995; 40:122-134.

[5] Bevers MM, Dieleman SJ, van der Hurk R, Izadyarf F. Regulation and modulation of oocyte maturation in the bovine. Theriogenology 1997; 47:13-22.

[6] Xu ZZ, Garverick HA, Smith GW, Smith MF, Hamilton SA, et al., Expression of FSH and LH receptor mRNA in bovine follicles during the first follicle wave. Biol Reprod 1995; 53:951-958.

[7] Erickson BH. Development and senescence of the post natal bovine ovarv. J Anim Sci 1966; 25:800-805.

[8] Johnson J, Canning J, Kaneko T, Pru JK, Tilly JL. Germline stem cells and follicular renewal in the postnatal mammalian ovary. Nature 2004; 428:145-150.

[9] Pfeifer LFM, Schneider A, Correa MN. Factors that affect the in vitro production of bovine embryos: A review. Rev Colomb Cienc Pecu 2008; 21:109-120.

[10] Lussier JG, Matton P, Dufour JJ. Growth rate of follicles in the ovary of the cow. J Reprod Fertil 1987; 81:301-307.

[11] Fair T, Hulshof SCJ, Hyttel P, Boland M, Greve T. Bovine oocyte trastructure in primordial to tertiary follicles. Anat Embryol 1977; 195:327-336.

[12] Fair T, Hyttel P, Greve T. Bovine oocyte diameter in relation to maturational competence and transcriptional activity. Mol Reprod Dev 1995; 42:437-442.

[13] Sunderland SJ, Crowe MA, Boland MP, Roche JF, Ireland JJ. Seldection dominantce and atresia of follicles during the oestrous cycle of heifers. J Reprod Fertil 1994; 101:547-555.

[14] Crowe MA, Bao B, Mihm M, Roche JF, Williams DH, et al., Effects of LH on gonadotropin receptor and steroid enzyme messenger RNA (mRNA) expression during normal and delayed dominant follicle (DF) selection in heifers. J Reprod Fertil 2000; abstract series 25, 35, (abstract no. 82).

[15] Gong JG, Bramley TA, Gutierrez CG, Peters AR, Webb R. Effects of chronic treatment with gonadotropin-releasing hormone agonist on peripheral concentration of FSH and LH and ovarian function in heifers. I Reprod Fertil 1995; 105:263-270.

[16] Gong JG, Campbell BK, Bramley TA, Gutierrez CG, Peters AR ete al., Suppression in the secretion of follicle-stimulating hormone and luteinizing hormone, and ovarian follicle development in heifers continuously infused with a gonadotropin-releasing hormone agonist. Biol Reprod 1996; 55:68-74.

[17] Abel MH, Wootton AN, Wilkins V, Huhtaniemi I, Kjight PG et al. The effect of a null-mutation in the follicle-stimulating hormone receptor gene on mouse reproduction. Endocrinology 2000; 141:1795-1803.

[18] Mihm M, Bleach ECL. Endocrine regulation of ovarian antral follicle development in cattle. Anim Reprod Sci 2003; 78:217-237.

[19] Luderer U. Ovarian Toxicity from Reactive Oxygen Species. In Gerald Litwack, editor: Vitamins and Hormones, Vol. 94, Burlington: Academic Press, 2014, pp. 99-127.

[20] Ryan KJ. The foeto-placental unit. In: Pe′cicle, A., Finzi, C. (Eds.), Theoretical Basis for Endocrine Control of Gestation-A Comparative Approach. Excerpta Medica Foundation, Amsterdam, 1969 pp. 120–131.

[21] Graham JD, Clarke, CL. Physiological action of progesterone in target tissues. Endocr. Rev. 1997; 18, 502–519.

[22] Niswender, G.D., Juengel, J.L., Silva, P.J., Rollyson, M.K., McIntush, E.W., 2000. Mechanisms controlling the function and life span of the corpus luteum. Physiol. Rev. 80, 1–29.

[23] Behrman HR, Kodaman PH, Preston SL., Gao S. Oxidative stress and the ovary. J. Soc. Gynecol. Investig. 2001; 8:S40–S42.

[24] Al-Gubory KH, Ceballos-Picot I, Nicole A, Bolifraud, P, Germain G, Michaud M, Mayeur C, Blachier F.Changes in activities of superoxide dismutase, nitric oxide synthase, glutathione-dependent enzymes and the incidence of apoptosis in sheep corpus luteum during the estrous cycle. Biochem. Biophys. Acta 2005; 1725:348–357.

[25] Al-Gubory KH, Camous S, Germain G, Bolifraud P, Nicole A, Ceballos-Picot I. Reconsideration of the proposed luteotropic and luteoprotective actions of ovine placental lactogen in sheep: in vivo and in vitro studies. J Endocrinol 2006; 188:559–568.

[26] Sugino N. Roles of reactive oxygen species in the corpus luteum. Anim Sci J 2006; 77.556–565.

[27] Sugino N, Takiguchi S, Kashida S, Karube A, Nakamura Y, Kato H. Superoxide dismutase expression in the human corpus luteum during the menstrual cycle and in early pregnancy. Mol Hum Reprod 2000; 6:19–25.

[28] Al-Gubory KH, Bolifraud P, Germain G, Nicole A, Ceballos-Picot I. Antioxidant enzymatic defence systems in sheep corpus luteum throughout pregnancy. Reproduction 2004; 128:767–774.

[29] Arianmanesh M, McIntosh R, Lea RG, Fowler PA, AlGubory KH. Ovine corpus luteum proteins, with functions including oxidative stress and lipid metabolism, show complex alterations during implantation. J Endocrinol 2011; 210:47–58.

[30] Al-Gubory KH, Garrel C, Faure P, Sugino N. Role of antioxidant enzymes in corpus luteum rescue from oxygen species-induced oxidative stress. Reproductive BioMedicine Online 2012; 25:551-560.

[31] Banfi G, Iorio EL, Corsi MM. Oxidative stress, free radicals and bone remodeling. Clin Chem Lab Med. 2008;46(11):1550-5. doi: 10.1515/CCLM.2008.302.

[32] Agarwal A, Gupta S, Sikka S. The role of free radicals and antioxidants in reproduction.. Curr Opin Obstet Gynecol. 2006;18(3):325-32.

[33] Halliwell B, Gutteridge JMC. The chemistry of oxygen radicals and other derived species. In: Halliwell B, and Gutteridge JMC eds. Free radicals in Biology and Medicine. 2nd edition Clarendon Press. Oxford. 1989; pp.22-85.

[34] Lykkesfeldt J, Svendsen O. Oxidants and antioxidants in disease: oxidative stress in farm animals. Vet J. 2007; 173(3):502-11. Epub 2006 Aug 17.

[35] Soriani M, Pietraforte D, Minetti M. Antioxidant potential of anaerobic human plasma: role of serum albumin and thiols as scavengers of carbon radicals. Arch Biochem Biophys. 1994; 312(1):180-188.

[36] Moran JH[1], Mitchell LA, Grant DFLinoleic acid prevents chloride influx and cellular lysis in rabbit renal proximal tubules exposed to mitochondrial toxicants.. Toxicol Appl Pharmacol. 2001 Nov 1;176(3):153-61.

[37] Lushchak VI. Glutathione Homeostasis and Functions: Potential Targets for Medical Interventions. Journal of Amino Acids 2012, pp.1- 26 doi:10.1155/2012/736837

[38] Meister A, Anderson ME. Glutathione. Annu Rev Biochem 1983;52:711-760.

[39] Sies H. Glutathione and its role in cellular functions. Free Radic Biol Med 1999; 27(9-19):916-921.

[40] Lushchak VI. Free radicals, reactive oxygen species, oxidative stress and its classification. Chemico-Biological Interactions 2014; 224:164–175.

[41] Foster M W, Hess D T, Stamler JS. Protein S-nitrosylation in health and disease: A current perspective. Trends in Molecular Medicine 2009; 15:391–404.

[42] Agarwal A, Aponte-Mellado A, Premkumar BJ, Shaman A, Gupta S. The effects of oxidative stress on female reproduction: a review.Reprod Biol Endocrinol 2012; 29;10:49. doi: 10.1186/1477-7827-10-49.

[43] Holland SL, Avery SV. Chromate toxicity and the role of sulfur. Metallomics 2011; 3(11):1119-23. doi: 10.1039/c1mt00059d.

[44] Lushchak OV, Kubrak OI, Nykorak MZ, Storey KB, Lushchak VI. The effect of potassium dichromate on free radical processes in goldfish: possible protective role of glutathione. Aquat Toxicol. 2008; 28, 87(2):108-14. doi: 10.1016/j.aquatox.2008.01.007.

[45] Cocchia N., Corteggio A., Altamura G., Tafuri S., Rea S., Rosapane I., Sica A., Landolfi F., Ciani F. Superoxide dismutase (SOD) addition to transport media during stor-

age of cat ovaries 4 °C. Reproductive Biology, 2015 Mar;15(1):56-64. doi: 10.1016/j.repbio.2014.10.002.

[46] Devine PJ, Perreault SD, Luderer U. Roles of reactive oxygen species and antioxidants in ovarian toxicity. Biol Reprod 2012;n86(2):27, 1-10 doi: 10.1095/biolreprod.111.095224.

[47] Bauer G. Targeting Extracellular ROS Signaling of Tumor Cells. Anticancer Research 2014; 34:41467-1482.

[48] Banerjee M, Vats P. Reactive metabolites and antioxidant gene polymorphisms in Type 2 diabetes mellitus. Redox Biol. 2013; 2C:170-177. doi: 10.1016/j.redox.2013.12.001.

[49] Ho YS, Xiong Y, Ma W, Spector A, Ho DS.Mice lacking catalase develop normally but show differential sensitivity to oxidant tissue injury. J Biol Chem; 2004; 279(31): 32804-32812.

[50] Sies H. Role of metabolic H2O2 generation: redox signaling and oxidative stress.J Biol Chem 2014; 289(13):8735-8741. doi: 10.1074/jbc.R113.544635. Epub 2014 Feb 10.

[51] Claeson K, Thorsén G, Karlberg B. Micellar electrokinetic chromatography separation and laser-induced fluorescence detection of the lipid peroxidation product 4-hydroxynonenal. J Chromatogr B Biomed Sci Appl. 2001; 763(1-2):133-8.

[52] Zimniak P. Relationship of electrophilic stress to aging. Free Radic Biol Med. 2011; 51(6):1087-105. doi: 10.1016/j.freeradbiomed.2011.05.039. Epub 2011 Jun 12.

[53] Lenz ML, Michael LH, Smith CV, Hughes H, Shappell SB, Taylor AA, Entman ML, Mitchell JR. Glutathione disulfide formation and lipid peroxidation during cardiac ischemia and reflow in the dog in vivo. Biochem Biophys Res Commun. 1989;164(2): 722-727.

[54] Wehr NB, Levine RL. Wanted and wanting: antibody against methionine sulfoxide. Free Radic Biol Med. 2012;53(6):1222-5. doi: 10.1016/j.freeradbiomed.2012.06.036. Epub 2012 Jul 3.

[55] Dröge W. Free Radicals in the Physiological Control of Cell Function. Physiological Reviews 2002; 82(1):47-95 DOI: 10.1152/physrev.00018.2001.

[56] Shkolnika K, Tadmora A, Ben-Dorb S, Nevoa N, Galiania D, Dekel N. Reactive oxygen species are indispensable in ovulation. PNAS 2011; 108 (4): 1462-1468.

[57] Bagavandoss P, Wiggins RC, Kunkel SL, Remick DG, Keyes PL. Tumor necrosis factor production and accumulation of inflammatory cells in the corpus luteum of pseudopregnancy and pregnancy in rabbits. Biology of Reproduction 1990; 42, 367–376.

[58] Brannstrom M, Giesecke L, Moore IC, Van Den Heuvel CJ, Robertson SA. Leukocyte subpopulations in the rat corpus luteum during pregnancy and pseudopregnancy. Biology of Reproduction 1994; 50, 1161–1167.

[59] Sugino N, Shimamura K, Tamura H, Ono M, Nakamura Y, Ogino K, Kato H. Progesterone inhibits superoxide radical production by mononuclear phagocytes in pseudopregnant rats. Endocrinology 1996; 137, 749–754.

[60] Suzuki T, Sasano H, Takaya R, Fukaya T, Yajima A, Date F, Nagura H. Leukocytes in normal-cycling human ovaries: immunohistochemical distribution and characterization. Human Reproduction 1998; 13, 2186–2191.

[61] Suzuki T, Sugino N, Fukaya T, Sugiyama S, Uda T, Takaya R, Yajima A, Sasano H. Superoxide dismutase in normal cycling human ovaries: immunohistochemical localization and characterization. Fertility and Sterility 1999; 72, 720–726.

[62] Olofsson J, Norjavaara E, Selstam G. In vivo levels of prostaglandin F2$\alpha$, E2 and prostacyclin in the corpus luteum of pregnant and pseudopregnant rats. Biology of Reproduction 1990; 42, 792–800.)

[63] Tanaka M, Miyazaki T, Tanigaki S, Kasai K, Minegishi K, Miyakoshi K, Ishimoto H, Yoshimura Y. Participation of reactive oxygen species in PGF2$\alpha$-induced apoptosis in rat luteal cells. Journal of Reproduction and Fertility 2000; 120, 239–245.

[64] Hayashi K, Miyamoto A, Konari A, Ohtani M, Fukui Y. Effect of local interaction of reactive oxygen species with prostaglandin F2$\alpha$ on the release of progesterone in ovine corpora lutea in vivo. Theriogenology 2003; 59, 1335–1344.

[65] Wu XM, Carlson JC. Alterations in phospholipase A2 activity during luteal regression in pseudopregnant and pregnant rats. Endocrinology 1990;127, 2464–2468.

[66] Nakamura T, Sakamoto K.. Reactive oxygen species up-regulates cyclooxygenase-2, 53, and Bax mRNA expression in bovine luteal cells. Biochemical and Biophysical Research Communications 2001; 284, 203–210.

[67] Freeman BA, Crapo JD. 1982. Biology of disease; free radicals and tissue injury. Laboratory Investigation 1982; 47, 412–426.

[68] Sugino N, Nakamura Y, Takeda O, Ishimatsu M, Kato H. Changes in activities of superoxide dismutase and lipid peroxide in corpus luteum during pregnancy in rats. Journal of Reproduction and Fertility 1993; 97, 347–351.

[69] Shimamura K, Sugino N, Yoshida Y, Nakamura Y, Ogino K, Kato H. Changes in lipid peroxide and antioxidant enzyme activities in corpora lutea during pseudopregnancy in rats. Journal of Reproduction and Fertility 1995; 105, 253–257.

[70] Carlson JC, Sawada M, Boone DL, Stauffer JM.. Stimulation of progesterone secretion in dispersed cells of rat corpora lutea by antioxidants. Steroids 1995; 60, 272–276.

[71] Sawada M, Carlson JC.. Intracellular regulation of progesterone secretion by the superoxide radical in the rat corpus luteum. Endocrinology 1996; 137, 1580–1584.

[72] Rapoport R, Sklan D, Wolfenson D, Shaham-Albalancy A, Hanukoglu I. Antioxidant capacity is correlated with steroidogenic status of the corpus luteum during the bovine estrous cycle. Biochimica et Biophysica Acta 1998; 1380, 133–140.).

[73] Behrman HR, Kodaman PH, Preston SL, Gao S. Oxidative stress and the ovary. J Soc Gynecol Investig. 2001; 8(1 Suppl Proceedings):S40-42.

[74] Forman HJ, Torres M. Reactive oxygen species and cell signaling: respiratory burst in macrophage signaling. Am J Respir Crit Care Med 2002; 166(12 Pt 2):S4-8.

[75] Shiotani M, Noda Y, Narimoto K, Imai K, Mori T, Fujimoto K, Ogawa K. Immunohistochemical localization of superoxide dismutase in the human ovary.Hum Reprod. 1991; Nov;6(10):1349-53.

[76] Tamate K, Sengoku K, Ishikawa M. The role of superoxide dismutase in the human ovary and fallopian tube. J Obstet Gynaecol (Tokyo 1995) 1995; (4):401-409.

[77] El Mouatassim S, Guérin P, Ménézo Y. Expression of genes encoding antioxidant enzymes in human and mouse oocytes during the final stages of maturation. Mol Hum Reprod. 1999; (8):720-725.

[78] Chun SY, Eisenhauer KM, Minami S, Billig H, Perlas E, Hsueh AJ. Hormonal regulation of apoptosis in early antral follicles: follicle-stimulating hormone as a major survival factor.] Endocrinology 1996; (4):1447-56.

[79] Tilly JL, Tilly KI. Inhibitors of oxidative stress mimic the ability of follicle-stimulating hormone to suppress apoptosis in cultured rat ovarian follicles. Endocrinology 1995;136(1):242-52.

[80] Jozwik M, Wolczynski S, Jozwik M, Szamatowicz M. Oxidative stress markers in preovulatory follicular fluid in humans. Mol Hum Reprod. 1999; (5):409-13.

[81] Agarwal A, Gupta S, Sharma RK. Role of oxidative stress in female reproduction. Reprod Biol Endocrinol 2005; 3:28. doi:10.1186/1477-7827-3-28.

[82] Matzuk MM, Dionne L, Guo Q, Kumar TR, Lebovitz RM. Ovarian function in superoxide dismutase 1 and 2 knockout mice. Endocrinology 1998; 139:4008–4011.

[83] Ho Y-S, Gargano M, Cao J, Bronson RT, Heimler I, Hutz RJ. Reduced fertility in female mice lacking copper-zinc superoxide dismutase. J Biol Chem 1998; 273:7765–7769.

[84] Wong PC, Waggoner D, Subramaniam JR, Tessarollo L, Bartnikas TB, Culotta VC, Price DL, Rothstein J, Gitlin JD. Copper chaperone for superoxide dismutase is essential to activate mammalian Cu/Zn superoxide dismutase. Proc Natl Acad Sci U S A 2000; 97:2886–2891.

[85] Matzuk MM, Dionne L, Guo Q, Kumar TR, Lebovitz RM. Ovarian function in superoxide dismutase 1 and 2 knockout mice. Endocrinology 1998; 139:4008–4011.

[86] Behrman HR, Kodaman PH, Preston SL, Gao S. Oxidative stress and the ovary. J Soc Gynecol Investig. 2001; 8(1 Suppl Proceedings):S40-S42.

[87] M.H.C. Cruz a, C.L.V. Leal, J.F. Cruz, D.X. Tan, R.J. Reiter. Essential actions of melatonin in protecting the ovary from oxidative damage. Theriogenology 2014;82:925–932.

[88] Tamura H, Takasaki A, Taketani T, Tanabe M, Kizuka F, Lee1 L, Tamura I, Maekawa R, Aasada H, Yamagata Y, Sugino N. The role of melatonin as an antioxidant in the follicle Journal of Ovarian Research. Endocr J. 2013; 60(1):1-13.

[89] R.J. Reiter, S. A. Rosales-Corral, L.C. Manchester, D.-X. Tan. Peripheral Reproductive Organ Health and Melatonin: Ready for Prime Time Int. J Mol Sci 2013, 14(4), 7231-7272. doi:10.3390/ijms14047231.

[90] Swanson W.F. Swanson, J.L. Brown International training programs in reproductive sciences for conservation of Latin American felids. Animal Reproduction Science 2004; 82–83:21–34.

[91] Ciani F, Cocchia N, Rizzo M, Ponzio P, Tortora G, Avallone L, Lorizio R. Sex determining of cat embryo and some feline species. Zygote. 2008; 16(2):169-77. doi: 10.1017/S0967199408004681.

[92] Ciani F, Cocchia N, Esposito L, Avallone L. (2012) Fertility Cryopreservation, Advances in Embryo Transfer, Dr. Bin Wu (Ed.), ISBN: 978-953-51-0318-9 InTech, DOI: 10.5772/38511. Available from: http://www.intechopen.com/books/advances-in-embryo-transfer/fertility-cryopreservation

[93] Cocchia N., Ciani F, Russo M, El Rass R, Rosapane I, Avallone L, Tortora G, Lorizio R. Immature cat oocyte vitrification in open pulled straws (OPSs) using a cryoprotectant mixture. Cryobiology. 2010;;60(2):229-34.. doi: 10.1016/j.cryobiol.2010.01.003.

[94] Salavati M, Ghafari F, Zhang T, Foladi-Nashta AA. Effects of oxygen concentration on in vitro maturation of canine oocytes in a chemically defined serum-free medium. Reproduction 2012; 144: 547-556.

[95] Gupta S, Choi A, Yu HY, Czerniak SM, Holick EA, Paolella LJ, Agarwal A, Combelles CM. Fluctuations in total antioxidant capacity, catalase activity and hydrogen peroxide levels of follicular fluid during bovine folliculogenesis. Reprod Fertil Dev 2011; 23(5):673-80. doi: 10.1071/RD10270.

[96] Jana SK KNB, Chattopadhyay R, Chakravarty B, Chaudhury K: Upper control limit of reactive oxygen species in follicular fluid beyond which viable embryo formation is not favorable. Reprod Toxicol 2010; 29:447–451.

[97] Sikka SC: Role of oxidative stress response elements and antioxidants in prostate cancer pathobiology and chemoprevention–a mechanistic approach. Curr Med Chem 2003; 10:2679–2692.

[98] Oyawoye O, Abdel Gadir A, Garner A, Constantinovici N, Perrett C, Hardiman P. Antioxidants and reactive oxygen species in follicular fluid of women undergoing IVF: relationship to outcome. Hum Reprod 2003; 18:2270–2274.

[99] Revelli A, Delle Piane L, Casano S, Molinari E, Massobrio M, Rinaudo P. Follicular fluid content and oocyte quality: from single biochemical markers to metabolomics. Reprod Biol Endocrinol 2009; 7:40.

[100] Jana SK KNB, Chattopadhyay R, Chakravarty B, Chaudhury K: Upper control limit of reactive oxygen species in follicular fluid beyond which viable embryo formation is not favorable. Reprod Toxicol 2010; 29:447–451.

[101] Takenaka M, Horiuchi T, Yanagimachi R: Effects of light on development of mammalian zygotes. Proc Natl Acad Sci U S A 2007; 104:14289–14293.

[102] Attaran M, Pasqualotto E, Falcone T, Goldberg JM, Miller KF, Agarwal A, Sharma RK: The effect of follicular fluid reactive oxygen species on the outcome of in vitro fertilization. Int J Fertil Womens Med 2000; 45:314–320.

[103] Martin-Romero FJ, Miguel-Lasobras EM, Dominguez-Arroyo JA, Gonzalez-Carrera E, Alvarez IS: Contribution of culture media to oxidative stress and its effect on human oocytes. Reprod Biomed Online 2008; 17:652–661.

[104] Ozkaya MO, Naziroglu M: Multivitamin and mineral supplementation modulates oxidative stress and antioxidant vitamin levels in serum and follicular fluid of women undergoing in vitro fertilization. Fertil Steril 2010; 94:2465–2466. doi:10.1186/1477.

[105] Rand JD, Grant CM. The thioredoxin system protects ribosomes against stress-induced aggregation. Mol Biol Cell. 2006;17(1):387– 401.

[106] Dovolou E, Clemente M, Amiridis GS, Messinis IE, Kallitsaris A, Gutierrez-Adan A, et al. Effects of guaiazulene on in vitro bovine embryo production and on mRNA transcripts related to embryo quality. Reprod Domest Anim 2011;46(5):862–869.

7

# Assisted Reproductive Technologies in Safeguard of Feline Endangered Species

Natascia Cocchia, Simona Tafuri, Lucia Abbondante, Leonardo Meomartino, Luigi Esposito and Francesca Ciani

**Abstract**

The growth of the human population and the escalating consumption of natural resources have reduced wild habitats, modifying the existing balance of biological cycles. Therefore, *ex situ* conservation efforts have received renewed attention as a potential safeguard for species with an uncertain future in the wild. Most wild felid species are classified as rare, vulnerable, or endangered due to poaching and habitat loss. Any directed action taken by humans to enhance animal reproduction results in assisted reproductive technologies (ART) development. These technologies have been included in programs for the conservation of endangered species. Therefore, ART provide a new approach in the safeguard programs of felid biodiversity. Currently, ART mainly include Artificial Insemination (AI); *In Vitro* Embryo Production (IVEP) consisting of *In Vitro* Maturation (IVM), *In Vitro* Fertilization (IVF), *In Vitro* Culture (IVC), Embryo Transfer (ET), and Intra Cytoplasmic Sperm Injection (ICSI); gamete/embryo cryopreservation; gamete/embryo sexing; gamete/embryo micromanipulation; Somatic Cell Nuclear Transfer (SCNT); and genome resource banking.

The domestic cat is used as a model for the ART development in *Felid* species and as a successful recipient of embryos from closely related, small, nondomestic cats. The Indian desert cat and African wildcat kittens have been born after IVF-derived embryo transfers.

The creation of the biological resource bank represents a complementary support tool for the application of ART in the *in situ* and *ex situ* conservation of endangered felids. Its chief purpose in the protection of endangered species is to preserve the maximum current genetic and biological diversity of the population by the processing and cryopreservation of germinal cells and tissues from dead animals so that these genetic recourses may be used in future reproductive projects. In humans and domestic species, it is usually possible to plan the place and time for gonad explants to recover germplasm, thereby enabling a reduction in the gonad storage time in the transport medium. In wild species, it is impossible to predict when and where the gonads can be collected. The gonads can be recovered postmortem, which entails the possibility that the collection place could be distant from a laboratory for IVEP.

In the present chapter, we will make an overview of the data from detectable literatures and focus our attention on analysis of methods utilized in ART for maximizing their efficiency in feline species.

**Keywords:** Assisted Reproductive Technologies (ART), In Vitro Embryo Production (IVEP), endangered feline species

---

## 1. Introduction

The growth of the human population and the escalating consumption of natural resources have reduced wild spaces, modifying the existing balance of the biological cycles. Therefore, *ex situ* conservation efforts have received renewed attention as a potential safeguard for species with an uncertain future in the wild. Assisted Reproductive Technologies (ART), which consist of various techniques such as Artificial Insemination (AI), In Vitro Fertilization (IVF), Embryo Transfer (ET), and cryopreservation of embryos, have greatly promoted animal reproductive efficiency and have become a potential means for the conservation and management of wildlife populations threatened with extinction. [1]. Several species, such as domestic cats, dogs, and ferrets are the most popular pets, while other carnivores, like minks and foxes, have an economic value to the industry of fur farming. Tigers, bears, and other large predators have a major effect on the health of natural ecosystems. Any directed action taken by humans to enhance animal reproduction has resulted in assisted reproductive technologies (ART) development. These technologies have been included in programs for the conservation of species threatened with extinction. ART, therefore, affords investigators a new approach that they can include in the safeguard programs of felid biodiversity. Although this technique has greatly improved animal reproduction, it has not advanced beyond the rudimentary stages for use in the conservation of felines threatened with extinction [1]. As several other more widely studied species, the earliest descriptions of successful production of embryos using in vitro fertilization (IVF) in the cat occurred in the 1970s [2, 3]. Meanwhile, as IVF studies in the most popular laboratory animals, economically important domestic animals, and humans literally exploded during the last two decades of the twentieth century, the field of cat IVF experienced no comparative proliferation in publications. Publications in human IVF area represent approximately 50% of the reports from 1970 through 2000 and approximately 50% from 2001 through 2012. The majority of the total citations listed in the search on "IVF in cats", were published in the current century [4]. Most wild felid species are classified as rare, vulnerable, or endangered due to poaching and habitat loss. A great deal of progress has been made in recent years toward the development of assisted reproductive techniques (ART) for species conservation [5, 6] In fact, ART have been included in the programs for the conservation of species threatened with extinction, but the effectiveness of this application to semi domestic, not domestic, and particularly endangered species such as felines, remains consistently low [4]. These ART tools are potentially important for the captive breeding programs of selected felid species. The domestic cat is often used as a model for developing these techniques in the felid species [5, 6]. In the last few years, the ART application in the domestic cat has allowed researchers to obtain 70% metaphase II oocytes after *in vitro* maturation (IVM) [7], and 80% cleaved embryos after IVF and 70–80% after Intra Cytoplasmic Sperm Injection (ICSI) [8]. However, only 10% cleaved embryos could develop to blastocyst [8-11]. Kittens have been born after embryo transfer [5]. *In vivo* embryo collection is the most popular technique for embryo production, in spite of the fairly rapid development and adoption of *in vitro* embryo production. The domestic cat could also be used as a successful recipient of embryos from closely related small nondomestic cats. In fact, some evidences have confirmed the birth of African wildcat and Indian desert cat kittens after the transfer of IVF-derived embryos in female domestic cats [12]. Recently, African wildcat kittens were produced after the transfer of embryos derived by fusion of adult somatic cells from one species with enucleated oocytes of a closely related species (domestic cat) [13]. However, the application of ART, which tries to produce a single viable offspring, unfortunately, cannot justify the expense, labor, and the handling of animals which is associated with stress. Thus, "ART" must be applied within the programs of population management established to have a real impact on conservation. The immediate value of ART is to assist those responsible for the maintenance of viable populations of felines in captivity. Its wider application will require the creation of a global network of qualified scientists and veterinarians willing to perform these procedures as a reproduction service for keeping cats themselves [1].

## 2. Reproductive cycles of wild felids

Knowledge of anatomical features and hormones and the cycles of wild reproductive feline is the ability to track feline reproductive activity. The hormone measure is a key technique to develop successful ex situ breeding programs to determine the reproductive activity of domestic feline. The ovaries in the wild felid and the domestic cat are caudal to the respective kidneys and connected proximally by the suspensor ligament and dorsally by the mesovaria. The oviducts are covered by the mesosalphinx that forms, laterally to the ovaries – an ovarian bursa. Each oviduct cranially is localized in the medial aspect of the ovarian bursa; caudally it is located in the lateral aspect before terminating at the uterotubal junction. The mesometrium suspends dorsally the horns of the uterus bicornuate. The uterine body is divided internally by an incomplete septum. The cervix is short, but it opens at an angle close to the vaginal orifice. The lips of the vulva are located just below the anus. After fertilization, the blastocysts are distributed evenly along the uterine horns, with an efficient result of transuterine migration. Cats have a zonary endotheliochorial type placenta. Regarding the hormone profile of wild felines, reasonable results were obtained by noninvasive monitoring of steroid [14]. Reproductive cycle models of ovarian steroids have now been published about half of nondomestic felid species, by analysis of fecal steroid metabolites. There are four phases of the oestrous cycle in the cat: proestrus, oestrus, diestrus, and anestrus (or interestrus) [15]. Proestrus usually lasts less than a day, and is associated with the presence of ovarian follicles, increased circulating estrogens, no sexual interest but occasionally there could be copulation with the male. Oestrous has maximum concentrations of follicular estradiol. It is characterized by coitus and, depending on the species, by special and typical behaviors such as vocalization, rubbing, rolling, lordosis, and foot stamping. The release of gonadotrophins-releasing hormone (GnRH) from the basal medial hypothalamus and successive waves of luteinizing hormone (LH) from the anterior pituitary gland, are considered necessary in most felines [16, 17]. This cascade of events will result in ovulation after mating. Surges of estrogens distinguish oestrous from interestrus periods, with cycles ranging from 2 to 4 weeks and oestrus lasting 3–10 days. Cats have historically been categorized as having "induced ovulation," that is, requiring mating to stimulate ovulation. Nevertheless, we now know that felids exhibit a range of ovulatory patterns, from almost exclusively induced to manifold combinations of induced and spontaneous ovulation. There are differences not only across species, but also between individuals within a species [14]. In fact, spontaneous increase in progestogens after oestrogen surges is rare or inexistent in the tiger (*Panthera tigris*), snow leopard (*Panthera uncia*), ocelot (*Leopardus pardalis*) puma (*Felis concolor*), tigrina (*Leopardus tigrinus*), cheetah (*Acinonyx jubatus*), and lynx (*Lynx pardinus, Lynx canadensi, Lynx lynx*). It happens, at least occasionally, in the lion (*Panthera leo*), Pallas'cat (*Otocolobus manul*), leopard (*Panther pardus*), fishing cat (*Prionailurus viverrinus*), and regularly in the margay (*Leopardus wiedii*), clouded leopard (*Neofelis nebulosa*), and domestic cat. In some species of certain taxonomy, the spontaneous ovulation occurs in a more prevalent way when the females are kept together, while in others the provoked ovulation occurs if they are kept in individual housings. Thus, within the same taxonomy, ovulatory mechanisms are regulated to different degrees depending on species and individual-specific responses to psychosocial and/or physical stimuli.

Several studies report the domestic cat be seasonally poly oestrous animal with positive photoperiod under natural [16]. In general, ovarian cyclic activity and reproductive functions are reduced under decreasing photoperiod and starts again after exposure to increasing light. In the cat, melatonin seems to regulate photoperiod-induced seasonality. The highest concentrations happen during the dark phase [17]. Reproduction is in someway seasonal in many nondomestic felids like the tiger, pallas'cat, clouded leopard, snow leopard, and lynx (Table 1). The follicular activity, conversely, is not influenced by season in lions, bobcats, pumas, leopards, margays, tigrinas, ocelots, jaguars, and fishing cats [14]. Progestogen concentrations during pregnant and nonpregnant luteal phases are quantitatively similar in nondomestic felids and domestic cats [15].

Felids express marked variations in reproductive mechanisms among species. Two characteristics impact both natural and assisted breeding efforts: effect of seasonality on reproduction and identifying the type of ovulation (induced *vs* spontaneous). Developing ovulation

| | Puberty | Seasonality | Induced Ovulation | Oestrus Length | Pregnancy Length |
|---|---|---|---|---|---|
| Domestic cat | 6–9 months | YES | YES | 3-16 days | 58–65 days |
| Cheetah | 2–3 years | NOT | YES | 2–6 days | 94 days |
| Pallas cat | 1 year | YES | OCCASIONALLY NOT | 3–14 days | 66–77 days |
| Clouded leopard | 2 years | YES | NOT (40%) | 3–6 days | 90 days |
| Tiger | 3–4 years | YES | YES | 7 days | 108 days |
| Leopardis species | 1–2 years | YES /NOT | NOT | 2–7 days | 75–85 days |
| Linx | 1–2 years | YES | YES | 7 days | 60–70 days |
| Lion | 3 years | NOT | NOT | 5–6 days | 108 days |

**Table 1.** Particularity of reproductive cycles of *domestic cat* and some *wild felids.*

induction protocol, with consistent responses, is high priority. Furthermore, it is important to ensure an optimal maternal environment for fertilization and embryo development. Down-regulating endogenous ovarian activity and synchronizing time of oestrus are steps of reproductive cycle that need to be controlled and reinforced [1, 18]. We also need a quick and reliable test for diagnosing pregnancy, preferably a noninvasive method.

## 3. Oestrus induction in felids

In the late of 1970s, various doses and single versus multiple treatments with either a pituitary extract of porcine FSH (approximately 10–20 mg) or eCG for stimulation of follicular development and induction of oestrus was evaluated [15]; 2.0 mg FSH per day until oestrus was observed to be the optimal dose of FSH despite the elevated average ovulation rate and the presence of residual follicles observed after treatment. Cats in the latter group were given the optimal dose of FSH as determined previously [15]: 2.0 mg/ day for 5 days ¼ 10 mg FSH. In the mid-1980s, the Center for Reproduction of Endangered Wildlife of the Cincinnati Zoo established a domestic cat colony model for developing assisted reproductive technologies to apply in conservation efforts for endangered species. The domestic cat, in addition to its prototypical role, was envisioned as a potential recipient of embryos from other species of similarly sized nondomestic cats, of which most are classified as threatened or vulnerable to extinction. In view of previous results in exogenous gonadotropins for oestrous induction, initial emphasis was directed at determining optimal FSH treatment regimes for ovarian follicular stimulation. In a 1987 published article [19] on ovarian response and embryo recovery after treatment with various doses of FSH (2.75–8.0 mg total) and hCG (0–1500 IU) and natural mating, the greatest average number of viable embryos (15.8 morulae and blastocysts) was recovered from the group receiving 4.0 mg FSH/750 IU hCG. Unexpectedly, there was no difference in the average number of viable embryos recovered from donors given the least amount of FSH (2.75 mg total) versus the greatest amount (8.0 mg total): 6.9 versus 7.9. Also, in 1988, we made our one and only attempt to apply the same methods to a species of nondomestic cat, the serval (*Leptailurus serval*). After daily FSH treatment, at the time of ovulation induction (with hCG), the female was paired with a male. Seven days later, both uterine horns were flushed, but only degenerating ova (>30) were recovered. The ova were examined microscopically, but no sperm were seen, either attached to or penetrating into the zona pellucida. The mating failure was persuasive evidence that, to achieve our goal of applying assisted breeding technology to nondomestic cats, a program to develop methods for in vitro fertilization/embryo culture in cats would be essential. Coincidently, the first report on the birth of kittens after transfer of IVF-derived embryos to recipient females was published at this time [20]. Moreover, repeated treatment of domestic cats with eCG and hCG may cause an immune-mediated refractoriness to ovarian stimulation, dictating that the suitability of these hormonal combinations should be further investigated [1]. Similarly, protocols using porcine FSH and LH resulted in reduced numbers of follicles at the second treatment as compared with the first, possibly due to a humoral immune response [4]. By considering the feasibility of fecal steroid analyses with radioimmunoassay [14] combined with sexual behavior and ultrasonographic images, it is possible to determine the more ideal time for oocyte recovery by laparoscopy, without the use of exogenous gonadotropins.

## 4. Gamete recovery from nondomestic felids

The first step for ART development is the gamete recovery. Several methods have been reported for semen collection in animals, such as the use of an artificial vagina [21], digital masturbation of the penile bulb and electroejaculation [22], but only electroejaculation method may be used for gamete recovery from wild felids. In any case, the application on nondomestic cats is based on learning how to use these methods in the domestic cats. Electroejaculation is to obtain both epidydimal spermatozoon and spermatogonial germ cells. In female, oocytes are retrieved and recovered from both antral and preantral follicles in ovarian tissue transplantation [23].

## 5. Male gamete recovery in felids

With wild carnivores, electroejaculation is the method of choice due to the difficulty and risks involved in handling these animals. Electroejaculation occurs after introducing of a transrectal probe with three electrodes, connected to an electric stimulator that provokes a controlled electric stimulation to allow the ejaculatory reflex to work. The nerves that supply the reproductive organs are stimulated by a weak electric current. The probe is inserted 7–9 cm into the rectum and the electrodes are directed ventrally. It is necessary to take care to evacuate any feces from the rectum for this kind of manipulation. [24]. Different protocols of electroejaculation have been used by many researchers [15]. The authors reported three series for a total of 80 electric stimulations. The three series were divided in: 30 stimuli (10 stimuli at 2–4 V series 01), 30 stimuli (10 stimuli at 3–5 V series 02), and 20 stimuli (10 stimuli at 5 and 6 V series 03) for the collection of semen from South African cheetahs (*Acinonyx jubatus*), with 5 min intervals between the series. The animal responds to the stimuli with a rigid extension of the hind legs. If this reaction is not seen in series 01 or if stronger stimulation is observed, the electrode may not be in the proper position in the rectum, or there may be interference in the current transmission due to the presence of feces. To collect semen, a gentle pressure applied at the penile base should allow for penile extrusion, and the ejaculate is collected into a prewarmed test tube that has been placed over the glans penis. Using electroejaculation has collected the semen from more than 28 cat species [25]. Moreover, some researchers have reported successful semen collection from wild felids by using electroejaculation, such as tigers (*Panthera tigris*), snow leopards (*Panthera uncia*), Indian leopards (*Panthera pardus*), caracals (*Caracal caracal*), jaguars (*Panthera onca*), ocelots (*Leopardus pardalis*), margays (*L. wiedii*), and tigrinas (*L. tigrinus*). The electroejaculation has been used to collect semen from nondomestic felids [4] and the semen has been cryopreserved. After thawing, in lions (*Panthera leo*), jaguars (*P. onca*), leopards (*Neofelis nebulosa*), cheetahs (*A. jubatus*), and leopard cats (*Felis bengalensis*) 25–50% sperm motility was preserved, and in the latter, a 70% sperm motility was maintained. Furthermore, they reported finding lesser values of sperm motility, ranging between 1 and 20% post-thaw, for Geoffroy's cats (*Felis geoffroy*), Indian tigers (*P. tigris*), and ocelots (*Felis pardalis*), but unfortunately, the spermatozoa from gold cats (*Felis aurata*) did not survive cryopreservation. In addition, 40% sperm motility post-thaw in Siberian tigers (*P. tigris*) was obtained, in semen collected with electroejaculation by [4]. The epididymis is an anatomical component of the male reproductive tract and is connected to the testicle. One of its main functions is the storage of spermatozoa for ejaculation [25]. Current technologies allow semen to be collected directly from the epididymis and this seems to be a viable alternative method for obtaining gametes from animals that have recently died or from animals unable to ejaculate (Figs. 1, 2, 3). It has been suggested that viable epididymal spermatozoa from Iberian deer (*Cervus elaphus*) could be collected in the 10–20 h postmortem period. However, it must be noted that this could vary depending on the temperature conditions and the weather where the procedure is being executed [26]. Comparing epididymal spermatozoa from domestic cats and ejaculated spermatozoa, it was verified that epididymal spermatozoa require less capacitating time as compared with those ejaculated and are able to penetrate feline oocytes 20 min after in vitro insemination [27, 28]. Fresh feline epididymal spermatozoa were able to fertilize oocytes in vitro, promoting 40.7% cleavage rate. After freezing, a 26% cleavage rate was obtained. After intracytoplasmic sperm injection (ICSI) using feline frozen epididymal spermatozoa, 34.9% of embryos have developed to the morale stage, indicating that spermatozoa with minimal motility could be used in assisted reproductive techniques [29]. Also, the unilateral intrauterine artificial insemination with frozen–thawed epididymal semen from cats may obtain 23% conception rate [30]. For nondomestic cats, [31] were able to collect spermatozoa from the finely minced cauda epididymus of leopards (*P. pardus*), tigers (*P. tigris*), lions (*P. leo*), pumas (*F. concolor*) and jaguars (*P. onca*). The samples were treated as described by [32], washing the spermatozoa in Hank's balanced salt solution and extended in medium M199 supplemented with 2.5 mmol/l sodium lactate and 0.4% bovine serum albumin. Progressively motile spermatozoa were 60–85% depending on the various felids. In the same study, the epididymal semen was frozen, and thawing motility is between 25 and 65% for the different species. The frozen semen was then submitted to in vitro fertilization and 18.5% developed to 8-cell embryo. Similarly, some evidences showed that frozen epididymal spermatozoa from jaguars were able to penetrate heterologous zona-free oocytes.

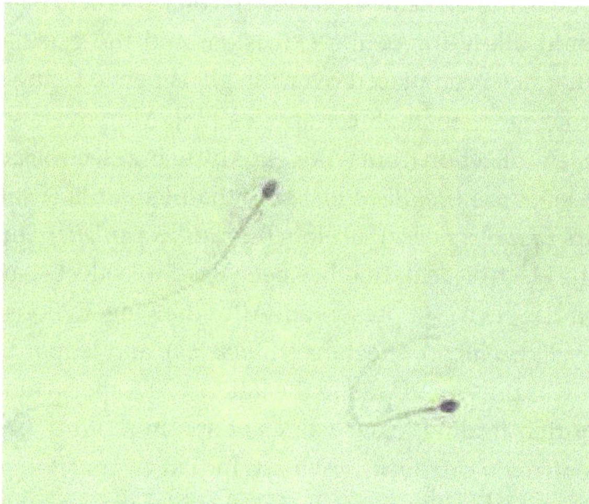

**Figure 1.** Epididymal sperms from dead *Panthera pardus*.

Spermatogenesis is a complex and very efficient process with the mitosis and the differentiation of spermatogonial stem cells in the basal membrane of seminiferous tubules where they are supported by Sertoli cells [33]. The spermatogonial stem cells in mammals are unique, and thus they can maintain their proliferation in adults: the genetic material can be passed from a generation to the subsequent one. Therefore, these cells are a valuable source for medical research, biological experimentation, agricultural biotechnology, and genetic modification of the species [34]. Recent studies on their recovery and cryopreservation showed the perspective of application in the conservation of genetic material from endangered animal species. Present methods described for spermatogonial isolation from fragments of collected testis consists of elutriation or sedimentation rate in a gradient of bovine serum albumin under gravity force action [35]. Some other isolation techniques have been proposed as immunological markers for posterior magnetic cellular separation [36]. After collection, germ cells can remain for several months in tissue culture media, only resuming spermatogenesis afterward in an environment that provides favorable conditions for their expansion and differentiation [37]. The favorable conditions are generally provided by transplant to other organisms [34]. The first success in the spermatogonial transplant was described by [38]. They showed that the microinjection of a cell heterogeneous suspension of mouse testis into the seminiferous tubules of a recipient sterile mouse resulted in spermatogenesis in the injected animal. After this study, several other researchers showed real possibilities such as the spermatogonial culture among different species: the xenograft [39]. It seems that cryopreservation of testis cell suspensions could be the greatest promise for the storage of germ cells to be used later in transplants. Indeed, after cryopreservation, spermatogenesis can continue [39]. In spite of the progress in this field, some elements remain to be controlled, such as the quantity of germ cells to be

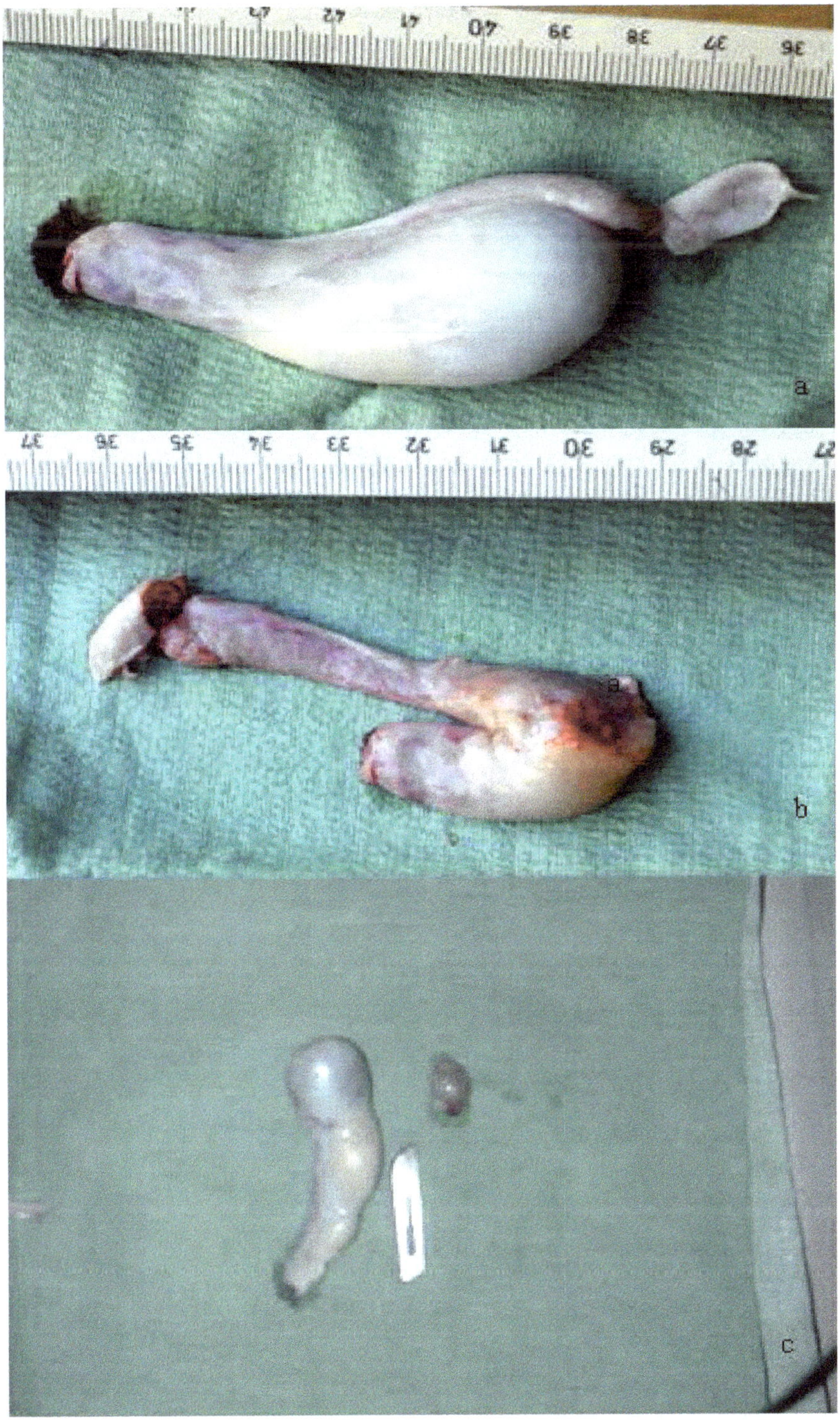


**Figure 2.** Testis and epididymus (a) and excised epididymus (b) of *Panthera pardus* collected 6 h postmortem; testis and epididymus of domestic cat and *Panthera onca* (c).

transplanted, formation of antibodies against spermatogonial cells by the recipient [40], and poor quality of cells that have developed using these procedures [41]. There is also a problem concerning xenograft related to the different time of spermatogenesis in each species [26, 42]. However, the complete spermatogenesis was observed after transplantation of testicular tissue fragments from species that are phylogenetically more distant, such as pigs and goats, into castrated immunodeficient mice. The new reproductive technologies on stem cells offer several potential advantages for carnivorous species. For example, the development of lines of embryonic stem cells in cats and dogs would allow the creation of a generation of transgenic animal models, which could be used to improve the health of both animals and humans. Techniques such as testis xenografting spermatogonial and stem cell transplantation offer new approaches to diffuse genetically valuable individual males, even if they should die before producing sperm. Therefore, these techniques could be applied to biomedical research, as well as to the programs for the conservation of endangered carnivore species. Recently, spermatogonial stem cell transplantation has been performed in a recipient able to produce sperm of donor genetic origin [26]. Sperm production, from prepubertal testis tissue from both ferrets and cats, was obtained from testis xenografting. These first steps reinforce the need for research on stem cell technologies and for complementary technologies of carnivore assisted reproduction, so clinical benefits and the largest array of research can be achieved [26].

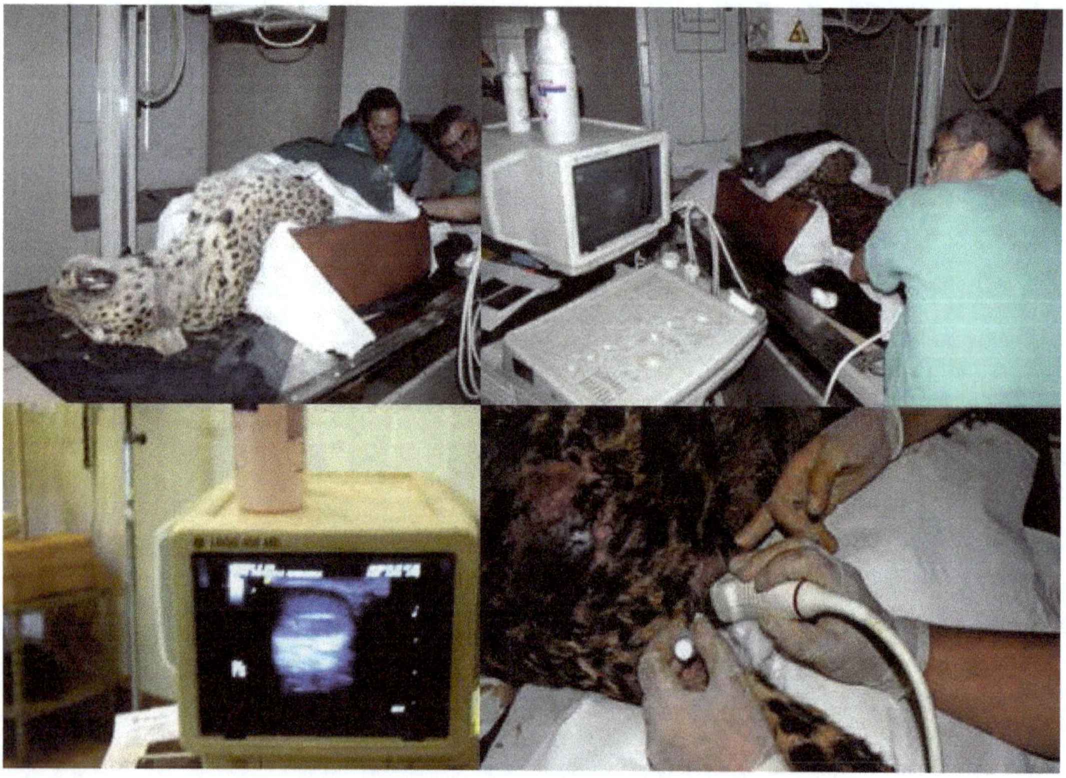

**Figure 3.** Ultrasound guided epididymal sperms collection in *Panthera pardus*.

## 6. Female gamete collection in felids

The ovarian follicular population seems to be made up of thousands of follicles in different mammalian females. Therefore, oocyte retrieval represents a rich source of genetic material to be used for genetic bank and assisted reproductive techniques in endangered species preservation, mainly in relation to the possibility of collecting material originated from postmortem or convalescent animals. The development of efficient methods for in vitro maturation (IVM) or fertilization (IVF) of oocytes collected postmortem or through ovariectomy is an important tool to prevent the species extinction [43-45]. Thus, IVM and IVF techniques are adjusted for several nondomestic animals [5] based on systematic studies in domestic animals [46] including wild carnivores. Moreover, application of oocyte and ovary tissue cryopreservation will help in the conservation of several animal species, with the objective of maintaining biodiversity [47]. Further, ultrasonographic images of the reproductive tract offer new opportunities for induction of sexual cycles and ovulation, adoption of superovulating regimens, as well as the ovum pickup application. Ovarian follicles are then visualized on a monitor, allowing oocyte collection by puncturing the follicles with a fine needle connected to a tube collector. The collected oocytes could be used in IVM and IVF [48, 49]. This technique is extensively used for oocyte collection in cattle and the findings indicate the possibility of repeated collections in both pregnant and nonpregnant females [50]. Concerning carnivorous species, ovum pickup using ultrasonography has yet to be reported. This may be due to the difficulty of ovarian visualization, because in bitches the ovary is surrounded by a pouch rich in conjunctive tissue [23]. Furthermore, there are no commercial probes developed for intravaginal use in either canids or felids. However, in spite of this difficulty, the presence of antral ovarian follicles can be detected by the fluid accumulation in the antral cavity [51]. A success in the follicular and corpora luteal visualization in ovaries of female African wild dogs (*L. pictus*) was reported by transrectal ultrasonography, suggesting the possibility of oocyte puncture in carnivores too [52]. The adaptation of this technique would be an important alternative, because it is a noninvasive procedure and it could allow oocyte collection without the risks involved with surgical procedures. The potential of ultrasonography is underestimated by researchers for assisted reproduction in endangered canid and felid species. Another possibility for oocytes retrieval is laparoscopy. It is the lowest invasive procedure commonly used for intrauterine deposition of frozen–thawed semen in domestic dogs [23] and cats [54]. For domestic cats, [27] reported the laparoscopic collection of oocytes, which were subject to fertilization in vitro with ejaculated semen. In this study, when the developing embryos reached the 4-cell stage, they were transferred to the oviduct of oocyte donors. Thus, five of the six cats receiving embryos became pregnant. According to [53], laparoscopy is effective in the evaluation of reproductive status, particularly the ovarian anatomy and function, direct visual biopsy of internal organs, and as a surgical means of fertility control. In wild felids, [55] reported the laparoscopic visualization of changes in the reproductive tract during ovarian stimulation by gonadotropins in the ocelot (*F. pardalis*). Moreover, the multiple laparoscopic oocyte retrievals was successfully performed in caracal (*C. caracal*) after repeated ovarian stimulation with equine (eCG) and human (hCG) chorionic gonadotropin [4]. Embryos could also be reliably produced in vitro using cryopreserved spermatozoa and live offspring could be produced after embryo transfer. It was suggested that the collection of ovaries from tigers (*P. tigris*), lions (*P. leo*), pumas (*F. concolor*), cheetahs (*A. jubatus*), leopards (*P. pardus*), and jaguars (*P. onca*) could be accomplished by ovary dissection up to 8 h after the death of these animals, by mechanical follicle isolation [56]. The best results were obtained with lion oocytes, fertilized by lion sperm, with a 31.6% (18/44) conception rate. It was demonstrated that leopard oocytes can be fertilized by domestic cat sperm and used in IVF procedures to produce 22% (2/9) 8-cell embryos. Otherwise, domestic cat oocytes can be fertilized by leopard spermatozoa, producing 19.5% (8/41) 8-cell embryos. Also oocyte collection from domestic and nondomestic cats by laparotomy and posterior ovary dissection was successfully performed. These oocytes were submitted to IVF and then transferred to recipient females [57]. The main result obtained in this study was the interspecies embryo transfer from an Indian desert cat (*Felis silvestris ornata*) embryo to a domestic cat (*F. catus*), which resulted in the birth of two kittens. Afterward, the oocyte collected from domestic cat ovaries after ovariectomy were used to demonstrate that morphology of the oocyte ooplasm can affect in vitro maturation, as well as the gonadotropin supplementation [12]. According to the morphological aspect by stereomicroscopic exam, cumulus–oocyte complexes were classified as mature, immature, or degenerated. Besides the successful embryo production by IVF using this approach, light and electron microscopic evaluations revealed that ovarian stimulation followed by follicular aspiration resulted in a heterogenous oocyte population with respect to meiotic maturation. The correct assessment of the oocyte maturation status is difficult to perform through stereomicroscopical exam [58]. Oocytes can be preserved if they are not immediately submitted to IVF. However, [59] observed that cooling could cause chromosomal anomalies in mature oocytes, as a consequence of the temperature decrease on meiotic fusion. [60] performed the IVM of domestic feline oocytes, previously kept under refrigeration at 4 °C for 24 h, and they did not observe deleterious effects of storage on oocyte meiotic progression. Moreover, [61] demonstrated that even brief (2–3 weeks) salt storage significantly affects cat oocyte penetration rate, and the penetration continues to decline as storage duration increases to 2–3 months. However, the authors hypothesized that the composition of the solution may have contributed to reduce sperm penetration. For canine species, [62] found that oocyte storage in hypertonic salt solution damages the zona pellucida, reducing the sperm penetration rates. In mice [63], rabbits [64], and bovines [65], it was possible to obtain the birth of normal offspring following IVF after thaw. In domestic felines, [66] demonstrated that the mature oocyte could be cryopreserved and, soon after, fertilized in vitro with success. The maturation of oocyte recovered from antral follicles is an efficient method for the use of haploid female material and the oocyte activation in initial phases of development is a possible tool that also increases the efficiency of the oocyte utilization [56]. The preantral ovarian follicles (PAF) represent 90% of the follicular population in mammals [67]. Small PAF recovered from the ovaries collected from postmortem animals or through ovariectomy, therefore, are a rich oocyte source, because they can mature in vitro (Fig. 4). [68] reported that feline PAF are capable of developing in vitro to the antral phase. Moreover, [69] demonstrated the isolation of PAF from domestic cats by mechanical ovary dissection. By adapting the methods described for domestic cats to nondomestic felid species, [70] accomplished the isolation and the ultrastructural characterization of PAF from cheetahs, jaguars, lions, and Sumatran, Siberian, and Bengal tigers that had died at local zoos. The similarity among domestic and nondomestic felid PAF was verified. The PAF collection was performed from ovary of several species of nondomestic felids [56] with a recovering of 1867±1144 PAF from each ovary, observing that the follicle growth is possible in the culture media for up to 14 days, with a 20% increase (40–50 mm) on the diameter of preantral follicles of the puma. These promising results suggest the possibility of future use of preantral follicles as a source of oocytes to be used in other biotechniques, and the foundation for germplasm banks. [70] reported that it is possible to maintain the viability of PAF from domestic cats after cryopreservation procedures.

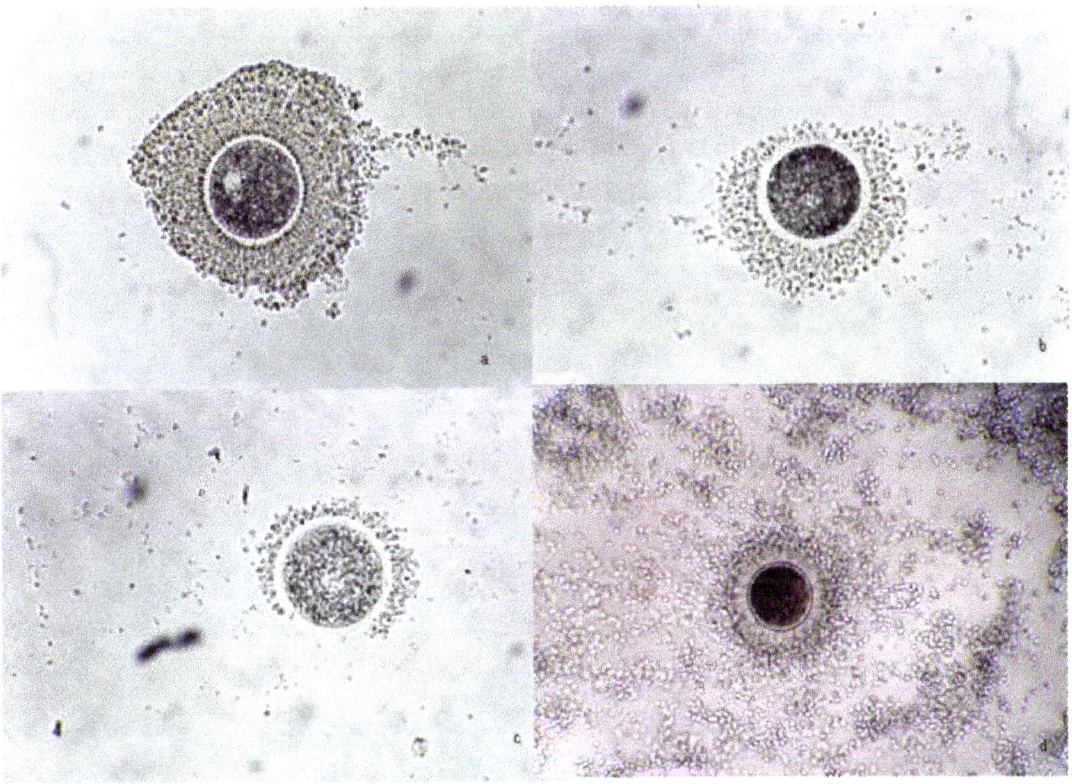

**Figure 4.** Cat Cumulus Oocyte Complex (COC) collected from Preantral Follicle (PAF); Cat COC grade: a) grade I: compact and integral and multistratified cumulus and dark ooplasm; b) grade II: compact but not integral and paucistratified cumulus and not homogeneous dark pigmentation of ooplasm; c) grade III: interrupted and incompact cumulus and clear ooplasm; d) expanded cumulus.

A further alternative is represented by the ovarian tissue transplantation. [71] was the first to report an ovarian transplantation. Only in the twentieth century was a significant improvement of the vascular anastomosis techniques of several transplanted organs including the ovary achieved [72]. According to [73], both whole ovary and ovarian fragment transplantations could be used for ovarian follicle cultures. Moreover, [74] was reported that a great advantage for the preservation and culture of ovarian tissue is due to the possibility of material collection not dependent upon the age or reproductive status of the donor. Moreover, [75] suggested that the term allotransplantation refers to the transplantation of an organ originating from one individual to another that is genetically different, but belonging to the same species. Ovarian cortex fragments transplantation was successfully performed from domestic cats to the renal capsules of severely immunedeficient infertile mice [76]. After 9 months, the necropsy of the recipient mice was accomplished, when the presence of follicles was verified in the grafts. These ovarian follicles reached a 3 mm diameter, had a normal antral cavity, and appeared to be cytologically normal as follicle in integer cat ovary (Fig. 5). However, ovulation was not observed in any of the grafts. Furthermore, [77] reported that xenotransplanting into the kidney capsule from severe combined immunedeficient mice freeze–thawed of cat ovarian cortex did not allow its surviving, but the follicles containing gonadotropin responsive granulosa cells were able to grow to antral stages. Conversely, [78] declared that oocyte and ovarian tissue cryopreservation is not yet fully established. There are still several obstacles to overcome for this technology to be routinely used. Even so, improvement in the cryopreservation techniques is seen as an important tool for the formation of ovarian tissue banks, with the purpose of conserving precious genetic material of endangered species [79].

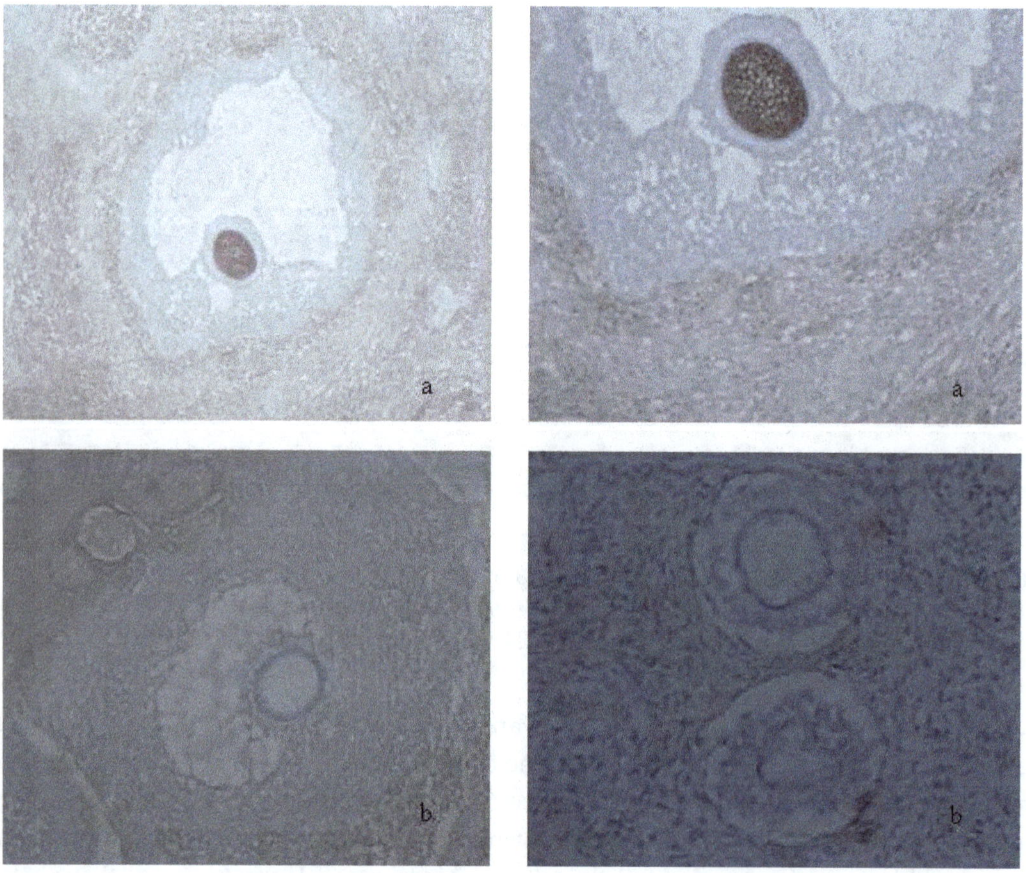


**Figure 5.** Histological section (O.M. 200X) of explanted cat ovarian tissue with follicle at different developmental stage: a) and a1) antral follicle; b) preantral follicle; b1) primary follicle.

## 7. Gamete cryopreservation in felids

Cryopreservation of gametes is an important tool in assisted reproduction programs. In fact, long-term storage of oocytes or spermatozoa is necessary for in vitro fertilization (IVF) or artificial insemination (AI) in the future. When geographical or temporal distance between donors and recipient results in nonsimultaneous availability of male and female gametes, cryopreservation is the only option. Maintenance of biodiversity has intrinsic value for the genetic preservation of valuable domestic cat breeds and an extrinsic value for conservation management of taxonomically related nondomestic feline species. New knowledge about felid reproductive physiology will enhance the development of techniques that are potentially applicable to nondomestic cats. Domestic cat spermatozoa and oocytes have peculiar physical characteristics that increase the difficulty of developing successful cryopreservation methods as compared to gametes of some other species. Therefore, even though a variety of procedures have been investigated, optimal cryopreservation techniques, either for spermatozoa or oocytes, are yet to be realized [80]. Cat semen was successfully cryopreserved, and kittens were born after AI with frozen–thawed semen [81]. Achievements in cryopreservation of felid semen and different protocols of freezing–thawing ejaculated and epididymal cat semen have been reviewed [80]. In our laboratory we cryopreserved epididymal sperm felines with the following protocol: epididymides were collected from 20 domestic cats during routine neutering procedure and from two wild felines at autopsy. The sperm samples, diluted with 4% glycerol/Tris/egg yolk, were loaded into 0.25 ml ministraws, exposed to nitrogen vapor and stored in liquid nitrogen. After 4 weeks, samples were thawed and reevaluated. The quality of each fresh and frozen–thawed sperm sample was tested by determining the motility (54.7±11.3% and 32±13.1%, respectively, for cat spermatozoa; 38.3±18.7% and 21.5±16.8%, respectively, for tiger spermatozoa), viability (74.3±8.6% and 45.2±9.4%, respectively, for cat spermatozoa; 42.4±14.5% and 33.5±12.9%, respectively, for wild felid spermatozoa), morphology, and acrosomal status. The present study showed that feline epididymal spermatozoa can be frozen in egg-yolk extender with 4.0% glycerol in 0.25 ml straws. The procedure used in the present study for epididymal cat sperm cryopreservation may be applied to bank for genetic resources of wild felid species. [82] Protocols for freezing/cryopreservation of cat oocytes [80] are established; nevertheless, this technology is still considered "experimental" because the survival rates of cat oocytes after freezing procedures are still low, but to date, there is evidence that some preantral follicles extracted from cat ovaries remain structurally intact and physiologically active after freezing/cryopreservation and subsequent thawing [80]. However, there is evidence that some preantral follicles from cat ovaries remain structurally intact and physiologically active after freezing/cryopreservation and subsequent thawing [70]. Domestic cat oocytes have high lipid droplet content in the ooplasm [83]; thus, oocyte permeability to cryoprotectant solutions may be lower than in oocytes of other species [84-87]. Only a few studies have investigated cat oocyte cryopreservation, and the few successes were only obtained for mature oocyte cryopreservation [80]. In the first study [80], mature and immature oocytes were cryopreserved by slow cooling, but no blastocysts were obtained after in vitro fertilization (IVF). In the second study [88], matured cat oocytes were vitrified in straws and, after IVF with frozen–thawed epididymal spermatozoa, the first two blastocysts were obtained [80]. In a recent study, the first attached cat blastocysts were obtained from matured cat oocytes that were vitrified using a cryo-loop system [89]. Another very recent study reported blastocyst production from vitrified germinal vescicle (GV) cat oocytes exposed to resveratrol (Res) in order to compact the decondensed chromatin contained in the large GV of cat oocytes [90]. Despite the importance of cryoprotectant penetration to avoid intracellular ice crystal formation, the greater cryoprotectant concentrations in vitrification solutions are toxic and may cause osmotic injury [91]. Suggestions for minimizing the toxicity of vitrification solutions include the use of less toxic substances, association with different cryoprotectants, previous exposure to lesser concentrations of cryoprotectants, and reduction of exposure time to vitrification solutions [92, 93]. The major penetrating cryoprotectants for oocyte cryopreservation are ethylene glycol (EG), glycerol (GLY), dimethylsulfoxide ($Me_2SO$), propylene glycol (PrOH), and acetamide [94]. Another common permeating CPA, 1,2-ethanediol (EG) [94], is also suitable for less permeable immature oocytes, as demonstrated in cattle [95]. A recent study investigating bovine oocyte vitrification demonstrated that a solution of EG + Me2SO is a favorable cryoprotectant combination, as the Me2SO (MW = 78.13) molecule is smaller and consequently more permeable than the glycerol molecule (MW = 92.1) [96]. In our laboratory for the first time we obtained blastocysts from egg vitrified at GV stage from cat [97]. The vitrification was performed in OPS into sucrose medium (1 M sucrose in HSOF + 6% BSA) containing dimethyl sulfoxide (DMSO) (16.5% final concentration) and ethylene glycol (EG) (16.5% final concentration) as cryoprotectants. This vitrification protocol ensured a development to blastocyst stage and it is the first report of development of vitrified GV COC and confirmed that the selection of an appropriate cryoprotectant mixture and sample volume reduction are two simple but important parameters in the study of a successful vitrification method for feline species. Ovarian tissue cryopreservation combined with the subsequent transplantation into immunocompromised recipients, in order to resuming follicular development, is considered to be a promising approach for cryobanking female gametes in nondomestic felid species [81].

## 8. *In vitro* embryo production in felids

Several laboratories have independently assessed the potential of maturing and fertilizing domestic cat oocytes, mainly using IVM /IVF. The biological competency of IVM/IVF domestic cat embryos has been demonstrated after embryo transfer. Nonetheless, it has become apparent that IVM/IVF success in the cat is generally less than that reported for other commonly studied species like the cow [4]. For example, it is not unusual for 60–80% of cow antral follicular oocytes to be fertilized and to cleave in vitro [9]. Techniques in the mouse have progressed even further to allow the growth, maturation, and successful fertilization of oocytes from primordial ovarian follicles. In contrast, only about 50–60% of cultured cat oocytes achieve nuclear maturation in culture and, after insemination, usually <40% oocytes are fertilized on the basis of embryo cleavage [9]. Even under optimal culture conditions, <20% of these cleaved embryos grow into blastocysts *in vitro* [9]. Nevertheless, in vitro embryo production has also been successful in felids. In vitro-derived embryos of the domestic cat were successfully frozen and developed to term kittens after cryopreservation and transfer. Various aspects of in vitro maturation of felid oocytes and in vitro culture of felid embryos have been comprehensively reviewed [81]. Cat oocytes can be collected from ovaries from sexually mature queens recovered following routine ovariohysterectomy. Feline oocytes can be collected from ovary explanted postmortem within 6 h from death. Within 3–6 h of excision, each ovary was sliced longitudinally with a scalpel blade followed by lateral mincing of the ovarian cortex in a 35 x 0.7 mm Petri dish, flushed by different media (e.g., HEPES synthetic oviductal fluid HSOF or HMEM or TCM199). Collected oocytes were graded (only oocytes exhibiting uniform, darkly pigmented ooplasm and an intact cumulus cell investment were chosen for culture), gently rinsed in a fresh dish of culture medium and immediately placed in 50 μl drops of culture medium under mineral oil or in 500 μl 4WD. In vitro maturation may be performed (25–50 oocytes/ml) in different media, for example, SOF synthetic oviductal fluid added with amino acids and 6 mg/ml BSA containing 0.1 IU of porcine follicle-stimulating hormone and porcine luteinizing hormone supplemented with 25 ng/ml EGF, 25 ml/ml insulin–transferrin–sodium selenite (ITS) and 1.2 mmol/l L-cysteine or Eagle's minimum essential medium containing 0.026 g pyruvate, 0.292 g L-glutamine, 0.4% (w/v) BSA, 100 IU penicillin, 100 IU streptomycin, 1 pg LH ml, 1 pg FSH and 1 pg oestradiol or MEM minimal essential medium containing Earle's salts and bicarbonate buffer supplemented with 0.4% (w/v) BSA, 2.0 mmol glutamine, 1.0 mmol pyruvate, 1 μg FSH, 1 μg LH ml, and 1 μg oestradiol (EMEM)] in a 5% $CO_2$ incubator at 38.5° C for 24 h. In vitro matured COC can be in vitro fertilized with fresh/cryopreserved epididymal or ejaculated spermatozoa. Briefly, in order to perform IVF, semen was diluted 1:1 in different media (SOF or Ham's FIO medium (HF10) supplemented with 1.0 mmol pyruvate, 2.0 mmol glutamine, and 5% (v/v) fetal calf serum or Tris extender (3.025% Tris(hydroxymethyl)aminomethane, 1.7% citric acid, 1.25% fructose, 0.06% Sodium Benzyl penicillin, 0.1% streptomycin sulphatee) and centrifuged at 300 g for 8 min. Supernatant was discarded and the remaining pellet overlaid with 100 μl HFlO and the sample maintained at room temperature undisturbed for 1 h. Next, 50 μl was removed from the top layer and evaluated for sperm motility, forward progression, and concentration. Cultured oocytes were washed twice in 90 μ fertilization drops of IVF media or in 500 μl FWD under oil in 5% $C0_2$ in air at 38°C. Processed sperm samples were diluted in IVF media in order to obtain a final concentration of 1 x $10^6$ spz/ml. After coincubation for 18 h, oocytes were washed to remove cumulus cells and loosely attached spermatozoa and returned to fresh 50 μ drops of IVC media (SOFaaBSA or F10). At 30 h after insemination, oocytes were evaluated at a stereomicroscope for survival, and those showing cytoplasmic degeneration were discarded. The cleavage to the two-cell stage was assessed as an index of fertilization. Subsequent embryonic development was assessed at intervals of 24 to 48 h. As explained, despite some past difficulties achieving in vitro development beyond the morale stage after IVF, more recently, several reports have shown blastocyst rates from approximately 50% to 80% on Day 6, Day 7, or Day 8 [98-100]. The frequency of blastocyst development is universally considered to be a useful measure of embryo developmental potential. In favorable in vitro culture conditions, cat blastocysts, like those of more widely studied species, undergo further growth, in cell numbers and in overall size. Thus, another widely accepted indication of blastocyst developmental potential is their ability to undergo expansion and "hatch" from the zona pellucida in vitro. Most of Day 8 blastocysts show noticeable expansion of the blastocyst cavity such that the zonal diameter is larger and its thickness is much thinner than at earlier stages. In addition, some of them are "hatching" because the embryonic cells are gradually extruded through one or more small apertures in the zona, rather than popping out through a large crack [4].

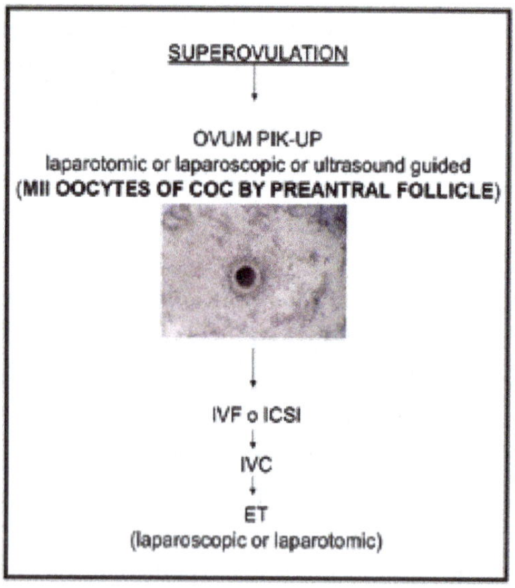


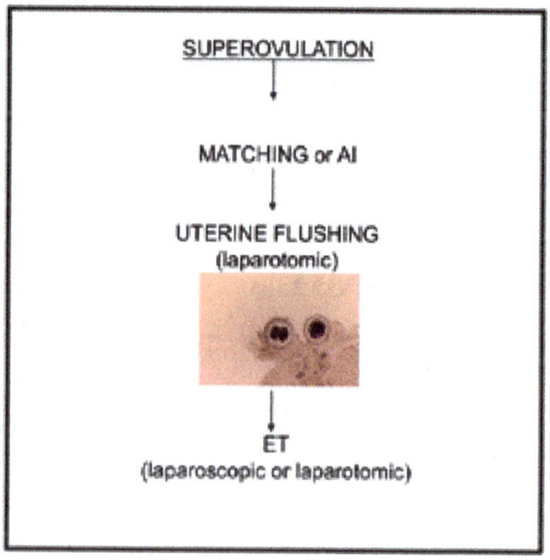


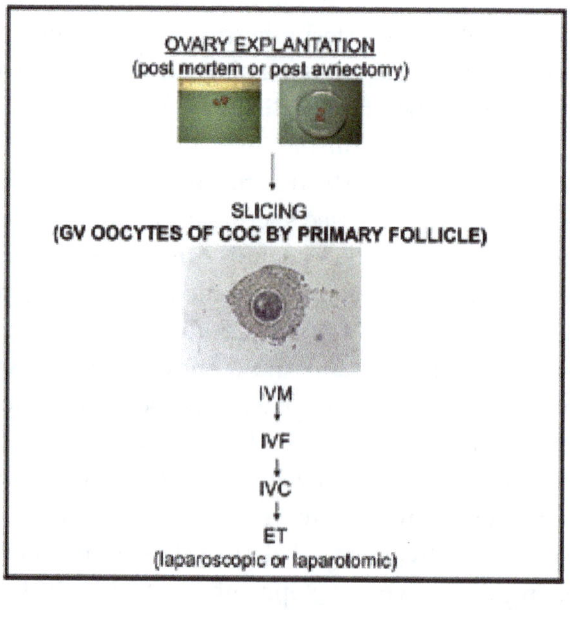

## 9. Artificial Insemination (AI) and Embryo Transfer (ET) in felids

Embryo transfer (ET) and artificial insemination (AI) are potentially important techniques for the propagation and management of genetically valuable domestic cat and endangered nondomestic cat populations. There are different AI techniques for cats [101]. In early studies, intravaginal insemination was exploited, but the success rate has not exceeded 43%. Later, this technique has been used with more effectiveness and a better success rate [102]. Another approach is intrauterine insemination, either surgical [103] or nonsurgical with the use of specially designed catheters [104]. They performed the first transcervical insemination with fresh or frozen semen in cats. This can be considered the method of choice in almost all cases; it is less invasive than the surgical approach, and a much smaller amount of semen is needed with respect to the intravaginal insemination. Recently, AI with semen cryopreservation has been applied in a number of wild felid species. Unfortunately, the teratospermia problem aggravates freezing/cryopreservation in many felid species [4]. In vitro embryo production has also been successful in felids. In vitro-derived embryos of the domestic cat were successfully frozen and developed to term kittens after cryopreservation and transfer. Various aspects of in vitro maturation of felid oocytes and in vitro culture of felid embryos have been comprehensively reviewed [4]. In 1979, the first successful embryo transfer (ET) in cats was reported [105]. The embryos, recovered from donors after mating during a natural cycle, were transferred into like recipients. Three litters of kittens were born from four pregnancies established in seven recipients. Nonetheless, in the following decade, in most ensuing reports on ET of in vitro-produced cat embryos, mixed morale and early blastocysts were deposited into the uterus of Day 4, 5, or 6 recipients [106-108]. This interval was used because it is the approximate length of time required for cat embryos to be transported through the oviduct and enter the uterus [109, 110]. To examine the effect of developmental stage, morula versus blastocyst, on pregnancy rate after ET, [111] recovered 1–4-cell embryos from gonadotropin-treated donors and cultured them in vitro (in 20% fetal calf serum) for 3–7 days before transfer into synchronous recipients. All four recipients of morulae (6–12 each) established pregnancies; two aborted before term, and two delivered a total of 10 kittens. Three of five recipients of blastocysts cultured for 4–6 days delivered a total of nine kittens, but none of the three recipients of blastocysts cultured for 7 days became pregnant. Although the zonal status of the blastocysts transferred after 7 days in vitro was not provided, most morulae had developed to the blastocyst stage by Day 7 of culture, with hatching starting to occur on Day 6 in blastocysts that were not fully expanded, which would suggest that most were either hatching or hatched when transferred. In their comments on failure of later-stage blastocysts (Day 8, 1 day in vivo, and 7 days in vitro) to establish pregnancies, the authors noted that further studies were needed "on in vivo development and hatching of transplanted embryos." [112] found that separate transfer of in vitro-produced Day 5 late morulae and Day 5 early blastocysts into synchronous gonadotropin-treated recipients resulted in equally high pregnancy rates of 71% (5/7) and 80% (8/10), respectively. Each recipient received six morulae or six blastocysts and the average litter size was 2.0 (1–3) and 3.0 (1–3), respectively. Possibly, the only pregnancy/birth after ET of in vitro-derived (IVM/IVF/IVC) Day 7 blastocysts is the single kitten born from 21 embryos transferred into two synchronous recipients [113]. All of the blastocysts were completely zona-intact when transferred. The transfer of fresh or frozen in vitro-derived embryos has proved to be successful in some wildlife felids. In the lion (*Pantera leo*), in vivo-derived oocytes were inseminated in vitro with fresh semen, and some of these embryos developed up to the blastocyst stage. In the tiger (*Panthera tigris*), term kittens developed after the transfer of in vitro-derived embryos [43], and one live kitten was born after the transfer of African wildcat (*Felis silvestris lybica*) frozen–thawed in vitro-derived embryos into three recipients [5]. Although the rate of success was low (4.5%), this result is important as this was the first kitten born after embryo cryopreservation in a wildlife felid species. Two term kittens born after transferring frozen–thawed embryos of ocelot (*Leopardus pardalis*) have also been reported [110]. Cleavage stage ocelot embryos were conventionally frozen with ethylene glycol and kept in liquid nitrogen [110]. More recently, three live ocelot kittens were born in Cincinnati Zoo after the thawing of ocelot embryos from a cryobank and the transfer of nine frozen–thawed embryos into eight synchronized recipients. The ocelot is an endangered species at least in some countries, and a cryobank is needed to secure its biodiversity [110]. The birth of live kittens produced by intracytoplasmic sperm injection of domestic cat oocytes matured in vitro has been reported [4]. Also noteworthy, there are experiments on "interspecies in vitro hybridization," when oocytes of nondomestic felid species were successfully fertilized in vitro by heterologous (domestic cat) spermatozoa. Cleavage stage "hybrid" embryos have resulted from in vitro fertilization of leopard (*Panthera pardus*) and puma (*Felis concolor*) oocytes with frozen–thawed domestic cat semen [4].

## 10. Cloning of domestic and wild cats and interspecies of felide

Along with these achievements with cryobanking, the domestic cat has been cloned by two independent groups [114,115]. Recently, a domestic cat recipient female has been reported to have given birth to African wildcat (*F. silvestris lybica*) cloned kittens and sand cat (Felis margarita) kittens [13]. Fibroblast nuclei of African wildcat were fused to domestic cat oocytes (interspecies nuclear transfer) and the cloned embryos were transferred into recipient domestic cat females; 17 kittens were born, but only 8 survived, after birth, up to 1 month. These African wildcat kittens represent the first wild Carnivora species to be produced by nuclear transfer [13]. This study showed the possibility of cloning other felid species beside the domestic cat, but it is also a big success in interspecies nuclear transfer/embryo transfer in felids. Earlier, an interspecies ET was performed between the Indian desert cat (*Felis silvestris ornata*) and the domestic cat [4]. Recently, transgenic clones have also been produced in the cat. Genetically modified adult or fetal fibroblasts have been used as donors of nuclei. These nuclei were moved into cat oocytes and then embryos were developed in vitro. After these embryos were transferred into appropriate recipients, three alive transgenic kittens were obtained [81].

## 11. Laparoscopic oviductal embryo transfer and artificial insemination in felids

The application of laparoscopy to reproductive studies in felids has been invaluable for helping to alleviate some concerns of animal welfare: sowing reproductive organs through the intraabdominal access through a minimally invasive and traumatic approach [116]. Likely, the extrapolation of ART to the genetic management of wild cats would be unattainable in the future without laparoscopy. The latter, for oocyte collection and intrauterine insemination, has been used largely with numerous cat species over the past 20 years. Recently, laparoscopic approaches have been developed and applied in cats for accessing the oviduct precisely to perform laparoscopic oviductal embryo transfer (LO-ET) and artificial insemination (LO-AI) procedures [117,118]. To our knowledge, just in eight cat hereditary disease models and two nondomestic cat species, the ocelot and sand cat, it has been possible to get viable offspring following LO-ET of nonfrozen and frozen–thawed IVF-derived embryos. LO-AI with low sperm numbers and LO-ET have been demonstrated to be similar in efficacy, resulting in high pregnancy percentages (50–70%) following insemination of domestic cats treated with gonadotrophins. Following LO-AI, multiple kittens have been produced in some hereditary disease models with frozen semen, and both Pallas' cat and ocelot kittens were born after LO-AI with freshly collected semen. The application of LO-ET and LO-AI to felids has brought important and effective improvement in the efficiency of ART for genetic management of these invaluable wild and domestic cat populations [119].

## 12. Conclusions

In the present chapter, we made an overview of the data and methods detectable in literature and focused our attention on analysis of methods utilized in ART for maximizing their efficiency in feline species. ART include mainly Artificial Insemination (AI); *In Vitro* Embryo Production (IVEP) consisting of IVM (*In Vitro* Maturation), IVF (*In Vitro* Fertilization), IVC (*In Vitro* Culture), ET (Embryo Transfer), and ICSI (Intra Cytoplasmic Sperm Injection); gamete/embryo cryopreservation; gamete/embryo sexing; gamete/embryo micromanipulation; Somatic Cell Nuclear Transfer (SCNT), and genome resource banking, which has been widely used in genetic improvement and industry in livestock animals. The domestic cat is used as a model for the development of ART in Felidae species and can serve as a successful recipient of embryos from closely related, small, nondomestic cats, as shown by the birth of the Indian desert cat and African wildcat kittens after in vitro fertilization (IVF)-derived embryo transfer. The creation of the Biological Resource Bank represents a complementary support tool for the application of ART in the in situ and ex situ conservation of endangered felids. The chief purpose of ART in the protection of endangered species is to preserve the maximum current genetic and biological diversity of the population by the processing and cryopreservation of germinal cells and tissues from dead animals, which can later be used in future reproductive projects. In humans and domestic species, it is usually possible to plan the place and time for gonadal explants to recover germplasm, thereby enabling a reduction in the gonadal storage time in the transport medium. In wild species, it is impossible to predict when and where the gonads can be collected. The gonads can be recovered postmortem, which entails the possibility that the collection place could be distant from a laboratory for IVEP.

## Author details

Natascia Cocchia, Simona Tafuri, Lucia Abbondante, Leonardo Meomartino, Luigi Esposito and Francesca Ciani*

*Address all correspondence to: ciani@unina.it

Department of Veterinary Medicine and Animal Productions, University of Naples Federico II, Naples, Italy

## References

[1] Swanson WF: Application of assisted reproduction for population management in felids: The potential and reality for conservation of small cats. *Theriogenology*. 2006;66:49–58.

[2] Hamner CE, Jennings LL, Sojka NJ: Cat (Felis catus) spermatozoa require capacitation. *J Reprod Fertil*. 1970;23:477–480.

[3] Bowen RA: Fertilization in vitro of feline ova by spermatozoa from the ductus deferens. *Biol Reprod*. 1977;17:144–147.

[4] Pope CE: Aspects of in vivo oocyte production, blastocyst development, and embryo transfer in the cat. *Theriogenology*. 2014;81:126–137.

[5] Pope CE: Embryo technology in conservation efforts for endangered felids. *Theriogenology*. 2000;53:163–174.

[6] Spindler RE, Crichton EG, Agca Y, Loskutoff N, Crister J, Gardner DK, Wildt DE: Improved felid embryo development by group culture is maintained with heterospecific companions. *Theriogenology*. 2006;66:82–92.

[7] Pope CE, Gómez MC, Dresser BL: In vitro production and transfer of cat embryos in the twenty-first century. *Theriogenology*. 2006;66:72–81.

[8] Comizzoli P, Wildt DE, Pukazhenthi BS: In vitro development of domestic cat embryos following intracytoplasmatic sperm injection with testicular spermatozoa. *Theriogenology*. 2006;66:1659–1663.

[9] Wood TC, Wildt DE: Effect of the quality of the cumulus–oocytes complex in the domestic cat on the ability of oocytes to mature, fertilize and develop into blastocysts in vitro. *J Reprod Fertil.* 1997;110:355–360.

[10] Wood TC, Bayers AP, Jennette BE, Wildt DE: Influence of protein and hormone supplementation on in vitro maturation and fertilization of domestic cat eggs. *J Reprod Fertil.* 1995;104:315–323.

[11] Freistedt P, Stojkovic M, Wolf E: Efficient in vitro production of cat embryos in modified synthetic oviductal fluid medium: Effects of season and ovarian status. *Biol Reprod.* 2001;65:9–13.

[12] Pope CE, McRae MA, Plair BR, Keller GL, Dresser BL: In vitro and in vivo development of embryos produced by in vitro maturation and in vitro fertilization of cat oocytes. *J Reprod Fertil.* Suppl. 1997;51:69–82.

[13] Gomez MC, Pope CE, Giraldo A, Lyons LA, Harris RF, King AL, Cole A, Godke RA, Dresser BL: Birth of African wildcat cloned kittens born from domestic cats. *Clon Stem Cells.* 2004; 6:247–258.

[14] Brown JL: Female reproductive cycles of wild female felids. *Anim Reprod Sci.* 2011;124:155–162.

[15] Wildt DE, Brown JL, Swanson WF: Reproduction in cats. In: Knobil, E., Neill, J. (eds.), *Encyclopedia of Reproduction,* 1st edn. Academic Press, 1998:497–510.

[16] Shille VM, Munro C, Farmer SW, Papkoff H: Ovarian and endocrine responses in the cat after coitus. *J Reprod Fertil.* 1983;69:29–39.

[17] Leyva H, Madley T, Stabenfeldt GH: Effect of light manipulation on ovarian activity and melatonin and prolactin secretion in the domestic cat. *J Reprod Fertil.* 1989;39:125–133.

[18] Pelican KM, Wildt DE, Pukazhenthi B, Howard JG: Ovarian control for assisted reproduction in the domestic cat and wild felids. *Theriogenology.* 2006;66:37–48.

[19] Dresser BL, Sehlhorst CS, Wachs KB, Keller GL, Gelwicks EJ, Turner JL: Hormonal stimulation and embryo collection in the domestic cat (Felis catus). *Theriogenology.* 1987;28:915–27.

[20] Goodrowe KL, Wall RJ, O'Brien SJ, Schmidt PM, Wildt DE: Developmental competence of domestic cat follicular oocytes after fertilization in vitro. *Biol Reprod* 1988;39:355–372.

[21] Jalkanen L: Embryonal development and embryo losses during the preimplantation period in the silver fox. *Norw J Agric Sci.* 1992;9:108–114.

[22] Wildt DE, Bush M, Morton C, Morton F, Howard JG: Semen characteristics and testosterone profiles in ferrets kept in a long-day photoperiod, and the influence of hCG

timing and sperm dilution medium on pregnancy rate after laparoscopic insemination. *J Reprod Fertil.* 1989;86:349–358.

[23] Silva A: The potential for gamete recovery from non-domestic canids and felids. *Anim Reprod Sci.* 2004;81:159–175.

[24] Platz CC, Wildt DE, Seager SWJ: Pregnancy in the domestic cat after artificial insemination with previously frozen spermatozoa. *J Reprod Fertil.* 1978;52:279-282.

[25] Howard JG, Brown JL, Bush M, Wildt DE: Teratospermic and normospermic domestic cats: ejaculate traits, pituitary–gonadal hormones, and improvement of spermatozoal motility and morphology after swim-up processing. *J Androl.* 1990;11:204–215.

[26] Travis AJ, KimY, Meyers-Wallen V: Development of new stem cell-based technologies for carnivore reproduction research. *Reprod Domest Anim.* 2009;44(Suppl 2):22–28.

[27] Goodrowe KL, Hay M: Characteristics and zona binding ability of fresh and cooled domestic cat epididymal spermatozoa. *Theriogenology.* 1993;40:967–975.

[28] Ciani F, Cocchia N, Rizzo M, Ponzio P, Tortora G, Avallone L, Lorizio R: Sex determining of cat embryo and some feline species *Zygote.* 2008;16:169 – 177.

[29] Bogliolo L, Leoni G, Ledda S, Naitana S, Zedda M, Carluccio A, et al.: Intracytoplasmic sperm injection of in vitro matured oocytes of domestic cats with frozen–thawed epididymal spermatozoa. *Theriogenology.* 2001;56:955–967.

[30] Tsutsui T, Tanaka A, Nakagawa K, Fujimoto Y, Murai M, Anzai M, et al.: Unilateral intrauterine horn insemination of frozen semen in cats. *J Vet Med Sci.* 2000;62:1247–1251.

[31] Jewgenow K, Penfold LM, Meyer HHD, Wildt DE: Viability of small preantral ovarian follicles from domestic cats after cryoprotectant exposure and cryopreservation. *J Reprod Fertil.* 1998;112:39–47.

[32] Lengwinat T, Blottner S: In vitro fertilization of follicular oocytes of domestic cat using fresh and cryopreserved epididymal spermatozoa. *Anim Reprod Sci.* 1994;35:291–301.

[33] Schlatt S, Kim SS, Gosden R: Spermatogenesis and steroidogenesis in mouse, hamster and monkey testicular tissue after cryopreservation and heterotopic grafting to castrated hosts. *Reproduction.* 2002;124:339–346.

[34] Brinster CJ, Ryu BY, Avarbock MR, Karagenc L, Brinster RL, Orwig KE: Restoration of fertility by germ cell transplantation requires effective recipient preparation. *Biol Reprod.* 2003;69:412–420.

[35] Bellvé AR, Cavicchia JC, Millette CF, O'Brien DA, Bhatnagar YM, Dym M: Spermatogenic cells of the prepuberal mouse. Isolation and morphological characterization. *J Cell Biol.* 1977;74:68–85.

[36] Shinohara T, Inoue K, Ogonuki N, Kanatsu-Shinohara M, Miki H, Nakata K, Kurome M, Nagashima H, Toyokuni S, Kogishi K, Honjo T, Ogura A: Birth of offspring following transplantation of cryopreserved immature testicular pieces and in-vitro microinsemination. *Hum Reprod*. 2002;17:3039–3045.

[37] Nagano M, McCarrey JR, Brinster RL: Primate spermatogonial stem cells colonize mouse testes. *Biol Reprod*. 2001;64:1409–1416.

[38] Brinster RL, Zimmermann JW: Spermatogenesis following male germ-cell transplantation. *Proc Natl Acad Sci USA*. 1994;91:11298–11302.

[39] Clouthier DE, Avarbock MR, Maika SD, Hammer RE, Brinster RL: Rat spermatogenesis in mouse testis. *Nature*. 1996;381:418–421.

[40] Ogawa T, Dobrinski I, Avarbock MR, Brinster RL: Xenogeneic spermatogenesis following transplantation of hamster germ cells to mouse testes. *Biol Reprod*. 1999;60:515–521.

[41] Russell LD, Ettlin RA, Sinha Hikim AP, Clegg ED: *Histological and Histopathological Evaluation of the Testis*. Cache River Press, Inc., St. Louis, MO 1990.

[42] Honaramooz A, Megee SO, Dobrinski I: Germ cell transplantation in pigs. *Biol Reprod*. 2002;66:21–28.

[43] Donoghue AM, Johnston LA, Seal US, Armstrong DL, Tilson RL, Wolf P, Petrini K, Simmons LG, Gross T, Wildt DE: In vitro fertilization and embryo development in vitro and in vivo in the tiger (Panthera tigris). *Biol Reprod*. 1990;43:733–744.

[44] Wildt DE: Fertilization in cats. In: Dunbar, BS, O'Rand, MG (eds.), *A Comparative Overview of Mammalian Fertilization*. Plenum Press, New York 1991;299–328.

[45] Luvoni GC, Oliva O: Effect of medium-199 and fetal calf serum on in vitro maturation of domestic cat oocytes. *J Reprod*. Fertil. Suppl. 1993;47:203–207.

[46] Wolfe BA,Wildt DE: Development to blastocysts from in vitro maturation and fertilization of domestic cat oocytes following prolonged cold storage ex situ. *J Reprod Fertil*. 1996; 106:135–141.

[47] Rodrigues APR, Amorim CA, Brasil AF, Figueiredo JRF: Criopreservação de oócitos mam´ıferos: Import^ancia, estado atual, limitações e perspectivas. *Ci Anim*. 2001;11:101–112.

[48] Hildebrandt TB, Hermes R, Jewgenow K, Göritz F: Ultrasonography as an important tool for the development and application of reproductive technologies in non-domestic species. *Theriogenology*. 2000;53:73– 84.

[49] Nibart M, Marquant Le Guienne B, Humblot P, Guerin B: The application of new reproductive technologies in France. *Arq FacVet*. UFRGS. 1997;25:21–35.

[50] Lacaze S, Marquant Le Guienne B, Delalleau N, Richef L, Maunas S, Nibart M, Humblot P: Centralized in vitro embryo production after ultrasound guided bovine oo-

cyte collection: Effects of parity and superovulation treatment. *Theriogenology*. 1997;47:161.

[51] Hayer P, Gunzel-Apel D, Luerssen D, Hoppen HO: Ultrasonographic monitoring of follicular development, ovulation and the early luteal phase in the bitch. *J Reprod Fertil Suppl*. 1993;47:93–100.

[52] Hermes R, Goritz F, Maltzan J, Blottner S, Proudfoot J, Fritsch G, Fassbeder M, Quest M, Hildebrandt TB: Establishment of assisted reproduction technologies in female and male African wild dogs (*Lycaon pictus*). *J Reprod Fertil Suppl*. 2001;57:315–321.

[53] Bush M, Wildt DE, Kennedy S, Seager SW: Laparoscopy in zoological medicine. *JAVMA* 1978;173:1081–1087.

[54] Farstad W, Hyttel P, Hafne AL, Nielsen J: Maturation and fertilization of blue fox (*Alopex lagopus*) oocytes in vitro. *J Reprod Fertil Suppl*. 2001;57:161–165.

[55] Swanson WF, Howard JG, Roth TL, Brown JL, Alvarado T, Burton M, Starnes D, Wildt DE: Responsiveness of ovaries to exogenous gonadotrophins and laparoscopic artificial insemination with frozen-thawed spermatozoa in ocelots (Felis pardalis). *J Reprod Fertil*. 1996;106:87–94.

[56] Jewgenow S, Blottner S, Lengwinat T, Meyer HHD: New methods for gamete rescue from gonads of non-domestic felids. *J Reprod Fertil Suppl*. 1997;51:33–39.

[57] Pope CE, Keller GL, Dresser BL: In vitro fertilization in domestic and non-domestic cats including sequences of early nuclear events, developments in vitro, cryopreservation and successful intra- and interspecies embryo transfer. *J Reprod Fertil Suppl*. 1993;47:189–201.

[58] Gjorret JG, Crichton EG, Loskutoff NM, Armstrong DL, Hyttel P: Ultrastructure of oocyte maturation, fertilization, and early embryo development in vitro in the Siberian tiger (Panthera tigris altaica). *Mol Reprod Dev*. 2002;63:79–88.

[59] Aman RR, Parks EJ: Effects of cooling and rewarming of the meiotic spindle and chromosomes of in vitro-matured bovine oocytes. *Biol Reprod*. 1994;50:103–110.

[60] Rodrigues FHG: Biologia e conservação do lobo guará na estação ecológica de Águas Emendadas, DF. Thesis, Instituto de Biologia, Universidade Estadual de Campinas, Campinas, Brazil 2002;96.

[61] Herrick JR, Swanson WF: Gonadotropin exposure, salt storage and storage duration affect penetration of domestic cat oocytes by homologous spermatozoa. *Theriogenology* 2003;59:1503–1513.

[62] Mastromonaco GF, Hay MA, Goodrowe KL:The effect of oocyte storage and cummulus cell presence on canine zone penetration by domestic dog spermatozoa. *Theriogenology*. 2002;57:1123–1134.

[63] Carrol J, Gosden RG: Transplantation of frozen-thawed mouse primordial follicles. *Hum Reprod*. 1993;8:1163–1167.

[64] Vicent C, Garnier V, Heyman Y, Renard JP: Solvent effects of cytoskeletal organization and in vivo after freezing rabbit oocytes. *J Reprod Fertil*. 1989;87:809–820.

[65] Fuku E, Kojima T, Shioya Y, Marcus GJ, Downey BR: In vitro fertilization and development of frozen-thawed bovine oocytes. *Cryobiology* 1992;29:485–492.

[66] Luvoni GC, Pellizzari P: Embryo development in vitro of cat oocytes cryopreserved at different maturation stages. Theriogenology 2000;53:1529–1540.

[67] Figueiredo JR, Rodrigues APR, Amorim CA: Manipulação de oócitos inclusos em fol 'ıculos ovarianos. In: Gonsalves, PBD, Figueiredo JR, Freitas, VJF (eds.), *Biotécnicas Aplicadas à Reprodução Animal*. Varella, São Paulo, 2002;227–260.

[68] Jewgenow K, Pitra C: Hormone-controlled culture of secondary follicles of domestic cats. *Theriogenology*. 1993;39:527–535.

[69] Jewgenow K, Stolt M: Isolation of preantral follicles from non-domestic cats-viability and ultrastructural investigations. *Anim Reprod Sci*. 1996;44:183–193.

[70] Jewgenow S, Penfold LM, Meyer HH, Wildt DE: Viability of small preantral ovarian follicles from domestic cats after cryoprotectant exposure and cryopreservation. *J Reprod Fertil*. 1998;112:39–47.

[71] Bert P: De la greffe animale. Thesis Medicale, Paris, France.1863.

[72] Carrel A, Guthrie CC: Technique de la transplantation homoplastique de l'ovarie. *C.R. Séances Soc* Brinster RL, Zimmermann JW: Spermatogenesis following male germ-cell transplantation. *Proc Natl Acad Sci USA*. 1994;91:11298–11302. *Biol*. 1906;6:466–468.

[73] Salle B, Demirci B, Franck M, Rudigoz RC, Guerin JF, Lornage J: Normal pregnancies and live birth after frozen-thawed hemi-ovaries autograft in ewes. *Fertil Steril*. 2002;77:403–408.

[74] Shaw JM, Oranratnachai JM, Trounson AO: Fundamental cryobiology of mammalian oocytes and ovarian tissue. *Theriogenology*. 2000;53:59–72.

[75] Bogliolo GBG, Pereira FEL, Vitela JEH, Bambirra EA, Barbosa AJA: Degenerações. In: Brasileiro GF, Pereira FEL, Pittela JEH, Bambirra EA, Barbosa AJA (eds.), *Patologia Geral*. Guanabara-Koogan, Rio de Janeiro. 1993; 51–59.

[76] Gosden RG, Boulton M, Grant K, Webb R: Follicular development from ovarian xenografts in SCID mice. *J Reprod Fertil*. 1994;101:619–623.

[77] Bosch P, Hernandez-Fonseca HJ, Miller DM, Wininger JD, Massey JB, Bracket BG: Cryopreservation and development of antral follicles in cat ovarian tissue after transplantation into Nod-Scid mice. *Theriogenology*. 2002;57:362.

[78] Ledda S, Leoni G, Bogliolo L, Naitana S: Oocyte cryopreservation and ovarian tissue bank. *Theriogenology*. 2001;55:1359–1371.

[79] Paris MCJ: Xenotransplantation and its potential role in assisted reproduction and animal conservation. In: *Proceedings of the Second International Symposium on Assisted Reproductive Technology for the Conservation and Genetic Management of Wildlife, Nebraska*. 2002;233–246.

[80] Luvoni GC: Gamete cryopreservation in the domestic cat. *Theriogenology*. 2006;66:101–111.

[81] Amstislavsky S, Lindeberg H, Luvoni GC: Reproductive technologies relevant to the genome resource bank in carnivora. *Reprod Domest Anim*. 2012;47:164–175.

[82] Cocchia N, Ciani F, ElRass R, Russo M, Borzacchiello G, Esposito V, Montagnaro S, Avallone L, Tortora G, Lorizio R: Cryopreservation of feline epididymal spermatozoa from dead and alive animals and its use in assisted reproduction. *Zygote*. 2010;18:1–8.

[83] Guraya SS: A histochemical analysis of lipid yolk deposition in the oocytes of cat and dog. *J Exp Zool*. 1965;160:123–136.

[84] Luciano AM, Franciosi F, Lodde1 V, Perazzoli F, Sleza´ kova M´, Modina S: Cryopreservation of immature bovine oocytes to reconstruct artificial gametes by germinal vesicle transplantation. *Reprod Dom Anim*. 2009;44:480–488.

[85] Massip A: Cryopreservation of bovine oocytes: Current status and recent developments. *Reprod Nutr Dev*. 2003;43:325–330.

[86] Papis K, Shimizu M, Izaike Y: Factors affecting the survivability of bovine oocytes vitrified in droplets. *Theriogenology*. 2000;54:651–658.

[87] Van der Elst J: Oocyte freezing: Here to stay? *Hum Reprod*. Update. 2003;9:463–470.

[88] Murakami OM, Karja NWK, Wongsrikeao P, Agung B, Suzuki T: Blastocysts derived from in vitro-fertilized cat oocytes after vitrification and dilution with sucrose. *Cryobiology*. 2004;48:341–348.

[89] Merlo B, Iacono E, Regazzini M, Zambelli D: Cat blastocysts produced in vitro from oocytes vitrified using the cryoloop technique and cryopreserved electroejaculated semen. *Theriogenology*. 2008;70:126–130.

[90] Comizzoli P, Wildt DE, Pukazhenthi BS: In vitro compaction of germinal vesicle chromatin is beneficial to survival of vitrified cat oocytes. *Reprod Domest Anim* (Suppl. 2) 2009;44:269–274.

[91] Arav A, Shehu D, Mattioli M: Osmotic and cytotoxic study of vitrification of immature bovine oocytes. *J Reprod Fertil*. 1993;99:353–358.

[92] Hotamisligil S, Toner M, Powers RD: Changes in membrane integrity, cytoskeletal structure, and developmental potential of murine oocytes after vitrification in ethylene glycol. *Biol Reprod*. 1996;55:161–168.

[93] Vajta G: Vitrification of the oocytes and embryos of domestic animals. *Anim Reprod Sci*. 2000;61:357–364.

[94] Pedro P, Yokoyama E, Zhu SE, Yoshida N, Valdez Jr DM, Tanaka M, Edashige K, Kasai M: Permeability of mouse oocytes and embryos at various developmental stages to five cryoprotectants. *J Reprod Dev*. 2005;51:235–246.

[95] Agca Y, Liu J, Peter AT, Critser ES, Critser JK: Effect of developmental stage on bovine oocyte plasma membrane water and cryoprotectant permeability characteristics. *Mol Reprod Dev*. 1998;49:408–415.

[96] Yamada C, Simoes R, Nicacio AC, Feitosa WB, Ortiz ME, D'A′ vila Assumpcao, Visintin JA: Immature bovine oocyte cryopreservation: Comparison of different associations with ethylene, glycol, glycerol and dimethylsulfoxide. *Anim Reprod Sci* 2007;99:384–388.

[97] N. Cocchia N, Ciani F, ElRass R, Russo M, Borzacchiello G, Esposito V, Montagnaro S, Avallone L, Tortora G, Lorizio R: Immature cat oocyte vitrification in open pulled straws (OPSs) using a cryoprotectant mixture. *Cryobiology*. 2010;60:229–234.

[98] Herrick JR, Bond JB, Magarey GM, Bateman HL, Krisher RL, Dunford SA, et al.: Toward a feline-optimized culture medium: impact of ions, carbohydrates, essential amino acids, vitamins, and serum on development and metabolism of in vitro fertilization derived feline embryos relative to embryos grown in vivo. *Biol Reprod*. 2007;76:858–870.

[99] Gómez MC, Pope CE, Harris RF, Davis A, Mikota S, Dresser BL: Births of kittens produced by intracytoplasmic sperm injection of domestic cat oocytes matured in vitro. *Reprod Fertil Dev*. 2000;12:423–433.

[100] Karja NW, Otoi T, Murakami M, Yuge M, Fahrudin M, Suzuki T: Effect of protein supplementation on development to the hatching and hatched blastocyst stages of cat IVF embryos. *Reprod Fertil Dev*. 2002;14:291–296.

[101] Zambelli D, Cunto M: Transcervical artificial insemination in the cat. *Theriogenology*. 2005;64(3):698–705.

[102] Tanaka A, Takagi Y, Nakagawa K, Fujimoto Y, Hori T, Tsutsui T: Artificial intravaginal insemination using fresh semen in cats. *J Vet Med Sci*. 2000;62(11):1163–1167.

[103] Howard FM: Breaking new ground or just digging a hole? An evaluation of gynecologic operative laparoscopy. *J Gynecol Surg*. 1992;8(3):143–158.

[104] Zambelli D, Buccioli M, Castagnetti C, Belluzzi S: Vaginal and cervical anatomic modifications during the oestrus cycle in relation to transcervical catheterization in the domestic cat. *Reprod Domest Anim.* 2004;39(2):76–80.

[105] Kraemer DC, Flow BL, Schriver MD, Kinney GM, Pennycook JW: Embryo transfer in the nonhuman primate, feline and canine. *Theriogenology.* 1979;11:51–62.

[106] Pope CE, Keller GL, Dresser BL: In vitro fertilization in domestic and nondomestic cats including sequences of early nuclear events, in vitro development, cryopreservation and successful intra- and interspecies embryo transfer. *J Reprod Fertil Suppl.* 1993;47:189–201.

[107] Pope CE, McRae MA, Plair BL, Keller GL, Dresser BL : Successful in vitro and in vivo development of in vitro-fertilized two- to four-cell cat embryos following cryopreservation, culture and transfer. *Theriogenology.* 1994;42:513–525.

[108] Kanda M, Miyazaki T, Kanda M, Nakao H, Tsutsui T: Development of in vitro-fertilized feline embryos in a modified Earle's balanced salt solution: Influence of protein supplements and culture dishes on fertilization success and blastocyst formation. *J Vet Med Sci.* 1998;60:423–431.

[109] Denker HW, Eng LA, Mootz U, Hamner CE: Studies on the early development and implantation in the cat: I. cleavage and blastocyst formation. *Anat Anz.* 1978;144:457–468.

[110] Swanson WF, Roth TL, Wildt DE: In vivo embryogenesis, embryo migration, and embryonic mortality in the domestic cat. *Biol Reprod.* 1994;51:452–464.

[111] Kanda M, Oikawa H, Nakao H, Tsutsui T: Early embryonic development in vitro and embryo transfer in the cat. *J Vet Med Sci* 1995;57:641–646.

[112] Kanda M, Miyazaki T, Kanda M, Nakao H, Tsutsui T: Development of in vitro-fertilized feline embryos in a modified Earle's balanced salt solution: influence of protein supplements and culture dishes on fertilization success and blastocyst formation. *J Vet Med Sci.* 1998;60:423–431.

[113] Pope CE, Gomez MC, King AL, Harris RF, Dresser BL: Embryos produced in vitro after recovery of oocytes from cat ovaries stored at 4 °C for 24 to 28 hours retain the competence to develop into live kittens after transfer to recipients. *Theriogenology.* 2003;59:308.

[114] Shin T, Kraemer D, Pryor J, Liu L, Rugila J, Howe L, Buck S, Murphy K, Lyons L, Westhusin M: A cat cloned by nuclear transplantation. *Nature.* 2002;415(6874):859. Epub 2002 Feb 14.

[115] Yin XJ, Lee Y, Lee H, Kim N, Kim L, Shin H, Kong I: In vitro production and initiation of pregnancies in inter-genus nuclear transfer embryos derived from leopard cat (Prionailurus bengalensis) nuclei fused with domestic cat (Felis silverstris catus) enucleated oocytes. *Theriogenology.* 2006;66(2):275–282. Epub 2005 Dec 27.

[116] Wildt DE, Kinney GM, Seager SWJ: Laparoscopy for direct observation of internal organs in the domestic cat and dog. *Am J Vet Res.* 1977;38:1429–1432.

[117] Conforti VA, Bateman HL, Vick MM, Lyons LA, Grahn RA, Deddens JA, Swanson WF : Improved fertilization success using laparoscopic oviductal artificial insemination with low sperm numbers in domestic cats. *Proc Soc Study Reprod.* 2011:40.

[118] Lambo C, Grahn RA, Lyons LA, Bateman HL, Newsom J, Swanson WF: Comparative fertility of freshly-collected versus frozen-thawed semen with laparoscopic oviductal artificial insemination in the domestic cat. International Symposium on Canine and Feline Reproduction. 2012.

[119] Swanson WF: Laparoscopic oviductal embryo transfer and artificial insemination in felids – challenges, strategies and successes Reprod Domest Anim. 2012;47(6):136–140.

8

# Human Embryology

Shigehito Yamada, Mark Hill and Tetsuya Takakuwa

**Abstract**

The study of human embryology has a very long history. Modern embryology owes its initial development to the key embryo collections that began in the 19th century. The first large collection was that of Carnegie, and this was followed later by the major 7 collections. The second role of the Carnegie collection was for researchers to establish a defined set of Carnegie stages based on embryo morphological features. Today, embryos are imaged three-dimensionally (3D) by a range of imaging modalities including, magnetic resonance microscopy (MRM), episcopic fluorescence image capture (EFIC), phase-contrast X-ray computed tomography (pCT), and optical projection tomography (OPT). Historically, embryo serial images were reconstructed using wax-plate and model techniques. The above new 3D imaging techniques now allow 3D computer reconstructions, analysis, and even 3D printing. This chapter will describe how the classical embryology collections and techniques have developed into today's imaging and analysis techniques, giving new insights to human embryonic development.

**Keywords:** Human Embryo, Embryo Collection, Developmental Stages, Imaging, 3D reconstruction, 3D printer

## 1. Introduction

Human embryology in the 19th century began by using human embryo samples derived from maternal deaths, abortion, or surgery. Nothing has been changed in the 21st century, because animal experimental biology developed in the 20th century could not and should not apply to human embryology on its ethical aspect. However, human embryology has progressed little during the last 100 years, with only recently some limited molecular studies on small numbers of human material. In contrast, recent studies using both nondestructive and destructive imaging techniques on existing collections have allowed many morphological measurements of these embryos using these novel imaging techniques.

Here we summarize the historic collections of embryos used in the study of human development, explain the criteria used for developmental staging, show sectioned and reconstructed images from newer three-dimensional (3D) imaging in high resolution, and discuss the future directions for the analyses of the human embryo.

## 2. Human embryo collections

During the history of human embryology the establishment and study of key human embryo collections has greatly contributed to our current understanding. In this section we briefly summarize the history of some of these collections, such as the Carnegie Collection, the Kyoto Collection, the Blechschmidt Collection, and the Madrid Collection (Table 1). More online information can be found on existing historic human collections (http://tiny.cc/Human_Embryo_Collections). The human embryo collections shown in Table 1, along with other collections, form part of the Digital Embryology Consortium (http://human-embryology.org), formed to electronically preserve and make available for research and education these irreplaceable historic collections.

Not included in this chapter will be descriptions of the smaller, less described human embryo collections, species comparative embryo collections, or collections that are of nonembryonic material, such as placenta. An example of one of the best and largest historic comparative embryo collections is the embryological collection of the Natural History Museum in Berlin, which includes many other species in the combined collections of Hubrecht, Hill, Dohrn, Bolk, and Kückenthal. An example of a mainly human placenta and early implanted uterus is the Hamilton-Boyd Collection in Cambridge. More recently, there are smaller collections of embryos used mainly for molecular studies, such as the Human Developmental Studies Network (HuDSeN) in Newcastle and London. Note that many anatomy departments hold their own small collections of human material that are not covered here.

A key factor in understanding the developmental morphological changes is the possession of human embryo samples at sequential developmental stages. The following are the major historic collections used in most research and textbook publications that have aided our understanding of human development.

| Collection | Place | Number | Characteristics | Establishment |
|---|---|---|---|---|
| Carnegie | Washington DC, USA | About 10,000 | Human fixed specimens and histology | 1887 |
| Madrid | Madrid, Spain | 100+ | Human histology | 1935 |
| Blechschmidt | Göttingen, Germany | About 120 | Human histology | 1950s |
| Kyoto | Kyoto, Japan | About 44,000 | Human fixed specimens and histology | 1961 |

**Table 1.** Comparison among major human embryo collections

### 2.1. Carnegie collection

Franklin P. Mall (1862–1917) began his human embryo at Johns Hopkins University in the early 1900s; these formed the beginnings of the Carnegie collection. He and Franz Keibel (1861–1929) used these embryos in their textbook *Manual of Human Embryology* [1, 2] and also in the Carnegie Institution of Washington Series *Contributions to Embryology* beginning in 1915. Organizing some of these human embryos form the first 8 weeks into a developmental sequence formed the basis of their "23 Carnegie Stages" staging criteria (see Figure 7), described in detail later in this chapter. The same staging criteria have been subsequently applied in the organizing of the other major human embryo collections. These stages will be described in detail from the Kyoto Collection later in this chapter. Reconstructions from histological sections of the collection embryos were the basis of the larger Carnegie models (Figure 1) and this technique has also been used in the development of other collection models, as in the Blechschmidt Collection.

Franklin P. Mall received his medical degree at the University of Michigan in 1883. He traveled to Germany to receive a clinical training, where he met the German embryologist Wilhelm His (1831–1904). This initiated his interest in studying human embryology, and he began collecting human embryos in 1887. His collection had reached several hundreds of specimens by the time he returned to the Anatomy department of the Johns Hopkins School of Medicine in Baltimore, Maryland. He received a Carnegie research grant in 1914 and became the first director of the Department of Embryology at the Carnegie Institution of Washington, in Baltimore, MD. The embryo collection grew at a rate of about 400 specimens a year, donated by clinicians and researchers, and the number of samples reached over 8,000 by the early 1940s. Researchers at the institute then began the complex task of organizing these embryos into a developmental sequence. Note that size alone was a difficult criterion due to the variable effects of fixation shrinkage. The solution was a "staging" system, developed by Mall, based instead on developmental ape embryo morphological features. Internal features were identified histologically from embryos that were serially sectioned, and also formed the basis of hundreds of 3D models and 700 wax-based reconstructions.

During Mall's era, several department members became renowned scientists. George L. Streeter (1873–1948) and Franz J. Keibel were also both former students of the important German embryologist Wilhelm His; Osborne O. Heard worked as an embryo modeler; and James D. Didusch as a scientific illustrator. Mall documented his research in a series of papers compiled in the *Contributions to Embryology* of the Carnegie Institution of Washington, published from 1915 to 1966. These articles even today are considered the core findings for studying human embryology. Mall unexpectedly died in 1917 and was replaced as director by Streeter. Streeter was then the first to define the 23 Carnegie Stages currently used to classify the developmental stages of the human embryo (see Table 2). The collection continued to grow by hundreds of specimens every year and included rare, very young normal specimens. At the time, induced abortions were illegal in the United States and miscarriages usually resulted from embryo abnormalities.

Streeter retired in 1940 and George W. Corner (1889–1981]) became the third departmental director. Corner was a former Johns Hopkins researcher who studied the menstrual cycle and identified the ovarian hormone progesterone. During his direction until 1956, many advances in human reproductive physiology were made and embryology research continued but came to an end with the succeeding director. Relocation of the collection began in 1973 to the University of California at Davis Medical School and was completed in 1976. Ronan O'Rahilly was the new director of the collection for the next 15 years, publishing many studies, often with Fabiola Müller, on human embryonic development. At the retirement of the director in 1991 the collection was relocated again to its current location at the Walter Reed Army Medical Center in Washington, D.C., forming part of the Human Developmental Anatomy Center 20 historic embryology collections and remains available for researcher study. In 2014, preliminary work began with the current curator on establishing a partnership with the Digital Embryology Consortium to eventually digitize, preserve, and make more widely available this collection. Further details of the embryo collection can be found in earlier publications [3, 4] as well as on the web (http://tiny.cc/HDAC_Collections), see also (http://tiny.cc/Carnegie_Collection).

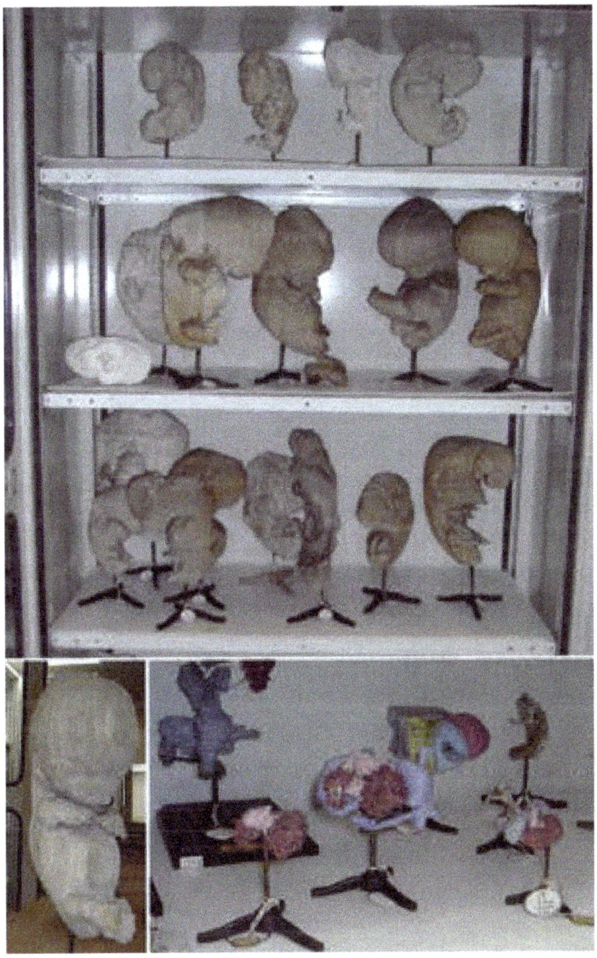

**Figure 1.** Carnegie models located at the Carnegie Collection. (Embryos shown in the bottom left-hand corner were laminated from individual layers and then painted.)

## 2.2. Harvard collection

Originally collected by Charles Minot (1852–1914), sometimes referred to as the Minot Collection, it now forms part of the larger Carnegie Collection. By 1905, the collection consisted of 937 histologically sectioned embryos from human and other species (Figure 2).

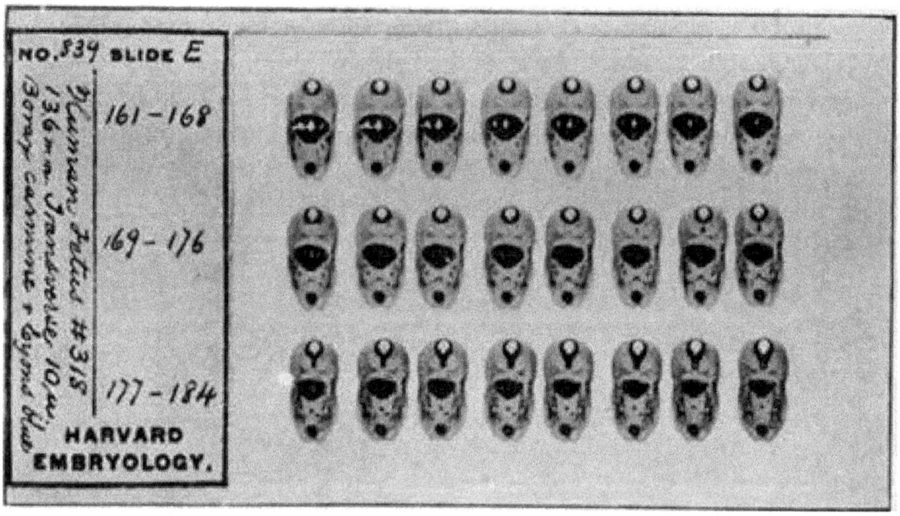


**Figure 2.** Harvard Collection histology slide No. 839 E, showing 10 micron serial sections from human embryo (No. 318) 13.6 mm in length.

## 2.3. Blechschmidt collection (University of Göttingen, Germany)

The Blechschmidt Collection is located in the Department of Anatomy and Embryology, Center of Anatomy, University of Göttingen. The University of Göttingen was founded in 1737, and has a long history in research that includes producing 45 Nobel Prize winners.

The human embryo collection is named after Erich Blechschmidt (1904–1992), who directed the Anatomical Institute from 1942 until 1973, and consists of two parts: firstly, a large histology collection of serial sections and, secondly, a model collection based upon these sections.

The histology collection is made up of about 120 human embryos that have been cut in a range of anatomical planes into some 200,000 serial sections. In 1972, some of the embryo serial section sets were temporarily incorporated into the Carnegie Collection and assigned Carnegie Nos. 10315 to 10434. These embryos have since been returned to their original home at the University of Göttingen.

The model collection (Figure 3) "Human embryologische Dokumentations sammlung Blechschmidt" forms a permanent exhibition housed at the Centre of Anatomy and consists of 64 large models, generated from 1946 to 1979. The models are available for viewing upon request and are arranged in perspex cases that allow each model to be observed from all directions. The models range from selected parts or systems of a specific embryo to whole embryos in surface view. In addition, parts of the embryos have been selectively removed or "windows" generated to observe internal system structures including: circulatory, respiratory, gastrointestinal, neural, and the musculoskeletal system.

The modeling method from the histological material used a technique based upon Blechschmidt's own method, described below. Each model illustrates whole embryo surfaces, some organic systems (including a circulatory organ, respiratory organs, a digestive organ, central nerve, and the skeletal system) in precision, in addition to the right-side out.

The embryo collection has probably the largest number of excellently preserved specimens of the latter half of the embryonic period (covering weeks 5–8 post conception). Detailed documentation on individual specimens of the collection is sparse and some of the specimens are also depicted as color drawings in Blechschmidt [5]. The high quality and standard of the histology material was achieved by a combination of a "state-of-the-art" embryo collection gynecological practice (mechanical curettage or hysterectomy) from operations including termination of pregnancy and development of a special fixation procedure. As a result, the quality of paraffin histological sections mounted on large glass microscope slides is unsurpassed and reveals valuable morphological detail of early organ development in the human embryo.

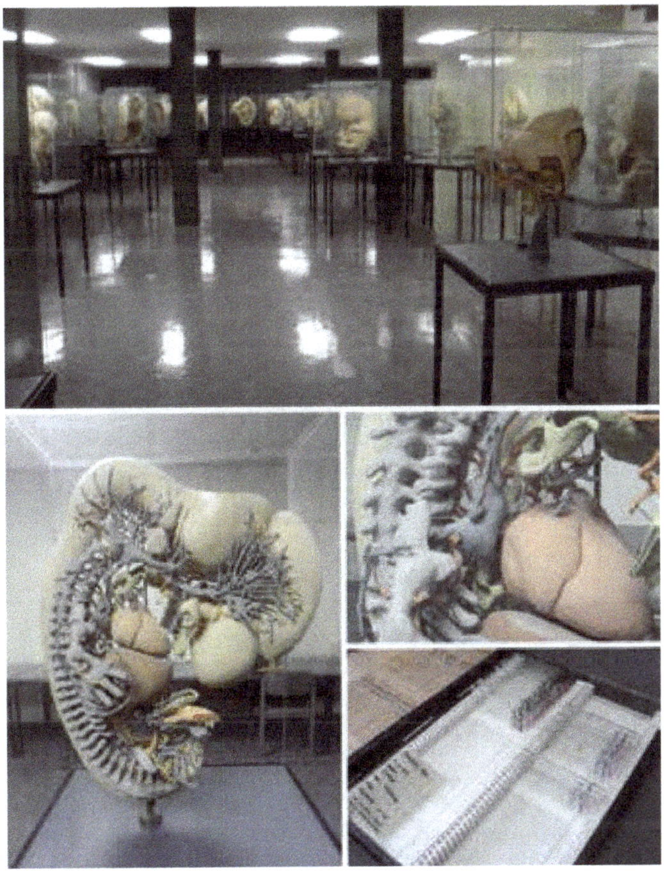

**Figure 3.** The Blechschmidt models and histology slides (photo by Saki Ueno).

Like many historic collections, even with optimal storage conditions, the slide histology has gradually deteriorated with evaporation of cover glass glue and bleaching of histological stains. Secondly, the large glass microscope slides are delicate and easily damaged during use. Both these issues highlight the pressing need for generating a "digital copy" of these historic collections.

Photomicrographs of individual histological sections from several specimens were included in Blechschmidt's embryology textbook [5]. At that time, the only way to preserve for posterity morphological information contained in these specimens consisted in building large-scale polymer plastic reconstruction models. These models were made from camera-lucida drawings at an intermediate magnification of regularly spaced histological sections [6]. Using the same series of serial sections several times over, Blechschmidt made reconstructions of the surface anatomy and the morphology of several organ systems of the same embryo, thereby enabling direct comparison of topographical characteristics and their dynamic changes during development, even though the cellular detail detectable at high magnification remained unexplored with this method. Currently, the way to preserve the collection in its current condition lies with the scanning and digital preservation of the histological material with the Digital Embryology Consortium.

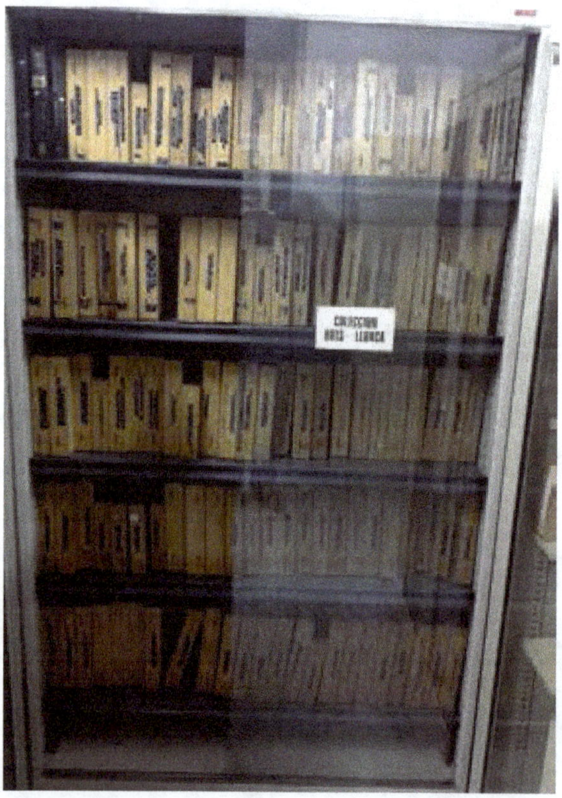

**Figure 4.** The Orts-Llorca Madrid Collection. Slides of serially sectioned embryos are stored in individual box sets. (Photo by Mark Hill)

### 2.4. Madrid institute of embryology human embryo collection

The human embryo histology collection was started in 1935 by the Spanish embryologist Francisco Orts-Llorca (1905–1993) and is located at the Embryology Institute of Complutense University of Madrid [7]. The collection consists of histological serial sections of more than 100 human embryos in thousands of serial sections covering the embryonic and fetal periods (Figure 4). The collection includes both normal and abnormal embryos. The sectioning is in a number of different anatomical planes and includes both normal and abnormal embryonic material. The collection has unfortunately suffered from the rigors of time, handling by many researchers, and fading of histological stains. The collection though still contains many very useful and unexplored embryos of a broad range of stages of development and the current head of department Professor José F. Rodríguez-Vázquez is determined to return this collection to a better condition and preserve this valuable research collection.

### 2.5. Hinrichsen collection (Bochum specimens)

Klaus V. Hinrichsen was a pupil of Blechschmidt and had the chair of Anatomy and Embryology at the Ruhr University Bochum in 1970. Many excellent specimens were collected by Hinrichsen's team between 1969 and 1994 and are now housed in the Department of Anatomy and Molecular Embryology at the Ruhr-Universität Bochum, Germany. The total number of the Hinrichsen Collection reached 70, and details of many of these specimens were published in Hinrichsen's textbook on human embryology [8] and in many original publications [9]. The reconstructions have not been attempted from these specimens and many specimens have likewise remained unexplored, to date.

### 2.6. Kyoto collection

Hideo Nishimura began this collection in 1961 and currently has over 44,000 human embryo specimens. It was further developed and managed by Kohei Shiota for a long period and is currently managed by Shigehito Yamada and all professors in the Department of Anatomy at Kyoto University School of Medicine.

Under the Maternity Protection Law of Japan, induced abortions were legal and in a great majority of cases pregnancies were terminated for social reasons during the first trimester. These provided Nishimura the beginning of the Kyoto collection. In 1975, he formed the Congenital Anomaly Research Center and the collection had now reached over 36,000 specimens. Currently, this collection is the largest in the world with over 45,000 specimens (Figure 5) and provides a key resource for international embryology researchers.

An important characteristic of the collection is inclusion of both normal and many abnormal embryos with severe malformations [10], including holoprosencephaly. Holoprosencephaly (HPE) is a rare newborn anomaly (1/10,000-20,000) occurring more frequently (1/250 or more) in the embryo, being the most common structural malformation of the human embryonic forebrain due to abnormal midline cleavage of the prosencephalon into cerebral hemispheres. This in turn leads to the characteristically abnormal facial development. [11]. Note that the estimation of embryonic frequency may be lower than the actual prevalence, as milder forms of holoprosencephaly also exist, but are more difficult to diagnose [12, 13].

Another unique feature of the Kyoto Collection is the associated maternal epidemiological data and detailed clinical information on the pregnancies that were collected with each specimen. The epidemiological data has been used for statistical analysis to determine potential causative links between maternal factors and congenital anomalies [14].

The collection has more recently been analyzed using several new advanced imaging technologies that allow 3D embryo imaging and subsequent generation of digital models. Firstly, magnetic resonance microscopy (MRM, see 4.1 in this chapter) of embryos has been carried out [15-18] and analyzed morphologically using 3D reconstruction [19-21]. Secondly, episcopic fluorescence image capture (EFIC) and phase-contrast X-ray computed tomography (pCT) techniques have also been applied to these embryos (18, 22, see 4.2 and 4.3 in this chapter). The current curator, Shigehito Yamada, has now commenced the lengthy process of digitizing all histological sections within this collection and is also a contributing partner in the new digital consortium. The Kyoto Collection is currently one of the largest and best catalogued human embryo collections, containing approximately equal numbers of both normal and abnormal specimens. The collection is also divided into whole wet specimens (see sub-heading 4.4 OPT) as well as about 1,000 serially, histological sectioned embryos (see 5.3, computer reconstructions). More recently, the current curator has digitized and made available online sections from some of the normal embryos in the collection (http://atlas.cac.med.kyoto-u.ac.jp).

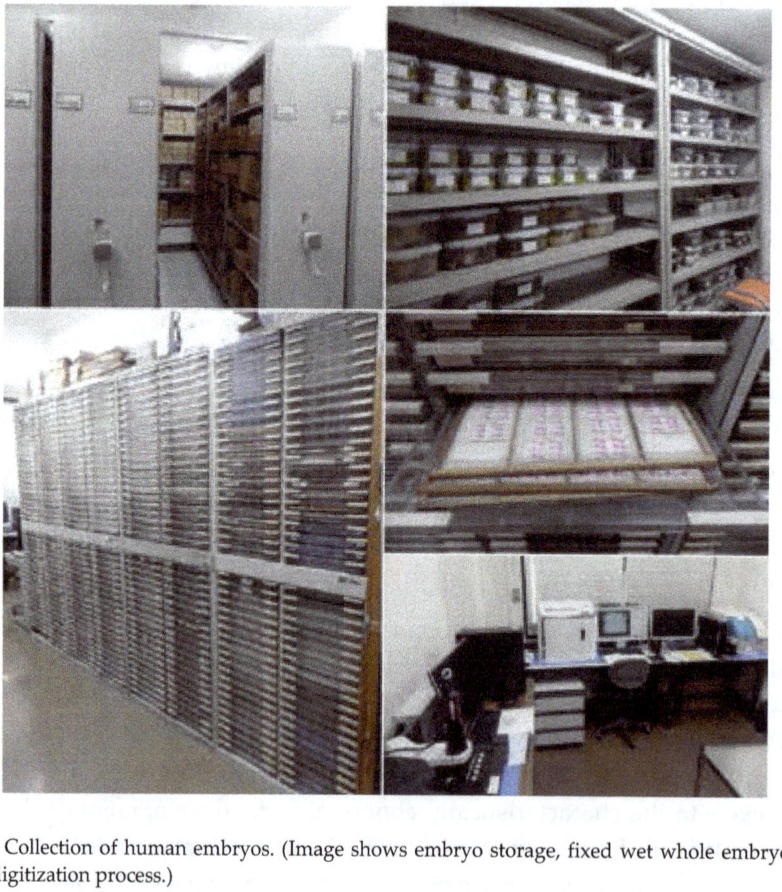

**Figure 5.** Kyoto Collection of human embryos. (Image shows embryo storage, fixed wet whole embryos, histological collection, and digitization process.)

## 2.7. Hubrecht collection

Ambrosius A.W. Hubrecht (1853–1915) was a Dutch embryologist who held a chair in comparative embryology at the University of Utrecht from 1910 and founded the "Institut Inteniational d'Embryologie" in 1911. This huge collection of comparative embryonic material from 600 vertebrate species consists of 3,000 wet specimens and 80,000 histological sections from many species including human [23]. There is also a significant collection of photographic material and documentation available. This collection along with the Hill Collection and other German collections forms the Embryological Collection at the Museum für Naturkunde in Berlin and is currently curated by Peter Giere (Figure 6). The collection is made available for researchers upon request. (http://tiny.cc/MfN_Berlin_Embryo)

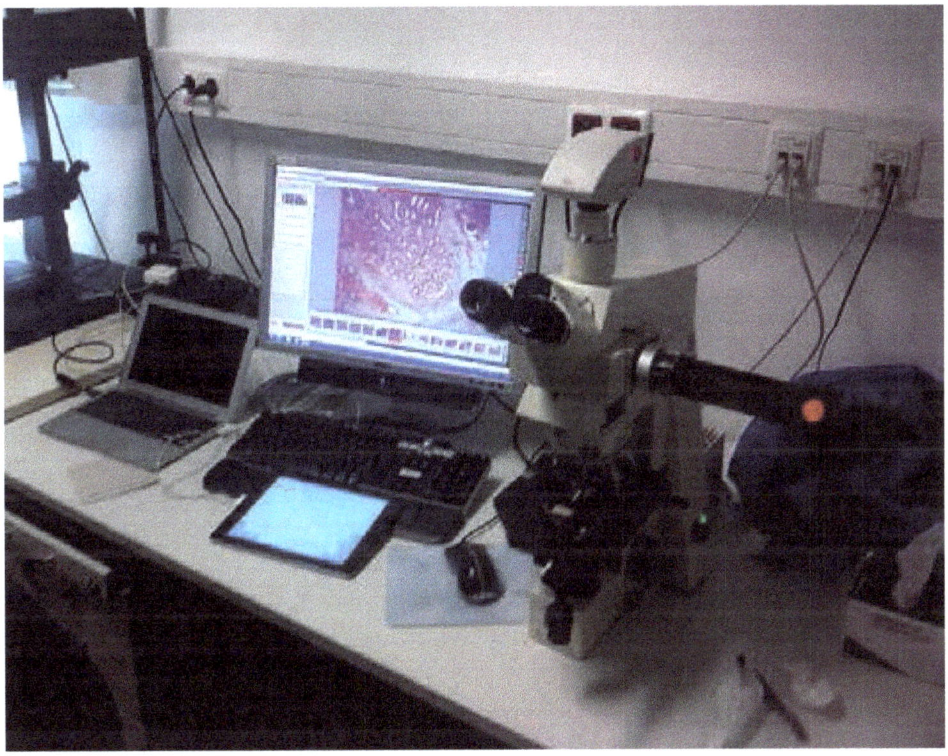

**Figure 6.** The Embryology Collection photomicroscopy setup at the Museum für Naturkunde. With permission, collection slides can be photographed and used for research purposes. (Photo by Mark Hill)

## 2.8. HUDSEN collection

The Human Developmental Studies Network (HuDSeN) atlas is based on 12 optical projection tomography (OPT) models covering the range of Carnegie stage 12–23 [24]. The Human Developmental Biology Resource (http://www.hdbr.org/) was established in 1999 in line with the ethical guidelines laid out in the Polkinghorne Report. There are also histological sections (hematoxylin and eosin stained) from human embryos covering these stages of development.

## 3. Human embryonic development

Classification into developmental stages is necessary to accurately describe prenatal growth. Embryonic staging of animals was introduced at the end of the 19th century [25], and was first applied to human embryology by Mall [26]. At first, human embryos were classified based on their length like "3-mm stage," but this approach was quickly obsolete because there are individual variations between each embryo. Subsequently, Streeter developed a 23-stage developmental scheme of human embryos in the 1940s called developmental "Horizons." Finally, stages 1–9 were established by O'Rahilly [1973], stage 10 was summarized by Heuser and Corner in 1957 from Streeter's note [27], and stages 11–23 were described in detail by Streeter [28–31].

### 3.1. Carnegie stages

The Carnegie stage is commonly known as a staging scheme which remains widely used today. Table 2 shows the relationship between embryonic ages from various researchers and the equivalent Carnegie stages proposed by O'Rahilly and Müller [32]. It is important to note that Streeter's human series included pathological specimens obtained from spontaneous abortion or ectopic implantation.

| Carnegie stage (CS) | Embryonic age (days) | | | | |
|---|---|---|---|---|---|
| | Streeter (28-31) | Nishimura (33, 34) | Jirásek (35) | O'Rahilly and Müller (32) | O'Rahilly and Müller (36) |
| 11 | 24 | 27 | 23-26 | 23-25 | 28-30 |
| 12 | 26 | 30 | 26-30 | 25-27 | 29-31 |
| 13 | 28 | 32 | 28-32 | 28 | 30-33 |
| 14 | 29 | 34-35 | 31-35 | 32 | 33-35 |
| 15 | 31.5 | 36 | 35-38 | 33 | 35-37 |
| 16 | 33 | 38 | 37-42 | 37 | 37-40 |
| 17 | 35 | 40 | 42-44 | 41 | 39-42 |
| 18 | 37 | 42 | 44-48 | 44 | 42-45 |
| 19 | 39 | 44 | 48-51 | 47-48 | 45-47 |
| 20 | 41 | 46 | 51-53 | 50-51 | 47-50 |
| 21 | 43 | 48 | 53-54 | 52 | 49-52 |
| 22 | 45 | 50 | 54-56 | 54 | 52-55 |
| 23 | 47 | 52 | 56-60 | 56-57 | 53-58 |

**Table 2.** Embryonic age (days) based on developmental stages (CS) of human embryos, according to various authors. Streeter [28-31], Nishimura [33, 34], Jirásek [35], and O'Rahilly and Müller [32] show the approximate ovulation age (days); O'Rahilly and Müller [36] show embryonic ages calculated from the greater length of embryo and ultrasound findings

### 3.2. Image and summary of each Carnegie stage (Figure 7)

Carnegie stage 1: Zygote

1 day after fertilization, cell size 120–150 μm in diameter.

At fertilization, the oocyte completes meiosis II, forming the female pronucleus. The spermatozoa nucleus in the oocyte cytoplasm decompresses, forming the male pronuclei. These two pronuclei fuse to form the first diploid cell, the zygote. The first mitosis occurs during the 24 h after zygote formation. The term "conceptus" is now used to describe all the cellular products of the zygote.

Carnegie stage 2: Morula.

1.5–3 days after fertilization, conceptus 0.1–0.2 mm in diameter.

The zygote forms two blastomeres. Mitosis of these blastomeres forms a solid ball of 16 cells, then 32 cells, still enclosed by the zona pellucida. This cleavage stage divides the large zygote cytoplasm into sequentially smaller cells. The term "morula" means berry, referring to the appearance of the solid ball of cells.

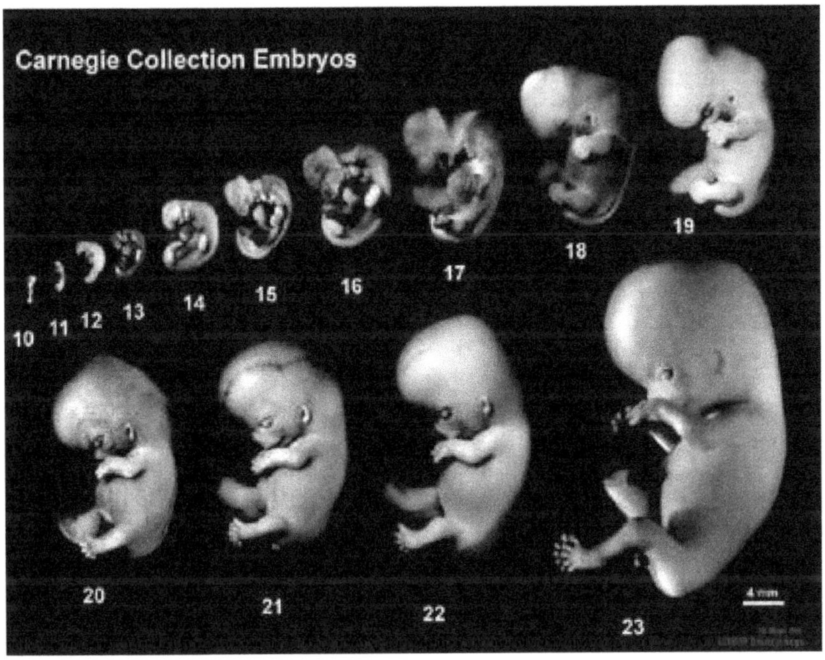


**Figure 7.** Examples of the Carnegie Collection embryos arranged into the classic Carnegie stages.

Carnegie stage 3: Free blastocyst

4 days after fertilization, conceptus 0.1–0.2 mm in diameter.

Cell division continues after the 32 cell stage occurring more rapidly at the surface and slower in the center cells. This and directional fluid transfer leads to a cavity, the blastocoel, in the conceptus. The surface cells form an outer squamous trophoblast layer linked by both tight and gap junctions. The larger inner cells form the inner cell mass or embryoblast.

Carnegie stage 4: Attaching blastocyst

5–6 days after fertilization, conceptus 0.1–0.2 mm in diameter.

The blastocyst hatches from the zone pellucida, still floating in uterine secretions of the secretory phase of the menstrual cycle. The surface trophoblast cells can now initially adhere to the endometrial epithelium at the site of implantation. The trophoblast cells proliferate and differentiate into two layers. The outer cells fusing to form syncytiotrophoblasts, the inner close remain as single cells, cytotrophoblasts.

Carnegie stage 5: Implanted but previllous

7–12 days after fertilization, conceptus 0.1–0.2 mm in diameter.

This stage was originally divided into three (a, b, and c) substages based on trophoblast differentiation status before outgrowth (villi) appears. 5a is the initial solid trophoblast cell layer; 5b, lacunar trophoblast with the appearance of spaces (lacunae) within the trophoblast layer; 5c, maternal blood-filled lacuna as capillaries and uterine glands are opened into the trophoblast spaces.

Carnegie stage 6: Chorionic villi and primitive streak

13 days after fertilization, conceptus 0.2 mm in size.

Trophoblast cells extend into the maternal uterine stroma (decidua) forming chorionic villi. The extra-embryonic mesoderm arises, lining the conceptus cavity and forming the chorionic cavity. Three separate cavities or extra-embryonic coeloms form outside the embryonic disc: the chorionic, amniotic, and yolk sac cavities. Toward the end of this stage, the primitive streak appears on the embryonic disc; this is the site of gastrulation.

Carnegie stage 7: Notochordal process

16 days after fertilization, embryonic disc 0.4 mm in length

The embryonic disc establishes axes and has an initial central primitive node (Hensen's node, primitive pit) with the primitive streak extending caudally to the disc edge where the connecting stalk will later form. Gastrulation occurs here forming endoderm and mesoderm that spread laterally and rostrally from the primitive streak. Above the primitive node, cranially, the notochordal process develops in the mesodermal layer. The length of this process increases from 0.03 to about 0.3 mm. The embryonic disc increases in size and the amniotic cavity enlarges over the yolk sac.

Carnegie stage 8: Primitive pit, neuenteric canal

18 days after fertilization, embryonic disc 1.0 mm in length

The embryonic disc is pyriform, tapering caudally, and now has cranio-caudal axis, measured from this stage onward by crown-rump length (CRL). The stage shows three key features: the primitive pit, the notochordal canal, and the neurenteric canal. The notochordal canal is marked by the cavity extending from the primitive pit into the notochordal process. The floor of the canal is lost to form a transient passage, neurenteric canal, between the amniotic cavity and the yolk sac. The notochord process will differentiate into the notochord or axial mesoderm. The remainder of new mesoderm layer has not yet segmented and is called the presomitic stage.

Carnegie stage 9: 1–3 pairs of somites

20 days after fertilization, embryo 1.5 mm in crown-rump length (CRL)

The mesoderm either side of the notochord now segments into paired somites. Segmentation of paraxial mesoderm only occurs at the level of the trunk, not the head, and proceeds in a cranial-caudal direction. Note that the sequential appearance of somite pairs can also be used as a criterion to stage the embryo. The embryonic disc resembles a shoe-sole, with the broad neural plate in the ectoderm layer positioned in the cranial region. The mid-line neural plate begins to fold forming a neural groove.

Carnegie stage 10: Neural folds begin to fuse, 4–12 pairs of somites

22 days after fertilization, embryo 1.8 mm in CRL

Somitogenesis continues increasing from 4 to 12 somite pairs. The neural groove continues to fold bringing the neural plate edges together to commence fusing. This fusion occurs in both cranial and caudal directions and at several sites. In the head region, the optic sulcus and first pharyngeal (branchial) arch appear. In the underlying trunk region mesoderm the cardiac tube appears.

Carnegie stage 11: Anterior neuropore closes

24 days after fertilization, 2.5–3 mm in CRL

Somitogenesis continues increasing from 13 to 20 somite pairs. The neural groove has formed an open-ended neural tube, and the upper head end (anterior, cranial or rostral) opening (neuropore) commences to close. Optic evagination is produced at the optic sulcus and the optic ventricle is continuous with that of the forebrain. The cardiac tube has formed a loop, with a sinus venosus region appearing. The second pharyngeal arch is visible. A ventral indentation (stomodeum) is present at the level of the first arch. The floor of the stomodeum forms the oral membrane (buccopharyngeal) that commences to degenerate. Dorsally at the level of the second arch, paired otic placodes fold inward to form the otic vesicles.

Carnegie stage 12: Posterior neuropore closes

28 days after fertilization, 4 mm in CRL

Somitogenesis continues with 21–29 somite pairs. The posterior (caudal) neuropore is starting to close or is closed. Three of the pharyngeal arches are now clearly visible. The upper limb buds appear, initially as lateral swellings at the level of the heart. Internally, the heart interventricular septum has begun to form, the liver is present and the lung buds appear.

Carnegie stage 13: Limb buds, optic vesicle

32 days after fertilization, 5 mm in CRL

Somitogenesis continues with more than 30 somite pairs. The numbers of somite pairs are now difficult to determine as staging criteria. Both upper and lower limb buds are visible. The optic vesicle is present, and the lens placode begins to differentiate.

Carnegie stage 14: Lens pit and optic cup

34 days after fertilization, 6 mm in CRL

The upper limb buds elongate and become tapering. Upper limb bud features appear about 2 days before the lower limb. The embryo cephalic and cervical flexures are prominent. Within the head, the future cerebral hemispheres and cerebellar plates are visible. On the head surface, the lens pit invaginates into the optic cup but is not yet closed and the otic vesicle endolymphatic appendage emerges. Within the trunk, pancreatic buds (ventral and dorsal) are present, the mesonephric duct forms the ureteric bud and at its tip is the metanephrogenic blastemal cap.

Carnegie stage 15: Lens vesicles, nasal pit and hand plates

36 days after fertilization, 8 mm in CRL

The upper limb hand plates are now visible. Lens vesicles are closed and covered by the surface ectoderm. The nasal plate invaginates to form a nasal pit. The auricular hillocks on pharyngeal arch 1 and 2 appear. Within the heart, the foramen secundum is present. Lung buds are now branched into lobar buds and the primary urogenital sinus is formed.

Carnegie stage 16: Nasal pit faces ventrally, retinal pigment, foot plate

38 days after fertilization, 10 mm in CRL

The upper limb hand plates are distinct and the foot plate has begun to form. On the trunk between the upper and lower limbs, a distinct mesonephric ridge is visible. On the head, the nasal pits deepen and face ventrally and the eye retinal pigment is visible externally. The nasolacrimal groove begins to form and lies between the frontal and maxillary processes.

Carnegie stage 17: Head relatively larger, nasofrontal groove, finger rays

40 days after fertilization, 11 mm in CRL

The upper limb hand plates have digital rays, and the foot has acquired a rounded digital plate. The head is now larger than previously and the trunk has begun to straighten. On the first and second pharyngeal arches the auricular hillocks are present and the nasolacrimal grooves are distinct.

Carnegie stage 18: Elbows, toe rays, eyelid folds

42 days after fertilization, 13 mm in CRL

The upper limb elbows are discernible and in the hand plates interdigital notches appear. Toe rays are observed in the foot plate. The trunk shape is more cuboidal and both cervical and lumbar flexures are denoted. On the head, eyelid folds appear and auricular hillocks are fusing to form specific parts of the external ear. Ossification commences in some skeletal structures.

Carnegie stage 19: Trunk elongation and straightening

44 days after fertilization, 16 mm in CRL

The upper and lower limbs are parallel, with preaxial borders cranially and postaxial borders caudally. On the head, eyes are now positioned in the front of the face, due to the growth of the brain, and the external ears have their definitive shape. The trunk continues to elongate and straighten. Within the trunk, the intestines have developed and herniated in the umbilical region.

Carnegie stage 20: Longer upper limb bent at elbow

46 days after fertilization, 19 mm in CRL

The upper limbs have increased in length and flexed at the elbows and hand joints. Fingers are curving slightly over the chest. The angle of cervical flexure becomes small, and the direction of the head goes upward. The head has a superficial scalp vascular plexus. The herniated intestines continue to elongate. Embryo spontaneous movements can occur at this stage.

Carnegie stage 21: Fingers are longer, hands approach each other

48 days after fertilization, 21 mm in CRL

The hands are slightly flexed at the wrists and nearly come together over the cardiac prominence. The head becomes round and the superficial vascular plexus has spread and now surrounds the head. The trunk tail now becomes rudimentary.

Carnegie stage 22: Eyelids and external ear are more developed

50 days after fertilization, 23 mm in CRL

The head vascular plexus is now very distinct. The eyelids have thickened and lie over the eyes. The external ear position is higher on the head and the tragus and antitragus regions are more definite. The trunk tail is almost lost.

Carnegie stage 23: End of embryonic period

52 days after fertilization, 30 mm in CRL

The head is now rounded out and the trunk has elongated to a more mature shape. The limbs have increased in length and the forearm is level or above the level of the shoulder. The head scalp vascular plexus is approaching the vertex of the head. The eyelids and ear auricles become definite. The external genitalia are developed but not sex-differentiated. The trunk tail has now gone.

## 4. Human embryo imaging

Rapid advances in medical imaging are facilitating the clinical assessment of first-trimester human embryos at increasingly earlier stages. To obtain data on early human development, we have used some micro-imaging modalities such as magnetic resonance microscopy, episcopic fluorescence capture, and phase-contrast X-ray computed tomography. The following sections describe and show the resulting embryo images from each of these imaging techniques.

### 4.1. Magnetic Resonance Microscopy (MRM)

Magnetic resonance (MR) imaging is now widely used as a tool for diagnostic medical imaging. In research, when scanning small samples this technique is called magnetic resonance microscopy (MRM). MRM was first applied to studying the human embryo in the 1990s [37, 38], and has now become a very powerful tool for 3D measurement of chemically fixed human embryos [15]. This research technique is still being developed and MRM images in higher resolution have been obtained using human embryos and a range of contrast agents [39]. The images shown in Table 3 were obtained using MRM equipped with a 2.34T magnet [15].

### 4.2. Episcopic Fluorescence Image Capture (EFIC)

Episcopic fluorescence image capture (EFIC) was devised and developed in the early 2000s [40, 41]. With EFIC imaging, tissue autofluorescence is used to image the whole embryo block face prior to histologically cutting each section. These individual sections can then be viewed or reconstructed into a 3D image [18], Figure 8. This technique has now been applied to staged human embryos from the Kyoto Collection. The first and only human embryo atlas developed from Kyoto embryos using EFIC can be accessed at website in University of Pittsburgh (http://apps.devbio.pitt.edu/HumanAtlas/; login ID and password are shown in [18]; the atlas also includes MRM images from similar staged embryos.

### 4.3. Phase-Contrast X-ray Computed Tomography (pCT)

Phase-contrast X-ray computed tomography (pCT) is a relatively newer technique of imaging. In this technique, the X-rays are used as electric waves characterized by amplitude and phase. Conventional X-ray imaging (radiography) is based on absorption-contrast (i.e., amplitude imaging) and represents the mass-density distribution of X-ray inside the sample.

In comparison, pCT uses the phase-shift, occurring when X-rays pass through samples [42]. The phase shift is converted into a change in X-ray intensity that is collected by a current-detecting device. There are some conversion methods such as interferometry with an X-ray crystal interferometer [42, 43], diffractometry with a perfect analyzer crystal [44-46], a propagation-based method with a Fresnel pattern [47, 48], and Talbot interferometry with a Talbot grating interferometer [49, 50]. Devices based on this principle have been developed [51, 52], and an image of human embryo at CS 17 obtained using a two-crystal X-ray interferometer (Yoneyama et al., 2011) is featured in Figure 9.

### 4.4. Optical Projection Tomography (OPT)

Optical projection tomography (OPT) was devised in 2002, using the principle of projection tomography [53, 54]. During the embedding process, the samples are dehydrated and cleared

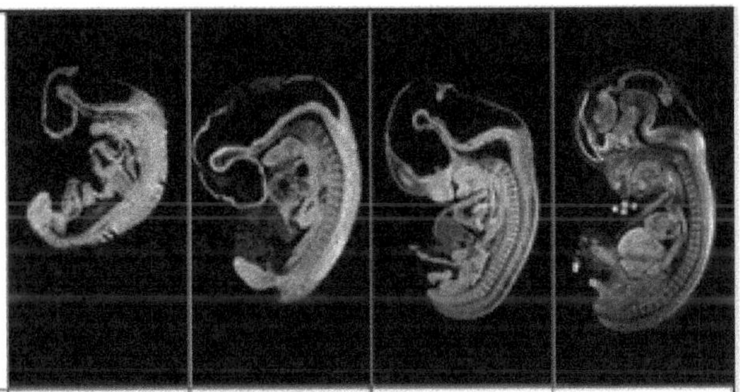

| Carnegie stage | 13 | 16 | 19 | 22 |
|---|---|---|---|---|
| Days after fertilization (Gestational weeks) | 32 (6w4d) | 38 (7w3d) | 44 (8w2d) | 50 (9w1d) |
| Cranio-rump length | 5.0mm | 10mm | 16mm | 23mm |
| Digital resolution | 40μm/pixel | 50μm/pixel | 100μm/pixel | 120μm/pixel |

**Table 3.** Result of MRM scanning using human embryos

with a mixture of benzyl alcohol and benzyl benzoate, allowing the light to pass through the specimen. This technique has also been applied into human embryo [55, 56], and the atlas regarding gene expression in the developing human brain has been established using OPT [24].

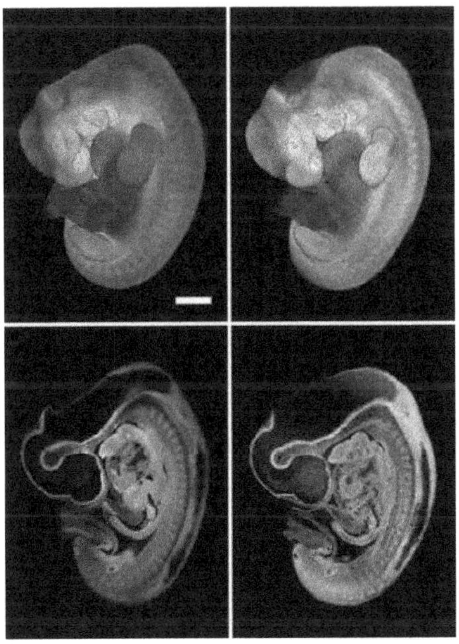

**Figure 8.** Comparison between imaging of the same stage embryo using two different techniques of EFIC (left) and MRM (right).

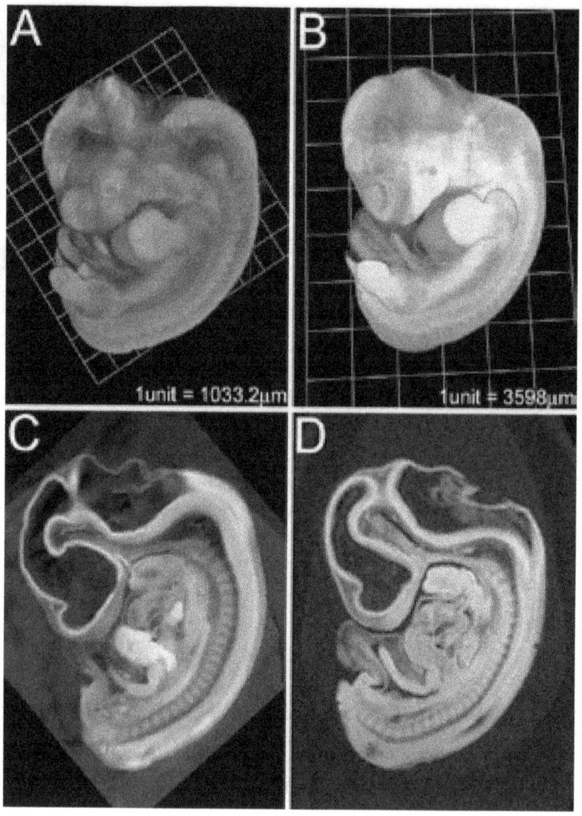


**Figure 9.** Comparison of human embryos (CS 17) imaged by pCT (A,C) and MRM (B,D). Note that Rathke's pouch can be seen in the embryo by pCT (C) but not detected by MRM (D).

## 5. Three-dimensional models and analyses of human embryos

In the 19th century, human embryo models were made manually based on macroscopic and microscopic observation. Wax plate technique was introduced into embryology in 1887, and the principle was used continuously until the computer era, although the material of the model has been changed from wax to plastics. Computer-assisted reconstruction started at the end of the 20th century. The reconstruction was made from the histological sections at first, followed by reconstruction from 3D image dataset. Recently, as 3D printers become cheaper and widespread, they are being applied in human embryology.

### 5.1. Ziegler models

By the middle of the 19th century, there had already been 2D illustrations of embryos and 3D embryo models were eagerly awaited, due to the difficulty of obtaining embryos, their fragility and size. Louis Auzoux, a French anatomist, made papier-mâché models in his Normandy workshop (Figure 10A). Later Adolf Ziegler started to render hand-shaped models after he returned to the University of Freiburg in 1854, and completed his first model series "The Development of the Frog." His modeling was applied in developmental biology, including human embryos. Adolf Ziegler retired in 1883 and his son Friedrich Ziegler took over the modeling operations. The "Ziegler models," including trout, sea urchin, beetle, frog, chick, and human embryos (Figure 10B) were displayed at the 1893 World's Columbian Exposition in Chicago, and there they attracted much attention.

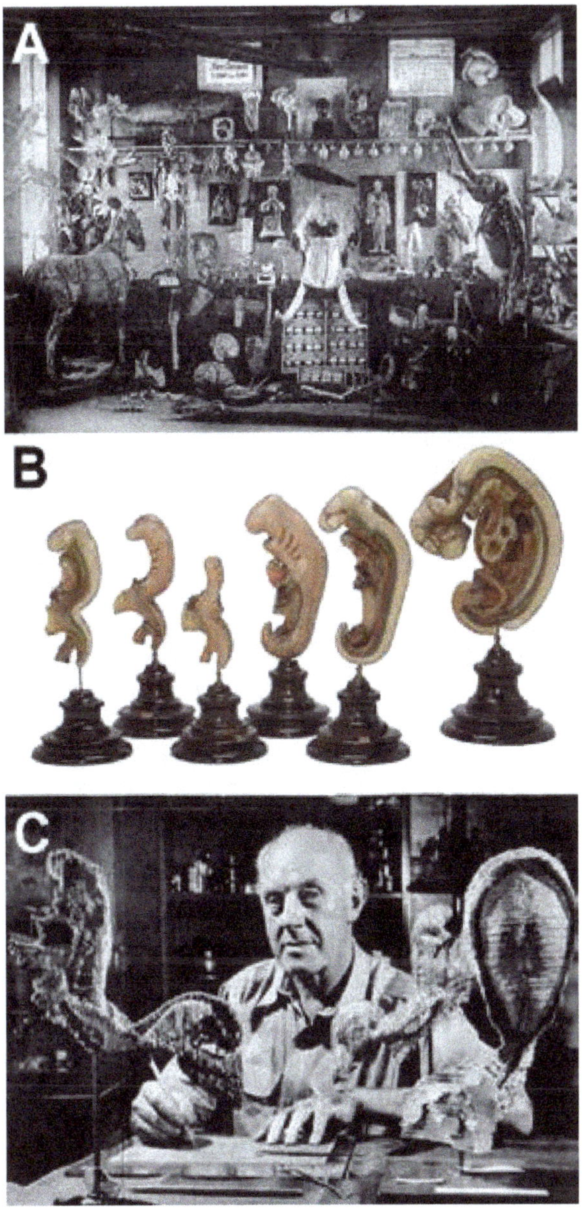


**Figure 10.** Examples of historic embryo models. Modeling workshop of Louis Auzoux (A), Ziegler human embryo models (B) and Carnegie Laboratory models and Osborne O. Heard (C).

### 5.2. Wax-plate model and its derivatives

In 1865, Wilhelm His Sr. invented the microtome [57], and he applied it to embryology. In 1883, Gustav Born devised the wax plate technique; 3D reconstruction from serial histological sections was made by wax plate [58]. This technique was applied to embryology [59] and later modified in the Carnegie Laboratory in Baltimore [60]. The material of model originally used was mainly wax (Figure 10C), and changed into plastic or its derivatives [61] in the 20th century. These new models were a significant improvement in detail and accuracy over the earlier Ziegler models. The technique was later further developed, with larger scale and detail, by Blechschmidt in his model series (see above, section 2.3].

### 5.3. Computer graphics from serial sections

Recent advancement in image technology and computer science has made computer-assisted reconstruction of embryonic structures more effectively, and the reconstructed images can be manipulated as desired on the viewing screen. This technique has been applied to human embryos in 1994, using the Madrid Collection [62], and 3D reconstruction of human embryo has also been established using the Kyoto Collection [62]. In the 21st century, the 3D models were colorized and elaborated [63, and see Figure 11]. In combination with the advance of web technique, some attractive web-based human embryo atlases have been constructed using the Kyoto Collection [18], http://apps.devbio.pitt.edu/HumanAtlas/), and the Carnegie Collection has been established and available freely [64], (http://www.ehd.org/virtual-human-embryo/).

### 5.4. 3D printer and scanner

A 3D printer is a tool for making 3D solid objects from digital data. Stereolithography was a technique developed at the end of the 20th century; in recent years, it has enabled the creation of inexpensive 3D models in engineering, medical and dental fields, as well as the academic area [65] and has been applied to human embryology [66], (see Figure 12).

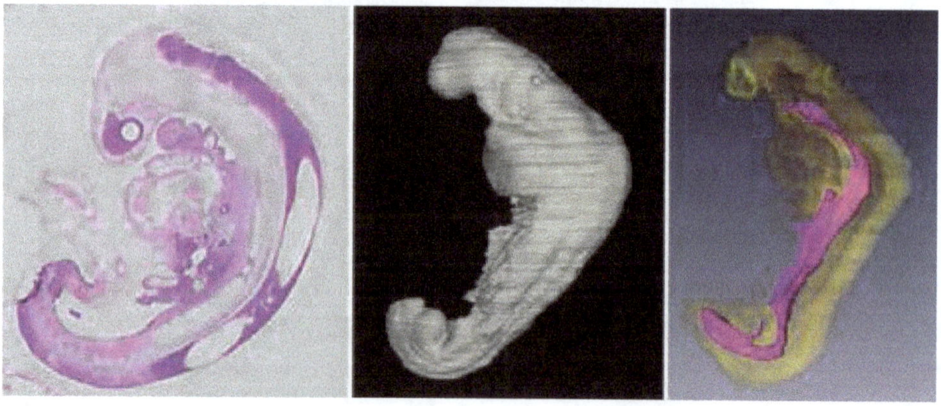

**Figure 11.** Histological section (left), embryo surface reconstruction (center) and a 3D reconstruction labeling of the gastrointestinal system (right) from a human embryo.

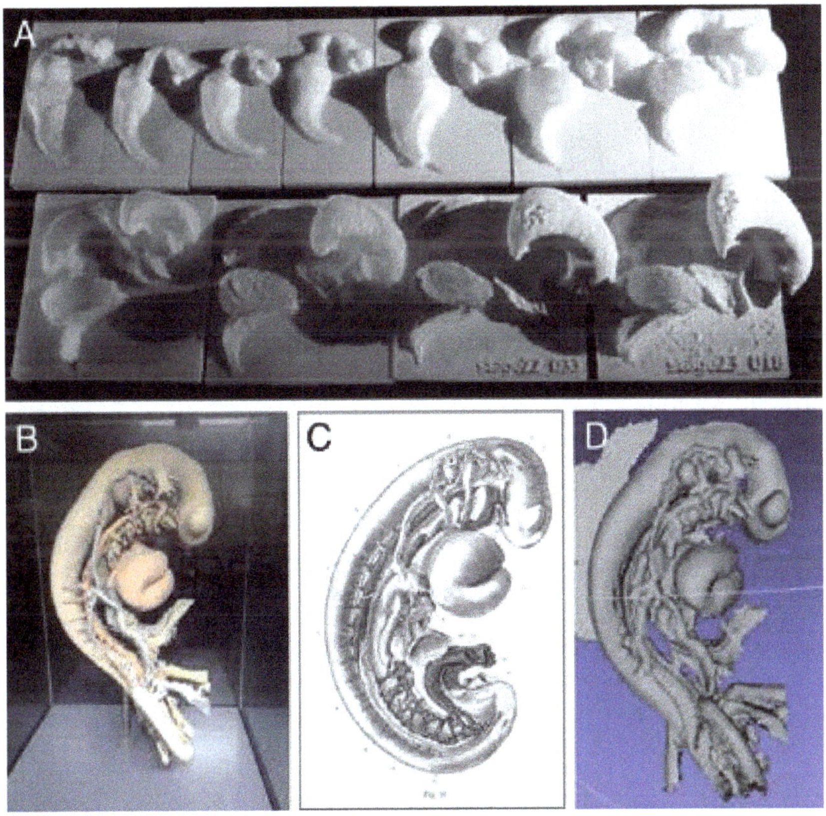

**Figure 12.** Images related with 3D printer and scanner. (A) The brain ventricle of human embryo ranging from CS13 to 23. (B) Solid reconstruction in the Blechschmidt Collection. (C) Drawing derived from B. (D) Image data of B converted by a commercially available 3D scanner (http://cubify.com/en/Products/Sense).

A 3D scanner is a tool for digitizing the surface of an object as data. Several groups are currently investigating its application to human embryology.

## Acknowledgements

We would like to thank Ms Chigako Uwabe at the Congenital Anomaly Research Center for technical assistance in handling human embryos; Prof. Katsumi Kose and Dr. Yoshimasa Matsuda at the Institute of Applied Physics at University of Tsukuba for technical help with MR imaging; Dr. Jörg Männer and Prof. Christoph Viebahn at the Department of Anatomy and Embryology, Georg-August-University of Göttingen for their generous cooperation using the Blechschmidt Collection; Prof. Tohoru Takeda at Allied Health Science, Kitasato University and Dr. Akio Yoneyama at Central Research Laboratory, Hitachi Ltd. For pCT scanning; Dr Peter Giere at the Museum für Naturkunde, Berlin for his generous cooperation with access to the Embryological collection. Research was financially supported by JSPS KAKENHI Grant Number #248055, #268044, #24790195, #25461642, 15H05270, and 15K08134 from the Japan Society for the Promotion of Science (JSPS), MEXT KAKENHI Grant Number #24119002 and

#26220004 from Grant-in-Aid for Scientific Research on Innovative Areas. Kyoto studies were approved by the Medical Ethics Committee, Kyoto University Graduate School of Medicine (Kyoto, Japan).

## Author details

Shigehito Yamada[1*], Mark Hill[2] and Tetsuya Takakuwa[1]

*Address all correspondence to: shyamada@cac.med.kyoto-u.ac.jp

1 Kyoto University Graduate School of Medicine, Japan

2 University of New South Wales, Australia

## References

[1] Keibel F. *Manual of Human Embryology*: JB Lippincott; 1910.

[2] Keibel F, Mall FP. *Manual of Human Embryology*: JB Lippincott Company; 1912.

[3] Brown DD. The Department of Embryology of the Carnegie Institution of Washington. *Bioessays*. 1987;6(2):92-6.

[4] O'Rahilly R. One Hundred Years of Human Embryology. In: Kalter H, editor. *Issues and Reviews in Teratology* 4. New York: Plenum Press; 1988. p. 81-128.

[5] Blechschmidt E. *The Stages of Human Development before Birth: An Introduction to Human Embryology*. Basel: Karger; 1960. 684 p.

[6] Blechschmidt E. (Reconstruction method by using synthetic substances; a process for investigation and demonstration of developmental movements). *Zeitschrift fur Anatomie und Entwicklungsgeschichte*. 1954;118(2):170-4.

[7] Arechaga J, Jimenez-Collado J, Ruano-Gil D. A glance at Spanish embryology and teratology during the XX century through the academic life of Francisco Orts-Llorca (1905-1993). *Int J Dev Biol*. 2009;53(8-10):1165-77.

[8] Hinrichsen KV. *Humanembryologie*. Berlin: Springer; 1990.

[9] Hinrichsen KV, Jacob HJ, Jacob M, Brand-Saberi B, Christ B, Grim M. Principles of ontogenesis of leg and foot in man. *Annf Anatomy = Anatomischer Anzeiger*: official organ of the Anatomische Gesellschaft. 1994;176(2):121-30.

[10] Shiota K. Development and intrauterine fate of normal and abnormal human conceptuses. *Congenit Anom Kyoto*. 1991;31:67-80.

[11] Matsunaga E, Shiota K. Holoprosencephaly in human embryos: epidemiologic studies of 150 cases. *Teratology*. 1977;16(3):261-72.

[12] Yamada S, Uwabe C, Fujii S, Shiota K. Phenotypic variability in human embryonic holoprosencephaly in the Kyoto Collection. *Birth Defects Res A Clin Mol Teratol*. 2004;70(8):495-508.

[13] Yamada S, Uwabe C, Nakatsu-Komatsu T, Minekura Y, Iwakura M, Motoki T, et al. Graphic and movie illustrations of human prenatal development and their application to embryological education based on the human embryo specimens in the Kyoto collection. *Developmental Dynamics*: an official publication of the American Association of Anatomists. 2006;235(2):468-77.

[14] Kameda T, Yamada S, Uwabe C, Suganuma N. Digitization of clinical and epidemiological data from the Kyoto Collection of Human Embryos: maternal risk factors and embryonic malformations. *Congenit Anom*. 2012;52(1):48-54.

[15] Matsuda Y, Ono S, Otake Y, Handa S, Kose K, Haishi T, et al. Imaging of a large collection of human embryo using a super-parallel MR microscope. *Magn Reson Med Sci*. 2007;6(3):139-46.

[16] Matsuda Y, Utsuzawa S, Kurimoto T, Haishi T, Yamazaki Y, Kose K, et al. Super-parallel MR microscope. *Magn Reson Med*. 2003;50(1):183-9.

[17] Haishi T, Uematsu T, Matsuda Y, Kose K. Development of a 1.0 T MR microscope using a Nd-Fe-B permanent magnet. *Magn Reson Imaging*. 2001;19(6):875-80.

[18] Yamada S, Samtani RR, Lee ES, Lockett E, Uwabe C, Shiota K, et al. Developmental atlas of the early first trimester human embryo. *Develop Dynam*: an official publication of the American Association of Anatomists. 2010;239(6):1585-95.

[19] Endo A, Ueno S, Yamada S, Uwabe C, Takakuwa T. Morphogenesis of the Spleen During the Human Embryonic Period. *Anat Rec* (Hoboken). 2015;298(5):820-6.

[20] Hirose A, Nakashima T, Yamada S, Uwabe C, Kose K, Takakuwa T. Embryonic liver morphology and morphometry by magnetic resonance microscopic imaging. *Anat Rec* (Hoboken). 2012;295(1):51-9.

[21] Shiraishi N, Nakashima T, Yamada S, Uwabe C, Kose K, Takakuwa T. Morphogenesis of lateral choroid plexus during human embryonic period. *Anat Rec* (Hoboken). 2013;296(4):692-700.

[22] Yoneyama A, Yamada S, Takeda T. Fine Biomedical Imaging Using X-Ray Phase-Sensitive Technique. In: Gargiulo DG, Mcewan A, editors. *Advanced Biomedical Engineering*: InTech; 2011. p. 107-28.

[23] Faasse P, Faber J, Narraway J. A brief history of the Hubrecht Laboratory. *Int J Dev Biol*. 1999;43(7):583-90.

[24] Kerwin J, Yang Y, Merchan P, Sarma S, Thompson J, Wang X, et al. The HUDSEN Atlas: a three-dimensional (3D) spatial framework for studying gene expression in the developing human brain. *J Anat.* 2010;217(4):289-99.

[25] Hopwood N. A history of normal plates, tables and stages in vertebrate embryology. *Int J Dev Biol.* 2007;51(1):1-26.

[26] Mall FP. On stages in the development of human embryos from 2 to 25mm long. *Anatomischer Anzeiger.* 1914;46:78-84.

[27] Heuser CH, Corner GW. Developmental horizons in human embryos. Description of age group X, 4 to 12 somites. Carnegie Institution of Washington publication 611, *Contributions to Embryology.* 1957;36:29-39.

[28] Streeter GL. Developmental horizons in human embryos. Description of age group XI, 13 to 20 somites, and age group XII, 21 to 29 somites. Carnegie Institution of Washington publication 541, *Contributions to Embryology.* 1942;30:211-45.

[29] Streeter GL. Developmental horizons in human embryos. Description of age group XIII, embryos about 4 or 5 millimeters long, abd age group XIV, period of indentation of the lens vesicle. Carnegie Institution of Washington publication 557, *Contributions to Embryology.* 1945;31:27-63.

[30] Streeter GL. Developmental horizons in human embryos. Description of age groups XV, XVI, XVII, and XVIII, being the third issue of a survey of the Carnegie Collection. Carnegie Institution of Washington publication 575, *Contributions to Embryology.* 1948;32:133-203.

[31] Streeter GL. Developmental horizons in human embryos. Description of age groups XIX, XX, XXI, XXII, and XXIII, being the fifth issue of a survey of the Carnegie Collection (prepared for publication by C. H. Heuser and G. W. Corner). Carnegie Institution of Washington publication 592, *Contributions to Embryology.* 1951;34:165-96.

[32] O'Rahilly R, Müller F. Developmental stages in human embryos: including a revision of Streeter's "horizons" and a survey of the Carnegie Collection. Washington, DC: Carnegie Institution of Washington Publication; 1987.

[33] Nishimura H, Takano K, Tanimura T, Yasuda M. Normal and abnormal development of human embryos: first report of the analysis of 1,213 intact embryos. *Teratology.* 1968;1(3):281-90.

[34] Nishimura H, Tanimura T, Semba R, Uwabe C. Normal development of early human embryos: observation of 90 specimens at Carnegie stages 7 to 13. *Teratology.* 1974;10(1):1-5.

[35] Jirásek JE. *Development of the Genital System and Male Pseudohermaphroditism.* Baltimore: Johns Hopkins Press; 1971.

[36] O'Rahilly R, Muller F. Developmental stages in human embryos: revised and new measurements. *Cells Tiss Org*. 2010;192(2):73-84.

[37] Smith BR. Visualizing human embryos. *Scientific Am*. 1999;280(3):76-81.

[38] Smith BR, Linney E, Huff DS, Johnson GA. Magnetic resonance microscopy of embryos. *Comput Med Imaging Graph*: the official journal of the Computerized Medical Imaging Society. 1996;20(6):483-90.

[39] Otake Y, Handa S, Kose K, Shiota K, Yamada S, Uwabe C. Magnetic Resonance Microscopy of Chemically Fixed Human Embryos with a Large Image Matrix. *Magnetic Resonance in Medical Sciences*. 2015;in press.

[40] Weninger WJ, Mohun T. Phenotyping transgenic embryos: a rapid 3-D screening method based on episcopic fluorescence image capturing. *Natur Genet*. 2002;30(1): 59-65.

[41] Rosenthal J, Mangal V, Walker D, Bennett M, Mohun TJ, Lo CW. Rapid high resolution three dimensional reconstruction of embryos with episcopic fluorescence image capture. *Birth Defects Res Part C, Embryo Today: Rev*. 2004;72(3):213-23.

[42] Momose A, Fukuda J. Phase-contrast radiographs of nonstained rat cerebellar specimen. *Med Phys*. 1995;22(4):375-9.

[43] Takeda T, Momose A, Itai Y, Wu J, Hirano K. Phase-contrast imaging with synchrotron X-rays for detecting cancer lesions. *Acad Radiol*. 1995;2(9):799-803.

[44] Davis TJ, Gao D, Gureyev TE, Stevenson AW, Wilkins SW. Phase-Contrast Imaging of Weakly Absorbing Materials Using Hard X-Rays. *Nature*. 1995;373(6515):595-8.

[45] Ingal VN, Beliaevskaya EA. X-Ray plane-wave topography observation of the phase-contrast from a noncrystalline object. *J Phys D Appl Phys*. 1995;28(11):2314-7.

[46] Chapman D, Thomlinson W, Johnston RE, Washburn D, Pisano E, Gmur N, et al. Diffraction enhanced x-ray imaging. *Phys Med Biol*. 1997;42(11):2015-25.

[47] Snigirev A, Snigireva I, Kohn V, Kuznetsov S, Schelokov I. On the possibilities of x-ray phase contrast microimaging by coherent high-energy synchrotron radiation. *Rev Sci Instrum*. 1995;66(12):5486-92.

[48] Wilkins SW, Gureyev TE, Gao D, Pogany A, Stevenson AW. Phase-contrast imaging using polychromatic hard X-rays. *Nature*. 1996;384(6607):335-8.

[49] Momose A, Kawamoto S, Koyama I, Hamaishi Y, Takai K, Suzuki Y. Demonstration of X-Ray Talbot interferometry. *Jpn J Appl Phys 2*. 2003;42(7B):L866-L8.

[50] Weitkamp T, Diaz A, David C, Pfeiffer F, Stampanoni M, Cloetens P, et al. X-ray phase imaging with a grating interferometer. *Opt Expr*. 2005;13(16):6296-304.

[51] Becker P, Bonse U. Skew-symmetric 2-crystal X-ray interferometer. *J Appl Crystallogr*. 1974;7(Dec1):593-8.

[52] Yoneyama A, Takeda T, Tsuchiya Y, Wu J, Thet-Thet-Lwin, Koizumi A, et al. A phase-contrast X-ray imaging system – with a 60 x 30 mm field of view – based on a skew-symmetric two-crystal X-ray interferometer. *Nucl Instrum Meth A*. 2004;523(1-2):217-22.

[53] Sharpe J. Optical projection tomography as a new tool for studying embryo anatomy. *J Anat*. 2003;202(2):175-81.

[54] Sharpe J, Ahlgren U, Perry P, Hill B, Ross A, Hecksher-Sorensen J, et al. Optical projection tomography as a tool for 3D microscopy and gene expression studies. *Science*. 2002;296(5567):541-5.

[55] Kerwin J, Scott M, Sharpe J, Puelles L, Robson SC, Martinez-de-la-Torre M, et al. 3 dimensional modelling of early human brain development using optical projection tomography. *BMC Neurosci*. 2004;5:27.

[56] Sarma S, Kerwin J, Puelles L, Scott M, Strachan T, Feng G, et al. 3D modelling, gene expression mapping and post-mapping image analysis in the developing human brain. *Brain Res Bull*. 2005;66(4-6):449-53.

[57] Roguin A. Wilhelm His Jr. (1863-1934) – the man behind the bundle. *Heart Rhythm*: the official journal of the Heart Rhythm Society. 2006;3(4):480-3.

[58] Born G. Die Plattenmodelliermethode. *Arch Mikr Anat*. 1883;22:584-99.

[59] His W. Über die Methoden der plastischen Rekonstruktion und über deren Bedeutung fur Anatomie und Entwickelungsgeschicht *Anat Anz*. 1887;2:382-94.

[60] Heard OO. A photographic method of orienting serial sections for reconstruction. *Anat Rec* (Hoboken). 1931;49(1):59-70.

[61] Boyer CC. The use of plastic in reconstructions from serial sections. *Anat Rec*. 1948;100(2):191-9.

[62] Komori M, Miura T, Shiota K, Minato K, Takahashi T. Virtual embryology: a 3D library reconstructed from human embryo sections and animation of development process. *MEDINFO*. 1995;8 Pt 2:1229-30.

[63] Yamada S, Itoh H, Uwabe C, Fujihara S, Nishibori C, Wada M, et al. Computerized three-dimensional analysis of the heart and great vessels in normal and holoprosencephalic human embryos. *Anat Rec* (Hoboken). 2007;290(3):259-67.

[64] Gasser RF, Cork RJ, Stillwell BJ, McWilliams DT. Rebirth of human embryology. *Develop Dynam*: an official publication of the American Association of Anatomists. 2014;243(5):621-8.

[65] Dimitrov D, Schreve K, de Beer N. Advances in three dimensional printing – state of the art and future perspectives. *Rapid Prototyping J*. 2006;12(3):136-47.

[66] Shiraishi N, Yamada S, Takakuwa T. Three-dimensional models once again: for research and teaching of early human development. Congenit Anom. 2013;53(1):58-9.

# 9

# Protein Kinase A and Protein Kinase C Connections: What Could Angiogenesis Tell Us?

Beatriz Veleirinho, Daniela Sousa Coelho,
Viviane Polli, Simone Kobe Oliveira,
Rosa Maria Ribeiro-Do-Valle,
Marcelo Maraschin and Paulo Fernando Dias

**Abstract**

The formation of embryonic blood vessels, defined as vasculogenesis, is a complex morphogenetic process ultimately related to tubulogenesis, carried out from *in situ* differentiation of mesoderm-recruited or proliferated progenitor endothelial cells (angioblasts) to endothelial cells for structuring a primary vascular plexus. Subsequent events involving apoptosis versus cell survival (remodeling) in the vessel network stabilizes the primordial microvasculature, which through the angiogenesis process yields new capillaries by sprouting from the preexisting ones. Methylxanthinic alkaloids such as caffeine (compounds present in a number of beverages consumed worldwide) exert some well-known effects upon heart and other cardiovascular structures, in part, by negatively interplaying with phosphodiesterase (PDEs) enzymes. Once caffeine as well as *Ilex paraguariensis* (yerba mate) infusion extract have shown to enhance the vessel formation (vasculogenesis and angiogenesis), we discuss the impact afforded by *I. paraguariensis* constituents on the (PDEs-related) quantities and stability of Protein kinase A (PKA) and Protein kinase C (PKC) enzymes. Besides, the text reflects on a suggested dual roles displayed by PKA and PKC enzymatic pathways in the developmental angiogenic events.

**Keywords:** Protein kinase A (PKA) and protein kinase C (PKC), Cyclases and phosphodiesterases, Methylxanthinic alkaloids, Vessels remodeling, Angiogenesis and vasculogenesis

## 1. Introduction

Angiogenesis and vasculogenesis are the better studied processes of vessel formation [1]. Angiogenesis starts from preexistent vasculature, these last structures being either the primitive vascular plexuses primordially formed by vasculogenesis in the embryo or the postcapillary venous compartment of the mature vascular systems [2, 3].

Vasculogenesis is defined as the formation of early embryonic blood vessels from *in situ* differentiation of mesoderm-recruited/proliferated progenitor endothelial cells (angioblasts) to endothelial cells [4, 5]. This process involves endothelial precursor cell clusters organization (blood islands), in the yolk sac membrane (YSM), laying down a primary vascular plexus [6–8]. A subsequent remodeling of this vascular network – a process that combines events of cell death or regression in some vessels and survival or enhancement in others – gives rise to a more refined and effective microvasculature [9–11].

Further proliferation of capillaries sprouting from preexisting vessels is referred to as angiogenesis [12], a process involving coordinated endothelial cell proliferation and migration as well as recovering of extracellular matrix (ECM), tubule formation (tubulogenesis), and expansion of the surrounding vascular tissues [13–15]. Despite angiogenesis in adults being a rare event, it plays a fundamental role in physiological processes, such as the reproductive cycle of fertile women and the wound healing process [16, 17].

There are evidences that the vasculogenesis process that works in the early embryo forming primary vessels at high rates to keep pace with the growth of the body has been adapted, under certain situations, in the adult [4, 18, 19], since bone marrow–derived endothelial progenitor cells in the peripheral blood of adult animals and humans have been shown to be incorporated into neovascularization [3, 20]. Under such conditions, cytokines can be produced to induce the formation of vascular networks alluding to vasculogenic mimicry [13, 21]. Thus, in accordance with this concept, the embryonic cellular mechanisms (proliferation and differentiation) underlying vasculogenesis process would be, in some level, recapitulated in adult life [21–23].

The cardiovascular system is susceptible to positive chronotropic and inotropic actions afforded by a class of compounds like xanthines which cause dilatation in a number of blood vessels (on lung and kidney, e.g.) and constriction in some others, such as the one occurring in brain vessels, revealing their controversial pharmacological features and biological targets diversity [24]. Methylxanthinic alkaloids, such as caffeine and theophylline are majoritarian compounds present in the coffee and cola beverages as well as in various tea extracts [25, 26]. Thus, in particular, caffeine may possibly be one of the most consumed substances all over the world. Its tropism on the cardiovascular structures and other organ systems is already reasonably known [27], as the specific-tissue mechanisms of action in some processes waits for further elucidation. Otherwise, methylxanthinic alkaloid interaction with protein kinase A (PKA) pathway has a remarkable effect on several vessel-related events. For example, Shafer et al. has verified that the treatment with caffeine and other methylxanthines increases cAMP level by inhibiting cAMP phosphodiesterase (PDE) [28]. As cAMP activates PKA, glycolysis is elevated which increases the amount of ATP available for muscle contraction and relaxation.

Caffeine, as well as *Ilex paraguariensis* St. Hill., Aquifoliaceae (e.g., mate) infusion extract (1.03–4.12 μM), have been shown to increase the microvessels number, due to the enhancement on vasculogenesis and angiogenesis rates, in the model of yolk sac and chorioallantoic membranes of chick embryos [29]. Moreover, an additional stimulant property on embryonic metabolism was evidenced by the increase in the body growth (defined by the body length). The pharmacological effects of caffeine and theophylline present in the mate drinks on the cardiovascular system are mainly addressed to PDEs inhibition, which directly impacts the quantity, stability, and cell activities of PKA and Protein kinase C (PKC) [30]. In fact, the relaxant effect in the smooth muscle is attributed to PDE inhibition, with the consequent increase in cyclic adenosine monophosphate (cAMP) concentration [27, 31]. Moreover, the heart muscle stimulation and the bronchial muscle relaxation are mediated by beta-adrenoceptors stimulation and adenylate cyclase (AC) stimulation. It is also suggested that the competitive antagonism exhibited by methylxanthines on the adenosine receptors ($A_1$ and $A_2$) determines some of its complex effects [32, 33].

The action mechanism of caffeine and mate extract/tea upon the processes of vessel formation remains unclear despite the important evidences of xanthine involvement-related biological targets (PDE–AC) on the cardiovascular physiology. Thus, it seems important to pay attention to the suggested dual roles of PKA and PKC enzymatic pathways in the angiogenesis.

## 2. Distinct roles of PKC and PKA in angiogenesis

PKC isoforms are key mediators in hormone, growth factor, and neurotransmitter-triggered pathways of cell activation [34]. Proteomic technologies (gel-based and gel-free analyses methods) and metabolomics have been successfully used in the study of protein kinases. The application of these novel tools and strategies in the field of kinase signaling has been focused on the role of PKC in the heart (for review, see [35]). Another recent review provides, with particular attention, information on the role of PKC isoforms in the cardiovascular complications [36]. A scheme of endothelial signaling pathways is displayed in Figure 1. As reported by Wright and co-workers, the DAG–PKC pathway activated by vascular endothelial growth factors (VEGFs) contributes to the vascular function in many ways, such as the regulation of endothelial permeability, vasoconstriction, extracellular matrix (ECM) synthesis/turnover, leukocyte adhesion, cytokine activation, cell growth, and ultimately, angiogenesis (Figure 1-1) [37]. In fact, such role of PKC on the angiogenesis activation was confirmed by *in vitro* and *in ovo* experiments.

An interesting study related with the PKA *versus* PKC actions on angiogenesis was performed by DeFouw and DeFouw [38]. These researchers showed that whereas the exogenous activation of cAMP by PKA pathway signaling acts decreases the macromolecules extravasation in the chick chorioallantoic membrane (CAM) during early angiogenesis (4.5-day CAM, i.e., 4.5 days of embryonic development; stage 24-HH) [39], the PKC activity contributes, at least in part, to CAM endothelial hyper permeability (a crucial pro-angiogenic event) at the 4.5-day chick embryo. Nevertheless, it was already reported [40] that the cyclooxygenase (COX-2)

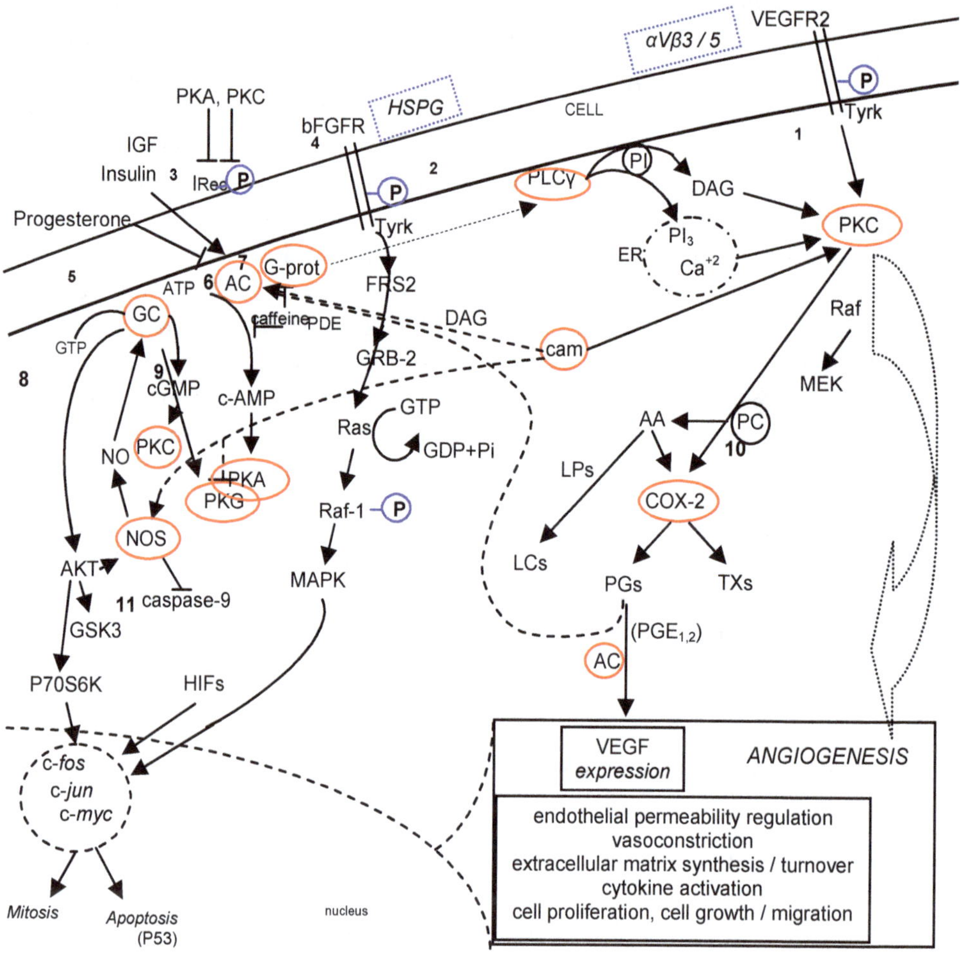


**Figure 1. Schemas of endothelial signaling pathways.** Basic fibroblast growth factor (bFGF) has been shown to activate a number of intracellular signaling pathways. Some well characterized processes that have been reported in endothelial cells and other cell types are shown. Many details in the steps of the processes were omitted for the sake of clearness and the numbers are included to enable the signals/effectors identification (then numbers not necessarily represent a sequence on transduction pathways, which are often non-exclusive). The autophosphorylation is activated by several tyrosine residues of FGFR and VEGFR. Some of the phosphotyrosine residues are binding sites for proteins with phosphotyrosine-binding domains such as FGF receptor substrate 2 (FRS2) that functions as docking protein and binds to the GRB2 which then can activate RAS. RAS may recruit RAF-1, a kinase whose action results in activation of a mitogen-activated protein kinases (MAPK) cascade. MAPK translocation to the nucleus proceeds activating transcription factors. PLC activation also plays a relevant role by causing the hydrolysis of phosphatidylinositol ($PIP_2$) to inositol-3-phosphate and diacylglycerol (DAG) leading to calcium release and activation of protein kinase C (PKC). These kinase/eicosanoid-mediated signal transduction pathways can lead to a number of biological responses on the cell housekeeping that involve cell proliferation, migration, and the other mechanisms related to the endothelial cell phenotype **(1–4)**. Guanylyl cyclase (GC) mediated survival promotion by means of AKT-NOS activation **(5–8)** and guaniline triphosphate/cyclic guaniline monophosphate (GC-cGMP)-PKC, as well as PKG activation pathways **(5–9)**. Phosphodiesterase (PDE) inactivation, as attained by xanthines (caffeine, for example), with the consequent up-regulation of cAMP-PKA signaling and the down-regulation of cGMP-PKG (6-7). A PDE compensatory role on the cAMP/PKA probable anti-proliferative (and/or anti-EC migration) effects afforded, as suggested, by a potent stimulus (from $PIP_2$, for example) on the PKC mitogenic pathway, with subsequent COX-2 activation **(10)**, or also by pro-vascular signals transmission contributions (11).

pathway, as well the AC–PKA signaling, enhances angiogenesis *in vivo* through induction by VEGF. Other studies have also indicated PKA as a positive angiogenesis regulator [41–45]. In this sense, PKA inhibition with H89 (PKA inhibitor) blocks vasoactive intestinal peptide-induced VEGF production and inhibits brain vascular endothelial cells proliferation [41], while PKA stimulation via Forskolin increases angiogenesis through PKA-dependent VEGF expression [42]. Also, Zhang et al. have demonstrated that the proinflammatory prostaglandin E2 (PGE2) promotes angiogenesis through activation of endothelial cell-expressed EP4 and PKA catalytic $\gamma$ subunits. Furthermore, suppressing the expression of PKA activated substrates (i.e., Rap1A, HSPB6, or endothelial NO synthase) inhibits the tube formation, while the knockdown of RhoA or glycogen synthase kinase 3β, that are inactivated after PKA phosphorylation, increases the tube formation of human microvascular endothelial cells [43].

In opposition to the concept of PKA-activated angiogenic events, some evidences have established a profile of angiogenesis inhibition and an endothelial cell survival decrease mediated by PKA [46]. However, these authors have also demonstrated that basic fibroblast growth factor (bFGF)-stimulated blood vessel branch points were non-abolished by concomitant treatments with cAMP or $PKA_{cat}$. A subsequent study [47] demonstrated, in human granulosa cells, the PKA-mediated negative regulation of vessel formation (as well as the modulation of endothelial cell survival) related to the increase on mRNA levels of angiopoietin-2 (ANG-2; a pro-apoptotic agent) by both PKA and PKC activators (8-Cl-cAMP and ADMB), whereas the respective inhibitors (GÖ 6983 and Rp-cAMP) markedly decreased the levels of ANG-2 mRNA. Concurrently, VEGF-induced human umbilical vein endothelial cells (HUVECs) migration and proliferation were decreased by PDE2 and PDE4 inhibitors [48]. Additionally, Jin et. al. have shown that PKA activation blocks pp60Src-dependent vascular endothelial–cadherin phosphorylation which stimulates cell–cell adhesion and inhibits endothelial cell polarization and migration, which consequently blocks sprouting in newly forming embryonic blood vessels [49]. In prostate tumor epithelial cells, the cAMP derivative 8-pCPT-2'-O-Me-cAMP, a weak agonist of PKA, acts via stimulation of that kinase that, in its turn, antagonizes Rap1 and hypoxic induction of 1$\alpha$ protein expression, VEGF production and, ultimately, angiogenesis [50]. More recently, Liu et al. have proposed that the major PKA function in physiological condition may be to inhibit angiogenesis through REG$\gamma$–proteasome mediated regulation. It has been shown that REG$\gamma$ interacts with protein kinase A catalytic subunit-$\alpha$ (PKAca reducing its intracellular stability) in HUVECs and mouse embryonic fibroblast cells (MEFs). The study has evidenced that REG$\gamma$ antagonizes PKA pathway and facilitates VEGF-induced expression of pro-angiogenic genes (e.g., vascular cell adhesion molecule-1 gene [*VCAM-1]* and endothelial-Selectin gene [*E-Selectin*]) through PKA-FoxO1 pathway. Nevertheless, authors empathize that the role of PKA on angiogenesis can vary depending upon different cell context and various signal cascades in physiological or pathological environments [51]. The anti-angiogenic role of PKA through different mechanisms represents useful tools to inhibit pathologic angiogenesis. Taken in the whole, the above cited results show contrasting actions upon angiogenesis, not only between PKA and PKC actions, but also involving each enzymatic pathway, *per se*.

## 3. How can xanthines interplay with vascular mediators?

As referred earlier [29], the treatments performed by 1.03–4.12 μM caffeine and mate extract, besides increasing vasculogenesis and angiogenesis concomitantly, have promoted embryonic growth as featured by increase in body total length of treated 4-day chick embryos. These findings may be better understood taking into consideration the findings previously reported by Shibley and Pennington [52]. These researchers have demonstrated that non-acute *in vivo* treatment of cultured 5-day-old chick embryo cells with 1 μM phorbol ester leads to down-regulation (instead of up-regulation as afforded by acute treatments) of PKC activity, significantly increasing the insulin-dependent amino acid intake/uptake and transport that are crucial processes for embryonic growth.

On the other hand, PKC has also been shown to be involved in the regulation of glucose (a well-known angiogenic activator and fetal weight and length-increasing factor) transport in adipocytes [53] and that this transportation activity was blocked by PKC inhibition. Indeed, hyperglycemia (15 mM glucose), as well as VEGF, are able, via VEGFR-2, to up-regulate PlGF (placental growth factor; a member of the VEGF family), which also acts as a survival factor for microvascular endothelial cells by preventing apoptosis [54, 55]. These evidences are concurrent with a time-dependent diacylglycerol (DAG)-mediated PKC activation event (Figure 1-2) in response to insulin and insulin-like growth factors activation [56].

Even though the impairment on nutrient transport related to PKC inhibition has been already demonstrated by Christensen et al. [53], possible remarkable compensatory responses exerted, for example, by insulin-like growth factor interaction with AC on the body length of the caffeine-treated embryos should be considered (Figure 1-3) [27].

## 4. What about phosphodiesterases?

Bearing in mind that the evidences of vasculogenesis and angiogenesis inhibition are related to PKC/PKA pathways, one could yet ponder that those effects not necessarily point to PDE-related action or additional AC-cAMP inhibitors, as the progesterone hormone, for example, It is plausible to assume that caffeine and mate effects might, at least in part, involve other angiogenic pathways than AC-cAMP-PKA inhibition, such as those related to phosphatidyl inositol-2-kinase (PI2K) and calcium/DAG-PKC activation, or its collateral induction by bFGF [57], which is a crucial angiogenic growth factor (Figure 1-4). Besides, the tumor necrosis factor-alpha (TNF-$\alpha$) and/or the guanylyl cyclase-cyclic guaniline monophosphate (GC-cGMP-PKC/PKG), pro-angiogenic activating pathways are also worth mentioning (Figure 1-5). Notwithstanding, the relevance of PDE involvement in vasculature development is evidenced by the concept which the differentiation of a restrictive angiogenic–endothelial barrier function *in vivo* would include inactivation of PDE III and PDE IV. This implies in up-regulation of cAMP-PKA signaling (Figure 1-6) and down-regulation on cGMP-PKG pathway [38]. Moreover, (1) PDE2, PDE3, PDE4, and PDE5 are expressed in HUVEC; (2) both EHNA (20 μM), a PDE2 selective inhibitor, and RP73401 (10 μM), a PDE4 selective inhibitor, are able to enhance the cAMP intracellular levels in HUVECs; (3) EHNA and RP73401 are able to inhibit cell proliferation, mitotic cycle progression and migration on HUVECs stimulated by VEGF; (4) HUVEC treatments with the cAMP analogue 8-Br-cAMP (600 μM) mimicry the cAMP *in vitro* inhibitory effects; and (5) only the association of EHNA and RP73401 (co-treatment by PDE2 and PDE4 selective inhibitors) blocks angiogenesis *in vivo*, indicating that to start antiangiogenic activity both migration and cell proliferation must be conjointly abolished [48].

In addition, the relevant study published by Netherton and Maurice [58] punctuates that human vascular endothelial cells (VECs) express variants of PDE2, PDE3, PDE4, and PDE5 families and demonstrate that the levels of these enzymes differ among VECs derived from aorta, umbilical vein, and micro vascular structures as those present in the yolk sac/chorioallantoic membrane (YSM/CAM) of chick embryos. As stated by those investigators, it is noteworthy that the selective inhibition of PDE2 does not only fail to increase cAMP in any VECs lineage, but also it did not inhibit migration in the VECs studied.

Otherwise, the inhibition of PDE4 activity decreased cell migration but, in association with forskolin (an AC/GC activator), increased cAMP in all VECs studied [58]. PDE3 inhibition potentiated forskolin-induced increases in cAMP and also inhibited migration in VECs derived from aorta and umbilical vein, but not on microvascular VECs. From these data, one should expect that methylxanthines had reduced vessel number in the early extra-embryonic membranes (YSM and CAM) in response to PDE inhibition (Figure 1-7), by antagonizing adenosine, or indeed by protecting cAMP from degradation. However, there are some evidences concerning the process of microvessels development where the opposite has just been found. The cAMP pathway truly "rivals" with the angiogenic microenvironment in complexity (for inhibiting inflammatory cytokines) and constitutes a kind of cross-junction to which converges a significant number of cell signaling ways. Then, during vessel formation, cAMP (and its distinct cellular roles) is surely under influence of factors as diverse as different time–space conditions, distinct main regulative pathways, and a number of second messengers/effectors in various signaling routs/cascades. Moreover, these events are dependent on each vascular endothelial cell lineage and the biological system or study model considered.

## 5. Focusing on the environment of developmental microvessels

Embryonic microvessels (such as those growing in the 4-day chick YSMs/CAMs) are structures physiologically under one primordial choice: that is potentially "life or death" [10]. Therefore, despite the proinflammatory cytokines blockade due to cAMP increase mediated by PDE inhibition in response to methylxanthines action, and also the presence of eventual apoptotic stimulus (such as insulin/IGFs-PKA interaction-mediated cell death), the embryonic endothelial cells may be concomitantly exposed to powerful survival stimuli, for example, vascular growth factors; survival factors (i.e., ANG-1), guanylyl cyclase (GC)-Akt (i.e., GC-PKB) [59] (Figure 1-8), pericyte-support; blood flow; and others. Besides, specific pro-angiogenic signals/conditions (NO-synthase/NO-GC, intermittent hypoxia, and GC-PKC, e.g.) would be preponderant to protect the ECs (Figure 1-9) [60, 61]. In the light of these evidences, it is still plausible to suggest that both caffeine and the *I. paraguariensis* extract may exert a compensatory role on the cAMP/PKA probable anti-EC proliferative effect and/or anti-EC migration effect, by means of potent stimuli (from $PIP_2$, $Ca^{2+}$, e.g.) to the PKC mitogenic pathway, with supplementary COX-2 prostaglandin-E ($PGE_{1,2}$) activation (Figure 1-10). Additionally, pro-vascular integrins/cytokines contributions and GC-Akt-P70SK-related *c-fos* and *c-jun* activation (Figure 1-11) should be considered. In the context of the dual effect between the AC-cAMP and GC-cGMP functions in the ECs (concerning the up-regulation of cAMP-PKA signaling against the down-regulation on cGMP-PKG pathway), it is possible to ponder on a non-improbable straightforward antagonist action of PKC on the PKA pathway. In fact, this idea is in part supported by evidences that PKC is able to phosphorylate also PKA-specific consensus sites of Tnl (troponin 1), a cardiac myofilament [62].

As an alternative hypothesis concerning a compensatory mechanism on angiogenesis, negative modulation by cAMP, we suggest the improvement of glucose (an angiogenic activator) uptake by ECs, possibly mediated by insulin/IGF-AC activation in response to methylxanthine administration. As support for this idea, data provided by Hashimoto et al. [63] have shown that inhibitors of PKA and PI3K completely attenuated the NO-induced *in vitro* endothelial tube formation (from human aortic endothelial cells). These findings strongly suggest that PKA (Figure 1-12) and PI3K might both be mediating the angiogenesis process.

## 6. Conclusion

In conclusion, we should not rescind from the importance of considering some apoptotic level *per se* on the endothelial cells lineages (*anoikis*) during the transition events from immature vasculature, yielded by vasculogenesis, to a more stable and sophisticated one attained by angiogenesis. In the context of angiogenic remodeling [64], some microvessels "have to die for others to survive" becoming stable/quiescent vascular structures [9]. Many "puzzle pieces" of kinases pathways appear to be, up to date, lacking. For example, how to begin solving the metabolome matter related to PKA *versus* PKC pathways in the angiogenesis? In accordance with Agnetti et al. [36], the "one protein at a time" approach is unlikely to provide a comprehensive picture of the cellular signaling due to the concerted action of "several molecular players at the same time." Thus, the activities of both PKC and PKA should not be considered so mutually exclusive characters in the scenery of developmental microvessel formation. However, the remarkable evidences on phosphodiesterases as possible pivotal target molecules for the angiogenic effects of caffeine and *Ilex paraguariensis* extract strongly suggest an antagonistic role of the protein kinases A and C in the same events.

## Acknowledgements

The authors are grateful to the Research and Extension Pro-Rectory of Federal University of Santa Catarina (PRPE/UFSC, Brazil) for their support.

## Author details

Beatriz Veleirinho[1], Daniela Sousa Coelho[2], Viviane Polli[2], Simone Kobe Oliveira[2], Rosa Maria Ribeiro-Do-Valle[1], Marcelo Maraschin[1] and Paulo Fernando Dias[1,2*]

*Address all correspondence to: paulo.fernando.dias@ufsc.br

1 NANOBIOMAT, Federal University of Santa Catarina, Florianópolis, Brazil

2 Department of Cell Biology, Embryology, and Genetics, Federal University of Santa Catarina, Florianópolis, Brazil

## References

[1] Murohara T. Therapeutic Angiogenesis: Cellular Approach from Bone Marrow. Cord Blood and Peripheral Blood. International Congress Series 2005;1262 332–338.

[2] Carmeliet P. Angiogenesis in Health and Disease. Nature Medicine 2003; 9 656–660.

[3] Rafii S., Lyden D. Therapeutic Stem and Progenitor Cell Transplantation for Organ Vascularization and Regeneration. Nature Medicine 2003;9(6) 702–712.

[4] Hanahan D., Folkman J. Patterns and Emerging Mechanisms of the Angiogenic Switch During Tumorigenesis. Cell 1996;86 353–364.

[5] Risau W., Sariola H., Zerves HG., Sasse J., Ekblom P., Kemler R., Doetchman T. Vasculogenesis and Angiogenesis in Embryonic-Stem-Cell-Derived Embryoid Bodies. Development 1998;102 471–478.

[6] Ruiter MC., De Poelmann E., Mentink MMT., Vaniperen L., Gittenberger-De-Groot AC. The Early Formation of the Vascular System in Quail Embryos. In: Ruiter MC. (ed.) Development of the Vascular System in the Embryo. A Concept of the Origin of Systemic-Pulmonary Collateral Arteries. The Netherlands: Leiden Univ Bibl.; 1992.

[7] Drake CJ., Larue A., Ferrara N., Little C. VEGF Regulates Cell Behavior during Vasculogenesis. Developmental Biology 2000;224 178–188.

[8] Asahara T., Isner JM. Endothelial Progenitor Cells for Vascular Regeneration. Journal of Hematotherapy and Stem Cell Research 2002;11 171–178.

[9] Yancopoulus GD., Davis S., Gale NW., Rudge JS., Wiegand SJ., Holash J. Vascular – Specific Growth Factors and Blood Vessel Formation. Nature 2000;407 242–247.

[10] Melino G. The Sirens' Song. Nature 2001;412(6842) 23–24.

[11] Jones N., Iljin K., Dumont DJ., Alitalo K. Tie Receptors: New Modulators of Angiogenic and Lymphangiogenic Responses. Nature Reviews Molecular Cell Biology 2001;2 257–267.

[12] Folkman J., Klagsbrun M. Angiogenic Growth Factors. Science 1987;235 442–447.

[13] Folkman J., Shing Y. Control of Angiogenesis by Heparin and other Sulfated Polysaccharides. Advances in Experimental Medicine and Biology 1992;313 355–364.

[14] Kalluri R. Basement Membranes: Structure, Assembly and Role in Tumour Angiogenesis. Nature Reviews Cancer 2003;3 422–433.

[15] Collinson DJ., Donnelly R. Therapeutic Angiogenesis in Peripheral Arterial Disease: Can Biotechnology Produce an Effective Collateral Circulation? European Journal of Endovascular Surgery 2004;28 9–23.

[16] Zygmunt M., Herr F., Münstedt K., Lang U., Liang OD. Angiogenesis and Vasculogenesis in Pregnancy. European Journal of Obstetrics and Gynecology and Reproductive Biology 2003;110 10–18.

[17] Bergers G., Benjamin LE. Tumorigenesis and the Angiogenesis Switch. Nature Reviews Cancer 2003;3 401–410.

[18] Ribatti D., Vacca A., Nico B., Roncali L., Cammacco F. Postnatal Vasculogenesis. Mechanisms of Development 2001;100 157–163.

[19] Zammarettia P., Zisch AH. Adult 'Endothelial Progenitor Cells' Renewing Vasculature. The International Journal of Biochemistry and Cell Biology 2005;37 493–503.

[20] Komarova NL., Mironov V. On the Role of Endothelial Progenitor Cells in Tumor Neovascularization. Journal of Theoretical Biology 2005;235 338–349.

[21] Maniotis AJ., Folberg R., Hess A., Seftor EA., Gardner LM., Pe'er J., Trent JM., Meltzer PS., Hendrix MJ. Vascular Channel Formation by Human Melanoma Cells *in Vivo* and *in Vitro*: Vasculogenic Mimicry. The American Journal of Pathology 1999;155(3) 739–752.

[22] Springer ML., Chen AS., Kraft PE., Bednarski M., Blau HM. VEGF Gene Delivery to Muscle: Potential Role for Vasculogenesis in Adults. Molecular Cell 1998;2 549–558.

[23] Shubik P., Warren BA. Additional Literature on 'Vasculogenic Mimicry' Not Cited. The American Journal of Pathology 2000;156 736–741.

[24] Rossing TH. Methylxanthines in 1989. Annals of Internal Medicine 1989;110 502–504.

[25] Mazzafera P. Caffeine, Theobromine and Theophylline Distribution in *Ilex Paraguariensis*. Brazilian Journal of Plant Physiology 1994;6 149–151.

[26] Hour TC., Liang YC., Chu IS., Lin JK. Inhibition of Eleven Mutagens by Various Tea Extracts, (-) Epigallocatechin-3-Gallate, Gallic Acid and Caffeine. Food and Chemical Toxicology 1999;37 569–579.

[27] Katzung BG. Cardiovascular-Renal Drugs. In: Katzung BG. (ed.) Basic and Clinical Pharmacology (10th ed.). San Francisco: McGraw-Hill; 2007.

[28] Shafer SH., Phelps SH., Williams CL. Reduced DNA Synthesis and Cell Viability in Small Cell Lung Carcinoma by Treatment with Cyclic AMP Phosphodiesterase Inhibitors. Biochemical Pharmacology 1998;56 1229–1236.

[29] Strassmann BB., Vieira AR., Pedrotti EL., Morais HNF., Dias PF., Maraschin M. Quantitation of Methylxanthinic Alkaloids and Phenolic Compounds in Mate (*Ilex Paraguariensis*) and their Effects on Blood Vessel Formation in Chick Embryos. Journal of Agricultural and Food Chemistry 2008;56 8348–8353.

[30] Lugnier C. Cyclic Nucleotide Phosphodiesterase (PDE) Superfamily: A New Target for the Development of Specific Therapeutic Agents. Pharmacology & Therapeutics 2006;109(3) 366–398.

[31] Persson CAG. The Pharmacology of Anti-Asthmatic Xanthines and the Role of Adenosine. Asthma Reviews 1987;1 61–93.

[32] Rang HP., Dale MM., Ritter JM., Flower RJ. Pharmacology (6th ed.). London: Churchill Livingstone; 2007.

[33] Riksen NP., Smits P., Rongen GA. The Cardiovascular Effects of Methylxanthines. The Handbook of Experimental Pharmacology 2011;200 413–437.

[34] Nishizuka Y. Studies and Perspectives of Protein Kinase C. Science 1986;233(4761) 305–312.

[35] Agnetti G., Kane LA., Guarnieri C., Caldarera CM., Van Eyk JE. Proteomic Technologies in the Study of Kinases: Novel Tools for the Investigation of PKC in the Heart. Pharmacological Research 2007;55 511–522.

[36] Das Evcimen N., King GL. The Role of Protein Kinase C Activation and the Vascular Complications of Diabetes. Pharmacological Research 2007;55 498–510.

[37] Wright PS., Cross-Doersen D., Miller JA., Jones WD., Bitonti AJ. Inhibition of Angiogenesis in Vitro and in Ovo with an Inhibitor of Cellular Protein Kinases, MDL 27032. Journal of Cellular Physiology 1992;152(3) 448–457.

[38] DeFouw LM., DeFouw DO. Differential Phosphodiesterase Activity Contributes to Restrictive Endothelial Barrier Function During Angiogenesis. Microvascular Research 2001;62(3) 263–270.

[39] Hamburger V., Hamilton H. A Series of Normal Stages in the Development of the Chick Embryo. Journal of Morphology 1951;88 49–92.

[40] Amano H., Haysahi I., Yoshida S., Yoshimura H., Majima M. Cyclooxygenase-2 and Adenylate Cyclase/Protein Kinase a Signaling Pathway Enhances Angiogenesis Through Induction of Vascular Endothelial Growth Factor in Rat Sponge Implants. Human Cell 2002;15(1) 13–24.

[41] Yang J., Shi QD., Song TB., Feng GF., Zang WJ., Zong CH., Chang L. Vasoactive Intestinal Peptide Increases VEGF Expression to Promote Proliferation of Brain Vascu-

lar Endothelial Cells Via the cAMP/PKA Pathway after Ischemic Insult *in Vitro*. Peptides 2013;42C 105–111.

[42] Namkoong S., Kim CK., Cho YL., Kim JH., Lee H., Ha KS., Choe J., Kim PH., Won MH., Kwon YG., Shim EB., Kim YM. Forskolin Increases Angiogenesis Through the Coordinated Cross-Talk of PKA-Dependent VEGF Expression and Epac-Mediated PI3K/Akt/Enos Signaling. Cellular Signaling 2009;21 906–915.

[43] Zhang Y., Daaka, Y. PGE2 Promotes Angiogenesis Through EP4 and PKA $C\gamma$ Pathway. Blood 2011;118(19) 5355–5364.

[44] Lu Y., Xiong Y., Huo Y., Han J., Yang X., Zhang R., Zhu DS., Klein-Hessling S., Li J., Zhang X., Han X., Li Y., Shen B., He Y., Shibuya M., Feng GS., Luo J. Grb-2-Associated Binder 1 (Gab1) Regulates Postnatal Ischemic and VEGF-Induced Angiogenesis Through the Protein Kinase A-Endothelial NOS Pathway. Proceedings of the National Academy of Science of the United States of America 2011;108 2957–2962.

[45] Venkatesh PK., Pattillo CB., Branch B., Hood J., Thoma S., Illum S., Pardue S., Teng X., Patel RP., Kevil CG. Dipyridamole Enhances Ischaemia-Induced Arteriogenesis Through an Endocrine Nitrite/Nitric Oxide-Dependent Pathway. Cardiovascular Research 2010;85 661–670.

[46] Kim S., Bakre M., Yin H., Varner JA. Inhibition of Endothelial Cell Survival and Angiogenesis by Protein Kinase A. The Journal of Clinical Investigation 2002;110(7) 933–941.

[47] Witt PS., Pietrowski D., Keck C. PKA- and PKC-Dependent Regulation of Angiopoietin 2 mRNA in Human Granulosa Lutein Cells. Hormone and Metabolic Research 2004;36 82–85.

[48] Favot L., Keravis T., Holl V., Le Bec A., Lugnier C. VEGF-Induced HUVEC Migration and Proliferation Are Decreased by PDE2 and PDE4 Inhibitors. The Journal of Thrombosis and Haemostasis 2003;90(2) 334–343.

[49] Jin H., Garmy-Susini B., Avraamides CJ., Stoletov K., Klemke RL., Varner JA. A PKA-Csk- Pp60src Signaling Pathway Regulates the Switch Between Endothelial Cell Invasion and Cell–Cell Adhesion During Vascular Sprouting. Blood 2010;116 5773–5783.

[50] Menon J., Doebele RC., Gomes S., Bevilacqua E., Reindl KM., Rosner MR. A Novel Interplay Between Rap1 and PKA Regulates Induction of Angiogenesis in Prostate Cancer. Plos One 2012;7 E49893.

[51] Liu S., Lai L., Zuo Q., Dai F., Wu L., Wang Y., Zhou Q., Liu J., Liu J., Li L., Lin Q., Creighton CJ., Costello MG., Huang S., Jia C., Liao L., Luo H., Fu J., Liu M., Yi Z., Xiao J., Li X. PKA Turnover by the REG$\gamma$-proteasome Modulates FoxO1 Cellular Activity and VEGF-induced Angiogenesis. Journal of Molecular and Cellular Cardiology 2014;72 28–38.

[52] Shibley IA., Pennington SN. Sodium Ion-Dependent (N-Methylamino)-$\alpha$-Isobutyric Acid Uptake by Embryonic Chick Cells Exposed to Ethanol in Ovo: Response to the

Stimulation/Downregulation of Protein Kinases. Alcohol Alcoholism 1998;33 451–456.

[53] Christensen RL., Shade DL., Graves CB., Mcdonald JM. Evidence that Protein Kinase C Is Involved in Regulating Glucose Transport in the Adipocyte. International Journal of Biochemistry 1987;19(3) 259–265.

[54] Adini A., Kornaga T., Firoozbakht F., Benjamin LE. Placental Growth Factor Is a Survival Factor for Tumor Endothelial Cells and Macrophages. Cancer Research 2002;62 2749–2752.

[55] Zhao B., Cai J., Boulton M. Expression of Placenta Growth Factor Is Regulated by Both VEGF and Hyperglycaemia Via VEGFR-2. Microvascular Research 2004;68 239–246.

[56] Bourne HR., Stryer L. G Proteins. The Target Sets the Tempo. Nature 1992;358(6387) 541–543.

[57] Nugent MA., Iozzo RV. Molecules in Focus. Fibroblast Growth Factor-2. The International Journal of Biochemistry & Cell Biology 2000;32 115–120.

[58] Netherton SJ., Maurice DH. Vascular Endothelial Cell Cyclic Nucleotide Phosphodiesterases and Regulated Cell Migration: Implications in Angiogenesis. Molecular Pharmacology 2005;67(1) 263–272.

[59] Datta SR., Brunet A., Greenberg ME. Cellular Survival: A Play in Three Akts. Genes & Development 1999;13 2905–2927.

[60] Mundel TM., Kalluri R. Type IV Collagen-Derived Angiogenesis Inhibitors. Microvascular Research 2007;74(2–3) 85–89.

[61] Toffoli S., Feron O., Raes M., Michiels C. Intermittent Hypoxia Changes HIF-1alpha Phosphorylation Pattern in Endothelial Cells: Unravelling of a New PKA-Dependent Regulation of HIF-1alpha. Biochimica et Biophysica Acta 2007;1773(10) 1558–1571.

[62] Burkart EM., Sumandea MP., Kobayashi T., Nili M., Martin AF., Homsher E., Solaro RJ. Phosphorylation or Glutamic Acid Substitution at Protein Kinase C Sites on Cardiac Troponin I Differentially Depress Myofilament Tension and Shortening Velocity. The Journal of Biological Chemistry 2003;278 11265–11272.

[63] Hashimoto A., Miyakoda G., Hirose Y., Mori T. Activation of Endothelial Nitric Oxide Synthase by Cilostazol Via a cAMP/Protein Kinase A- and Phosphatidylinositol 3-Kinase/Akt-Dependent Mechanism. Atherosclerosis 2006;189(2) 350–357.

[64] Peng J., Zhang L., Drysdale L., Fong GH. The Transcription Factor EPAS-1/Hypoxia-Inducible Factor 2alpha Plays an Important Role in Vascular Remodeling. Proceedings of the National Academy of Science of the United States of America 2000;97(15) 8386–8391.

# Permissions

All chapters in this book were first published by InTech Open; hereby published with permission under the Creative Commons Attribution License or equivalent. Every chapter published in this book has been scrutinized by our experts. Their significance has been extensively debated. The topics covered herein carry significant findings which will fuel the growth of the discipline. They may even be implemented as practical applications or may be referred to as a beginning point for another development.

The contributors of this book come from diverse backgrounds, making this book a truly international effort. This book will bring forth new frontiers with its revolutionizing research information and detailed analysis of the nascent developments around the world.

We would like to thank all the contributing authors for lending their expertise to make the book truly unique. They have played a crucial role in the development of this book. Without their invaluable contributions this book wouldn't have been possible. They have made vital efforts to compile up to date information on the varied aspects of this subject to make this book a valuable addition to the collection of many professionals and students.

This book was conceptualized with the vision of imparting up-to-date information and advanced data in this field. To ensure the same, a matchless editorial board was set up. Every individual on the board went through rigorous rounds of assessment to prove their worth. After which they invested a large part of their time researching and compiling the most relevant data for our readers.

The editorial board has been involved in producing this book since its inception. They have spent rigorous hours researching and exploring the diverse topics which have resulted in the successful publishing of this book. They have passed on their knowledge of decades through this book. To expedite this challenging task, the publisher supported the team at every step. A small team of assistant editors was also appointed to further simplify the editing procedure and attain best results for the readers.

Apart from the editorial board, the designing team has also invested a significant amount of their time in understanding the subject and creating the most relevant covers. They scrutinized every image to scout for the most suitable representation of the subject and create an appropriate cover for the book.

The publishing team has been an ardent support to the editorial, designing and production team. Their endless efforts to recruit the best for this project, has resulted in the accomplishment of this book. They are a veteran in the field of academics and their pool of knowledge is as vast as their experience in printing. Their expertise and guidance has proved useful at every step. Their uncompromising quality standards have made this book an exceptional effort. Their encouragement from time to time has been an inspiration for everyone.

The publisher and the editorial board hope that this book will prove to be a valuable piece of knowledge for researchers, students, practitioners and scholars across the globe.

# List of Contributors

**Hiroshi Fujiwara**
Department of Obstetrics and Gynecology, Kanazawa University Graduate School of Medical Science, Japan

**Yoshihiko Araki**
Institute for Environmental and Gender-specific Medicine, Juntendo University Graduate School of Medicine, Japan

**Shigeru Saito**
Department of Obstetrics and Gynecology, Faculty of Medicine, University of Toyama, Toyama, Japan

**Kazuhiko Imakawa**
Laboratory of Animal Breeding and Reproduction, Veterinary Medical Sciences, Graduate School of Agricultural and Life Sciences, University of Tokyo, Japan

**Satoru Kyo**
Department of Obstetrics and Gynecology, Faculty of Medicine, Shimane University, Japan

**Minoru Shigeta**
Advanced Fertility Center of Fuchu Nozomi, Osaka, Japan

**Akihito Horie**
Department of Gynecology and Obstetrics, Kyoto University Graduate School of Medicine, Japan

**Takahide Mori**
Academia for Repro-Regenerative Medicine, Tokyo, Japan

**Daniele Conte and Giorgio R. Merlo**
Department of Molecular Biotechnology and Health Sciences, Università degli Studi di Torino, Italy

**Luisa Guerrini**
Department of Biosciences, Università degli Studi di Milano, Italy

**Simona Tafuri, Francesca Ciani, Danila d'Angelo, Luigi Esposito and Natascia Cocchia**
Department of Veterinary Medicine and Animal Productions - University of Naples Federico II, Naples, Italy

**Eugenio Luigi Iorio**
International Observatory of Oxidative Stress, Salerno, Italy

**Néstor Isaías Tovío Luna, Arturo Duica Amaya and Henry Alberto Grajales Lombana**
Groups Researchers Biologia de la adaptacion de los animales al tropico, Facultad de Medicina Veterinaria y de Zootecnia, Universidad Nacional. UYWAY, Facultad de Ciencias Agrarias, programa de Zootecnia, Fundacion Universitaria Agraria de Colombia, Bogota, Columbia

**Bin Wu and Hai Wang**
Arizona Center for Reproductive Endocrinology and Infertility, Tucson, Arizona, USA
Yunnan Jiuzhou Hospital, Kunming, Yunnan, China

**Linsen Zan**
College of Animal Science and Technology, National Beef Cattle Improvement Center, China

**Fusheng Quan**
College of Veterinary Medicine, Northwest A&F University, Yangling, Shaanxi, China

**Masahide Shiotani**
Hanabusa Women's Clinic, Kobe, Japan

**Natascia Cocchia, Simona Tafuri, Lucia Abbondante, Leonardo Meomartino, Luigi Esposito and Francesca Ciani**
Department of Veterinary Medicine and Animal Productions, University of Naples Federico II, Naples, Italy

**Shigehito Yamada and Tetsuya Takakuwa**
Kyoto University Graduate School of Medicine, Japan

**Mark Hill**
University of New South Wales, Australia

**Beatriz Veleirinho, Rosa Maria Ribeiro-Do-Valle and Marcelo Maraschin**
NANOBIOMAT, Federal University of Santa Catarina, Florianópolis, Brazil

**Daniela Sousa Coelho, Viviane Polli and Simone Kobe Oliveira**
Department of Cell Biology, Embryology, and Genetics, Federal University of Santa Catarina, Florianópolis, Brazil

**Paulo Fernando Dias**
NANOBIOMAT, Federal University of Santa Catarina, Florianópolis, Brazil
Department of Cell Biology, Embryology, and Genetics, Federal University of Santa Catarina, Florianópolis, Brazil

# Index

## I



## L



## M



## O



## P



## R



## S



## T



## V

www.ingramcontent.com/pod-product-compliance
Lightning Source LLC
LaVergne TN
LVHW062234200926
848484LV00006B/1541
* 9 7 9 8 8 8 7 4 0 2 4 9 9 *